Tuberculosis: A Clinical Guide

Tuberculosis: A Clinical Guide

Editor: Ralphie Clark

MURPHY & MOORE
www.murphy-moorepublishing.com

www.murphy-moorepublishing.com

MURPHY & MOORE

Cataloging-in-Publication Data

Tuberculosis : a clinical guide / edited by Ralphie Clark.
p. cm.
Includes bibliographical references and index.
ISBN 978-1-63987-542-9
1. Tuberculosis. 2. Tuberculosis--Treatment. 3. Tuberculosis--Diagnosis. I. Clark, Ralphie.
RC311 .T83 2022
616.995--dc23

Murphy & Moore Publishing,
1 Rockefeller Plaza,
New York City, NY 10020, USA

ISBN 978-1-63987-542-9 (Hardback)

Contents

Preface

The main aim of this book is to educate learners and enhance their research focus by presenting diverse topics covering this vast field. This is an advanced book which compiles significant studies by distinguished experts in the area of analysis. This book addresses successive solutions to the challenges arising in the area of application, along with it; the book provides scope for future developments.

Tuberculosis is an infectious disease that generally affects the lungs and is caused by bacterium Mycobacterium tuberculosis. When the infection does not show any symptom, it is known as latent tuberculosis infection. Sometimes, the latent tuberculosis progresses as an active infection and can be fatal if left untreated. Symptoms of active tuberculosis are fever, chronic cough with blood containing mucus, weight loss and night sweats. It can spread from one person to others through air when the infected person speaks, spits, coughs or sneezes. People who have latent tuberculosis infection do not spread the disease to other people. Diagnosis of active infection is based on microscopic examination and culture of body fluids, and chest X-rays. This book contains some path-breaking studies in the field of tuberculosis. It consists of contributions made by international experts. Researchers and students in this field will be assisted by this book.

It was a great honour to edit this book, though there were challenges, as it involved a lot of communication and networking between me and the editorial team. However, the end result was this all-inclusive book covering diverse themes in the field.

Finally, it is important to acknowledge the efforts of the contributors for their excellent chapters, through which a wide variety of issues have been addressed. I would also like to thank my colleagues for their valuable feedback during the making of this book.

Editor

1

The Impact of Tuberculosis among Immigrants: Epidemiology and Strategies of Control in High-Income Countries

Carlo Contini, Martina Maritati,
Marachiara di Nuzzo, Lorenzo Massoli,
Sara Lomenzo and Anastasio Grilli

Abstract

A significant reappearance of tuberculosis (TB) was observed in industrialized countries during the last two decades. This is due to the spread of HIV infection itself and to today's migratory phenomenon as a consequence of wealth disparity, poverty, wars and political persecutions. This proportion is expected to increase and represents an important cause of the overall resurgence of the TB epidemic and drug-resistant TB in Western Europe and the USA. TB is currently one of the leading causes of death worldwide and a health problem in high-income countries. Although WHO global TB report 2015 with its "STOP TB" strategy has the goal to eliminate TB as a public health problem by 2050, TB shows no signs of disappearing despite some decline in high-income countries. In order to intensify the fights against this deadly disease, further efforts should be aimed to improve examination/detection processes to accurately determine all kinds of TB, and how best to enhance TB control through a coordinated medical screening program of migrants for active TB. Migration in itself is not a definitive risk for TB. Stressful living condition, social isolation, poverty, political fear/persecution, and difficulties to access to health care can expose these individuals to the risk of TB infection during and after the migration process. This chapter aims to discuss and highlight all these issues.

Keywords: tuberculosis (TB), latent tuberculosis infection (LTBI), migrants, documented migrants, undocumented migrants, asylum seekers, refugees, Europe (EU)

1. Introduction

Tuberculosis (TB) currently represents one of the leading causes of death worldwide and, despite globally the TB incidence fell by an average of 1.5% per year since 2000 and is now

18% lower than the level of 2000, it has been declared a global health emergency in high-income countries [4]. TB is also the primary killer due to a single infectious disease and, after HIV/AIDS, is the second single disease which causes more deaths in the world [2]. The World Health Organization (WHO) estimates that one-third of the world population harbors latent TB infections (LTBI), 14.1 million people have active cases, 9 million are newly diagnosed per year (9.6 million new TB cases in 2014, of which 58% in the Southeast Asia and Western Pacific regions), and 1.5 million deaths are attributable to TB annually [1–4]. This death toll equals 2% of global mortality, even if it is a disease for which a cure has existed for 70 years.

In relation to HIV infection, more than 48% of TB patients globally had a documented positive HIV test result. In the African region, which has the highest TB/HIV burden, three out of four TB patients knew their HIV status [4].

Although the general decrease [1, 4] of TB cases (globally, the TB mortality rate fell by an estimated 45% between 1990 and 2013 and the TB prevalence rate fell by 41% during the same period) in recent decades has led the medical profession to pay less attention to the presence of high-risk patients, TB continues to be a public health concern in high-income countries, primarily among the foreign-born and migrant population [5]. In fact, a reappearance of this disease was observed since the early 1990s due to other than the spread of HIV infection and the increase in poor living conditions and immunosuppression; it is due to the migratory phenomenon, and an interplay of various push and pull factors are a consequence of wealth disparity, poverty, wars, and political persecutions [6, 7].

There are 244 million migrants worldwide, which is 41% more since 2000. Note that 76 million are in Europe, the continent with the highest number of migrants, followed by Asia (75 million), United States (54 million), Africa (21 million), Latin America and the Caribbean (9 million), and Oceania (8 million), according to the calculations of the latest International Migration Report of the United Nations [8]. Of all the immigrants living in Europe, Germany and Russia have 12 million, the United Kingdom has 9 million, France has 8 million, Spain and Italy have 6 million; while Saudi Arabia has 10 million and Canada and Australia have 7 million, respectively. According to the previous report of the UN [8], the largest number of citizens migrated abroad come mainly from India (16 million), Mexico (12 million), Russia (11 million), China (10 million), Bangladesh (7 million), Pakistan and Ukraine (6,000,000), and the Philippines and Syria with about 5 million migrants.

Immigrants from TB endemic countries account for a significant proportion of TB cases in industrialized countries. It can be anticipated that this proportion will continue to increase, and will represent an important cause of the overall resurgence of the TB epidemic in Western EU and the USA. Most migrants are healthy, but conditions surrounding the migration process can pose health risks such as inequalities in accessing health services, substandard quality of care, marginalization, and discrimination. Thus, the particular condition of "immigrant" predisposes to an increased risk of developing TB, either for increased incidence rates in their countries of origin, or the high rate of LTBI which predisposes to TB for conditions of social fragility and complexity related to the process of migration and multiculturalism found in the host country.

The chapter is structured as follows:

- Overview and epidemiological features of TB among immigrants in low-TB burden countries.
- Definition of LTBI and risk of progression toward TB.
- Management of LTBI among immigrants and screening practices.
- Essentials of diagnosis of infectious TB among immigrants in low TB burden countries.
- Management and treatment of drug-resistant TB.
- Conclusions and social issues.

2. Overview and epidemiological features of TB among immigrants in low-TB burden countries and screening practices

2.1. Overview and epidemiological features of TB among immigrants in low-TB burden countries[1]

Many migrants originating from countries where TB has a high incidence, including tropical areas [9], have a high risk of acquiring TB before migration. Much of TB burden is concentrated in high-burden settings of Africa and Asia (28 and 58%, respectively) where TB continues to be a cause of morbidity and mortality [5]. Some areas of tropical countries, such as Haiti, Perù, Bolivia, and Suriname, have the highest TB incidence in the Americas (between 100 and 200 per 100,000 inhabitants) [10], whereas Brazil has a high TB burden, but this is not uniformly distributed. In sub-Saharan Africa and in some regions of India, HIV-coinfection and poverty affecting housing conditions, ventilation, nutritional status, education, and access to health care, other than growing urbanization with the consequent overcrowded living conditions, are the most important determinants of TB epidemic in tropical countries [9].

TB remains one of the major public health challenges in North Africa with decreasing gradient incidence from Morocco (the highest) with more than 27,000 new cases per year, to intermediate in Algeria and lowest in Tunisia and Egypt (30 and 17 cases per 100,000, respectively) [11]. In the European Economic Area (EEA), the majority of subjects of foreign origin with TB in 2009 originated from Asia, Africa, and other European countries (34, 28, and 9.5%, respectively) [9, 10, 12]. This proportion continues to increase, and represents an important cause of the overall resurgence of the TB epidemic in the USA and Western Europe (EU) [12]. It can be anticipated that, despite efforts of the industrialized countries to conquer the disease, the incidence of new TB cases in EU varies from very low rates in Scandinavian countries (6–8 cases/100,000 population) to rates as high as 231 cases/100,000 populations in Tajikistan; the Russian Federation is eleventh among the 22 high-burden TB countries [12]. In Italy, where

[1]Low TB burden or low TB incidence countries are defined as those with a TB notification rate of ≤100 cases (all forms) per million population a year. The high-TB burden or incidence countries are countries with the highest estimated numbers of incident TB cases that account for 80% of the global total.

over the last decade the TB notification has been stable at approximately 7 cases per 100,000 people annually, the immigrant population has a relative risk of suffering from TB, 10–15 times higher than the Italian-born population [4]. In fact, the proportion of TB cases of foreigners increased from 22% in 1999 to 46% in 2008 of the total [13]; at the same time, the proportion of drug-resistant TB cases rose to 83% [14]. Almost two-thirds of the cases of TB in foreigners in 2008 occurred in northern Italy, where immigration is more prominent than in other areas of the country [13]. The most affected age group was of young adults [13]. Concurrently in Italy, while the proportion of African-born persons with TB decreased from 51 to 30%, the proportion of cases with TB born in Eastern EU, including former Soviet Union countries, increased from 16 to 33% [14, 15]. In the Italian population, the two most affected population groups are the elderly and the foreign born. The elderly population, due to progressive weakening of both, their general conditions and their immune system, caused by the aging process itself, is at increased risk of reactivation of LTBI. Foreign-born residents, which are at increased risk of developing TB either because of the high incidence rates of TB in their countries of origin or because of the social fragility deriving from the migration process itself [16], account for the increase of TB in people less than 65 years of age and for the great majority of drug-resistant TB cases.

Summarizing, the European countries share a TB epidemiology which is characterized by a decrease of TB incidence in natives but an increasing incidence in foreign-born persons; occurrence of the majority of TB cases in recent migrants and younger age groups, especially those experiencing inadequate living and health conditions; and high percentage of drug-resistant TB among immigrants and previously treated patients [11].

Factors that influence the risk of TB reactivation among immigrants in low TB burden countries include the prevalence of TB in the country of origin, the duration of residence in the host country, and the efficiency and quality of curative and preventive services. As mentioned previously, after the actual migration process, immigrants are exposed to additional risk of acquiring reactivated TB infection because of stressful living in overcrowded conditions, social isolation, poverty, malnutrition, unemployment, and difficulties to access to health care. Generally, TB in immigrants in low-burden countries arises from an active TB infection which occurred overseas. There are also reactivations of remotely acquired LTBI, which occurs months to years after settlement in the host country, or acquired TB as new infection postarrival in the host county through local transmission or during a return travel to the country of origin [17]. Second-generation migrants, who often keep a link with their country of origin, or international travellers including visiting friends and relatives (VFR), especially children, are known to represent high-risk groups for TB [18]. Finally, homeless immigrants and other deprived groups in low-burden countries can have transmission rates as high as some high-burden countries [19].

2.2. Screening practices among adults

Migrants currently play an important role in determining the current epidemiology of TB in low TB burden countries where they are settled. As a consequence, although reports from different high-income countries with well-performing immigration medical screening have demonstrated that foreign-born TB patients do not contribute to the transmission of TB in the native population [20], there is an increasing interest on how best to enhance TB control through coordinated medical screening of documented as well as undocumented migrants such as migrants or refugees that are arriving presently at the Greek and Italian coasts. Undocumented migrants have been shown to be at higher TB risk than other migrants, as their entry and TB infection is often more recent and their migration and living conditions are worse than those of documented migrants [21].

Immigration TB screening programs for high immigration and low TB incidence countries vary according to the national legislation, resource availability, and public health risk management practices. Moreover, programs differ by whether screening is done for active TB or LTBI, or both. The programs also differ in relation to arrival in the host country, i.e., the migrants' status, such as refugees or asylum seekers, the countries of origin, and tools used to screen for active TB or LTBI [22, 23]. The rationale of these programs is the early detection and treatment of active and often contagious TB cases in order to prevent *Mycobacterium tuberculosis* transmission to the host population of a low-burden country and reduce the burden of imported TB in low-incidence countries. Methods of TB control in migrant populations have historically focused on identifying active TB with accompanying contact tracing, but the yields for this remain relatively low. In this setting, screening can occur before entry (pre-entry screening), at entry (sometimes called port of entry screening), or after entry [24].

In most of cases, active TB immigrant medical screening in high-income industrialized countries for both documented migrants, refugees, or asylum seekers is performed on or soon after the entry (borders such as airport, reception centers/holding camps, migrant centers); 36% (9 of 25 countries including Australia, Canada, Israel, Jordan, New Zealand, France, the UK, and the USA) have a pre-entry TB screening in country of origin for people who intend to migrate; 20% (5 of 25 countries including Norway, Sweden, Switzerland, the Netherlands, and the UK) perform screening at entry [24, 25]. Literature shows that 88% of countries use chest X-rays (CXR) alone or in combination with clinical examination or TST [5, 24]. The sensitivity and specificity of CXR vary from 86–97% to 75–89%, respectively, and according to the criteria of imaging interpretation. CXR alone does not detect extrapulmonary TB (EPTB) which is increasing in comparison to pulmonary TB, especially in low-burden and high immigrant receiving countries [26], and in HIV-positive persons that have higher rates of EPTB compared with those who are HIV-negative.

Sputum smear and culture follow CXR only if this is found to be abnormal. The destiny of migrants to enter the host country depends on the outcome of these tests.

An interesting and original active TB finding approach was recently investigated by Schepisi [27] in Italy, a country where there is no TB national screening policy for new entrants [28]. Italy is a country with a TB incidence rate of 5.3/100,000 persons with 3.153 cases in 2013 [29]. TB cases are especially concentrated among high-risk TB groups, including migrants from high-incidence countries, homeless people, and drug and alcohol abusers. The study analyzed TB case finding intervention based on verbal symptoms screening,[2] conducted at primary centers for undocumented migrants, refugees, and asylum seekers in different Italian sites.

[2]Presence of cough, fever, fatigue, hemoptysis and weight loss.

Although only a limited number of TB cases was detected, of those screened and evaluated, the study, based on its feasible cost approach and reduced burden of medical procedures, contributed to the diagnoses and control of TB, especially among subpopulations that have difficulties to access specialized healthcare centers [27].

2.3. TB screening of migrant children

Although many countries have developed and documented immigration TB screening programs to suit the needs of adults, attention to migrant children lacks intensive studies.

Screening migrant children for TB is particularly important, as they have a higher risk of developing active disease due to recent infection. Furthermore, due to its "paucibacillary" nature, which makes it rarely infectious, when they develop the disease, it is more severe, resulting in increased morbidity and mortality compared with adults. Thus, TB screening in high-risk children from high-incidence countries should form part of all immigration TB screening programs. A recent survey compared various screening tools (history, physical examination, TST, interferon-gamma release assays (IGRAs), CXR,[3] and MTB (*M. tuberculosis*) bacteriology) among migrant children [30]. The screening programs varied considerably between the various participating countries. History and physical examination was often normal in children with active TB disease, and TST emerged as a better predictor of TB infection or disease [30]. Sociocultural and behavioral factors have shown to be involved in the acceptance of LTBI treatment in these populations [31]. In pediatrics, although TB may not be of immediate public health concern, individual morbidity and mortality is high. The goal of TB screening is to identify children with LTBI who are at risk for progression to active TB, as early LTBI treatment prevents extended and disseminated disease.

3. Definition of LTBI and risk of progression toward TB

Although the word LTBI should be "reconsidered" considering that both "latent" and "infection" terms indicate lack of disease and thus are redundant [32], LTBI is defined as a state of persistent immune response to previously acquired TB antigens without evidence of clinically manifested active TB disease. It is an asymptomatic and nontransmissible condition that is maintained for the lifetime of the infected person. Current tools are insufficient to measure the global prevalence of LTBI, but investigations carried out a decade ago estimated that approximately one-third of the world population (>2 billion people) is latently infected with *M. tuberculosis*.

A relatively small proportion, 5–15% of screen-test-positive patients of the estimated >2 billion people with LTBI will develop TB disease (TB reactivation) within the first 5 years after initial infection, with the remaining risk distributed over the rest of the life span [33, 34]. The likelihood of progression from LTBI to active clinical TB disease is determined by bacterial,

[3]Mainly employed in children ages from 11 to 16 years.

host, and environmental factors, potentially favoring TB evolution. A schematic diagram showing TB evolution following exposition is illustrated in **Figure 1**.

The risk factors for acquiring LTBI infection involve people at increased risk which include infants, children (<5 years), and adolescents who have intimate contact with high-risk adults, as well as persons who have had close contact with someone known or suspected to have active TB, health care workers, high-risk racial and ethnic minorities, prisoners, residents in nursing homes, hospitals, and homeless shelters [34]. LTBI also occurs in the migrant population coming from low-income countries with a high burden of disease, especially from the Indian subcontinent and sub-Saharan Africa (the highest burden in the world), as well as in asylum seekers and refugees, a subgroup of immigrants at particular risk for TB. Persons coming from tropical areas are also at an increased risk for developing TB. The probability of developing TB is much higher among people with cellular immunity impairment due to: human immunodeficiency virus (HIV) infection, tumor necrosis factor α inhibitors, glucocorticoids administration, and organ or hematologic transplantation. Diabetes mellitus and chronic kidney disease are also more common in migrant populations and significantly increase the risk of reactivation from LTBI to active TB [34, 35].

Among all the considered conditions, HIV infection is the most potent risk factor for progression from LTBI to active TB disease [36]. TB in fact is the leading cause of death among people living with HIV, estimated to account for around 33% of all HIV-related deaths globally [4] and individuals with both, LTBI and HIV infection, have a risk of reactivation of 10% per year of life compared with 10% for life for those who do not have an HIV infection [23]. Many HIV-positive people in developing countries develop TB as the first manifestation of AIDS [4]. The major risk factors for progression from latent infection to active disease are wide ranging and are listed in **Table 1**.

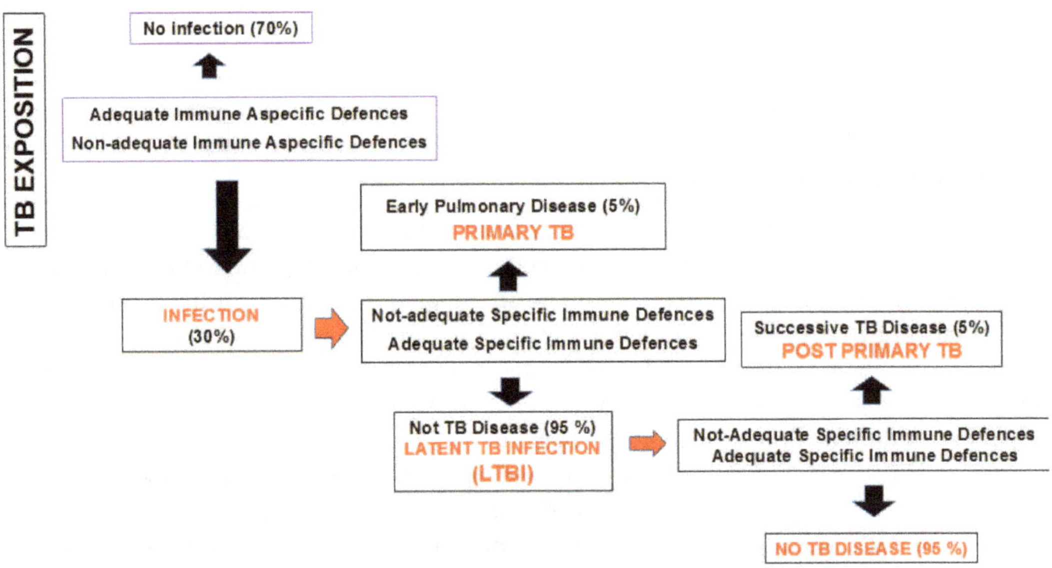

Figure 1. Evolution of TB from latent infection to active disease following exposition.

- Children younger than 5 years
- Persons with immunocompromising conditions (HIV, leukemia, lymphoma)
- Persons infected with *M. tuberculosis* within the past 2 years; persons who inject illicit drugs or use other locally identified high-risk substances (e.g., crack cocaine), tobacco, or alcohol abuse (risk of infection and active disease)
- Persons with a history of untreated or inadequately treated TB, including those with CXR findings consistent with previous tuberculosis (e.g., apical fibronodular changes on CXR)
- Homeless adults, elderly, health care workers, and medical students
- Persons with recent conversion of a negative tuberculin skin test to a positive test
- Persons with the following clinical conditions or other conditions compromising immunity: disorders requiring long-term use of corticosteroids or other immunosuppressant medications (including tumor necrosis factor-alpha antagonists), body weight 10% or more below the ideal, chronic renal failure, and end-stage renal disease requiring dialysis, diabetes mellitus*, gastrectomy or intestinal bypass, malignancy (cancer of the head, neck, or lung), silicosis
- Tropical parasitic diseases including helminthic infestations**
- Black race, black skin individuals***

*Diabetes can increase the relative TB risk (range 1.16–7.83) [37].
**These can negatively impact on TB disease inducing immunological weakening throughout Th1 impairment [38].
***Black skin individuals are constitutively more susceptible than white skin persons owing to environmental and genetic factors [39].

Table 1. Groups at increased risk of progression from LTBI to active tuberculosis.

4. Management of LTBI among immigrants and screening practices

Given that the majority of active TB in foreign-born persons in low-incidence countries arises from reactivation of LTBI, acquired many years previously in the country of origin, as also demonstrated by epidemiological studies based on *M. tuberculosis* strain isolates by molecular genotyping that found that 55-90% of TB cases in foreign-born persons are due to LTBI reactivation [40–41]. Screening new entrants for LTBI remains the cornerstone for controlling imported TB. While most developed countries screen for active TB, screening for LTBI is much less commonly performed [24, 42].

Guidelines for LTBI screening among immigrants are not homogenous and vary among regions; moreover, evidence supporting their effectiveness is lacking and identifying models of best practice remains difficult, so that there are no perfect methods for the diagnosis and management of LTBI [43–45] whose identification provides opportunity for early treatment and the prevention of significant health sequelae for the individual. Diagnosis of TB is currently based on a positive result of either a tuberculin skin test (TST) or IGRA test indicating an immune response to *M. tuberculosis*. The TST is widely used and inexpensive, but requires a repeat visit to the physician and has low performance in persons recently vaccinated with BCG (e.g., immigrants arriving in industrialized countries), or who are infected with HIV. With the TST, an induration of 15 mm or more is considered positive in persons without risk factors, 10 mm or more is positive for those at higher risk, such as immigrants from high TB-endemic countries with no history of TB, and 5 mm or more is positive for certain high-risk persons (e.g., immunocompromised patients, those exposed to active TB). The more expensive IGRAs overcome some of the TST performance issues [46]. IGRAs require a single patient visit to conduct the test and results can be available within 24 hours. IGRAs, however, are not the preferred testing method for use in children younger than 5 years old, persons recently exposed to TB, immunocompromised persons, and those who will be tested repeatedly [47]. To test immigrant and refugee children with LTBI who are probably vaccinated with BCG, IGRAs may limit the number of children targeted for preventive therapy [48]. The use of one-step IGRA has also demonstrated to be the best option for young migrants [9]. Although in the last decade, IGRAs have increasingly replaced the use of TST, these tests have also limitations, both cannot verify the presence/ absence of dormant bacteria still able to reactivate and thus they do not reliably predict who will progress to active TB [2, 3]. Moreover, strong positive tests do not suggest a higher TB risk reactivation, and in children under 5 years of age and immunocompromised patients, including HIV-infected subjects, the test performances are particularly poor, thus needing a better detection test for LTBI [49, 50]. The comparative performance of the TST and IGRAs also varies between high-incidence and low-incidence countries, possibly because of the effects of BCG vaccination and reinfection [51]. In this setting, WHO strongly recommend that either TST or IGRA be used to test for LTBI in special risk populations (i.e., HIV persons, transplant patients, patients initiating anti-TNF treatments, household members or close contacts, including children of pulmonary TB cases). A positive IGRA or TST test is required to diagnose LTBI and to start specific therapy according WHO guidelines [4]. In high TB burden countries a LTBI test is not required prior to LTBI treatment, but it is encouraged for HIV-positive persons.

4.1. Screening practices

Individuals should be asked about symptoms of TB before being tested for LTBI. In this setting, WHO guidelines [4] suggest an algorithm for targeted diagnosis and treatment of LTBI in individuals of risk groups (**Figure 2**).

A recent survey found that only 55.2%, 16 out of the previously mentioned 29 countries (see p. 6), screen for LTBI most frequently postarrival in their country using TST in 68.8% of cases, TST plus a confirmatory IGRA in 25%, and IGRA alone in 18.8%. In 11 of these countries, the screening is compulsory for documented migrants [5, 24, 25].

The screening may decrease the period of infectiousness by as much as 33% in some situations [5]. LTBI screening is effective in persons at risk of contracting *M. tuberculosis* or of progressing from LTBI to active TB. It is generally thought that routine screening outside these high-risk groups wastes resources and leads to high false-positive test rates. According to the WHO 2015 Guidelines on the Management of LTBI [4], systematic testing and treatment of LTBI is highly recommended in immigrants from high TB burden countries; prisoners, homeless persons, and illicit drug users should be treated according to TB epidemiology and resource availability. This procedure has shown to lead to early detection of cases, resulting in a shorter duration of symptoms, and fewer hospitalizations.

The decision to screen for TB is a decision to treat. LTBI can be effectively treated in order to prevent progression to active TB, thus resulting in a substantial benefit for both the individual and the community. Currently available treatment options allow to reduce the risk of

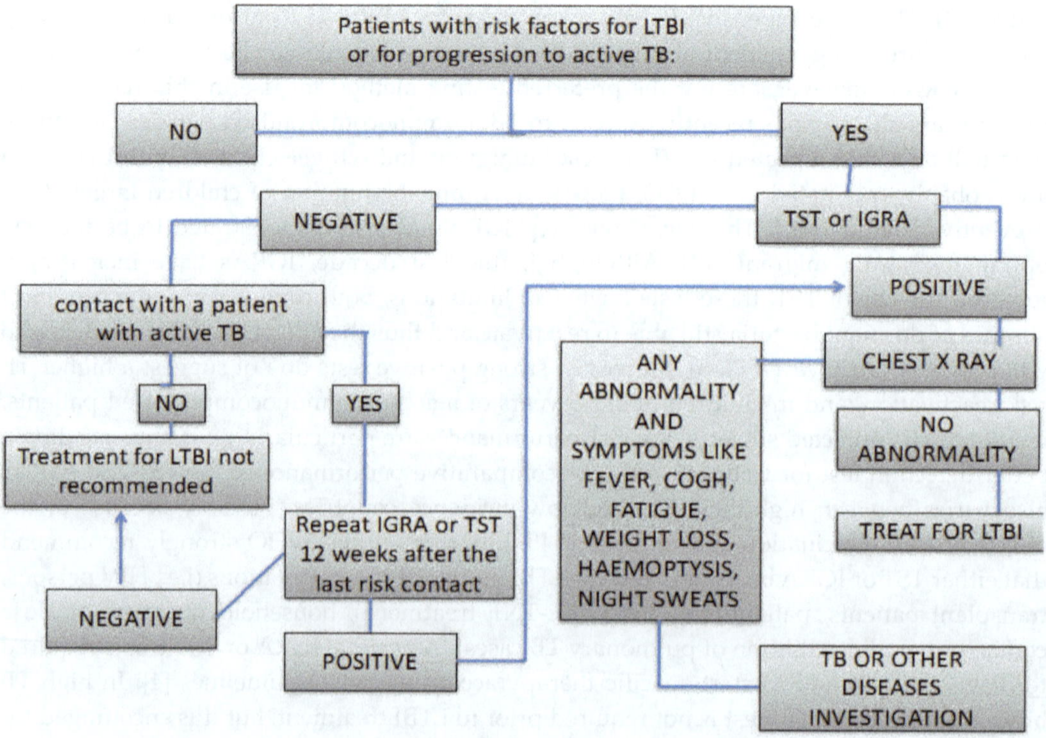

Figure 2. Algorithm for the management of LTBI in individuals at risk for TB. Modified and adapted from Guidelines on the Management of Latent Tuberculosis Infection. Available from: www.who.int/tb/areas-of-work/preventive-care/ltbi/en/

developing active TB by at least 60%. However, safety concerns exist, mainly related to the development of drug-related adverse events including hepatotoxicity. The following regimens recommended by the WHO TB Report 2015 [4] for the treatment of LTBI are: daily therapy with INH for 6–9 months; 12 weeks rifapentine plus INH weekly; 3–4 months INH plus rifampicin daily; rifampicin plus pyrazinamide for 2 months or 3–4 months RIF alone. While the safety of 2 months of RIF and PZA has shown to be acceptable in HIV-infected persons and children, in non-HIV-infected adults, this regimen has demonstrated a high rate of severe liver toxicity [52].

Identification of latently infected individuals and their treatment has lowered TB incidence in rich, advanced countries. Similar approaches also hold great promise for countries with low to intermediate rates of TB incidence. Wide variations are observed for the cost of screening of eligible candidates for LTBI treatment and the costs for treatment. For reasons of practicality and cost effectiveness, most high-income countries consider and check as eligible population refugees or asylum seekers or those individuals arriving from high TB burden settings. The available evidence suggests that screening for and treatment of LTBI may be a cost-effective intervention in population groups characterized by high prevalence of LTBI and/or high risk of progression to active TB, such as persons migrating from high TB incidence countries, contacts with active TB cases, and persons living with HIV.

5. Essentials of diagnosis of infectious TB among immigrants in low TB burden countries

Owing difficulties in access to health system, TB diagnosis and treatment are lower in migrant populations compared to native subjects. This is in part due the fact that migrants, in general, have a longer patient diagnostic delay for TB (time elapsed from the onset of symptoms and the first medical visit) possibly due to a combination of reasons including language barriers, unemployment, or interruption due to lack of medical insurance that hinder migrants from using the available health TB services, while natives have a longer health care diagnostic delay (defined as the time elapsed between the first medical consultation and the initiation of treatment) [53]. Although the reliability of epidemiological assessments has progressively improved in recent years, no more than 30% of the estimated number of people suffering from TB, including migrants, is actually diagnosed with a method of proven efficacy [54]. Moreover, current diagnostic tests have poor performance on forms of TB which are intrinsically difficult to diagnose, such as childhood TB, smear-negative pulmonary TB and EPTB, TB in HIV/AIDS patients, and drug-resistant TB.

5.1. Conventional diagnostic methods

To date, the most common methods for diagnosing TB worldwide which constitute the backbone of TB diagnosis remain the "old" sputum smear microscopy test and bacteriological culture which is also the test necessary for monitoring patients' response to treatment [2, 3]. These methods, however, represent a major constraint even in high-tech, high-resources western countries, when the mycobacterial load is low or the district of infection is not easily accessible. TB diagnosis includes suspicion as first step. All patients with TB, including migrants, can present with almost any symptom including cough, shortness of breath, chest pain, hemoptysis, together with the presence of constitutional symptoms (weight loss, fever, fatigue, and night sweats) which meet the definition of a suspected TB case according to WHO [55]. These symptoms must be considered in differential diagnosis in patients with epidemiologic risk (exposure to infectious patients, travel to or residence in a high prevalence area, previous TB) [2, 54]. The clinical suspicion of TB is then investigated through radiographic imaging, microbiology, and histopathology. Radiology could also have an important role in the diagnosis of TB in low-resource countries, especially as pre-entry TB screening in country of origin for those migrants who intend to migrate and refugees. However, the equipment is expensive and it needs qualified and experienced staff to be able to interpret the radiological signs—they are not always available in these settings [23, 45, 56, 57]. Moreover, CXR cannot provide a conclusive diagnosis on its own and needs to be followed by sputum testing. Although inexpensive and potentially easy to perform, conventional smear microscopy has a number of limitations including the variable (from 20 to 80%) sensitivity which is low, particularly among all persons coinfected with TB and HIV, including migrants and children, due to the reduced pulmonary bacillary load in these subjects [58]; it cannot distinguish between MBT complex and non-TB mycobacteria and it does not provide information on the resistance profile of the bacilli. In this setting, phenotypic drug-susceptibility testing (DST) on cultured specimens is the conventional method used to detect resistance to first- and SLD-TB drugs in

MDR-TB and monitoring patients' response to treatment [4]. Finally, the challenge of TB diagnosis in the low-income countries including the tropics, must also take into account the differential diagnosis with a wide spectrum of microbial agents causing respiratory infections of which migrants can be affected and include viruses, bacteria (*Actynomicetes*), and parasites (*paracoccidioidomycosis, paragonimiasis, dirofilariosis*), which can mimic TB [2, 3, 9], and other diseases such as sarcoidosis and cancer. In these settings, basic radiography and other analyses are of considerable use but are not available in all centers [9].

5.2. Advanced diagnostic techniques

Current-generation MTB-specific nucleic acid amplification tests (NAATs) can be a valid surrogate to direct observation or isolation of tubercular bacilli and to replace culture [33] and detect new TB cases within few hours. Although NAATs are widely used in Europe [33, 59], their high cost and level of technical support hindered the widespread adoption in TB endemic countries. Improving diagnosis in high-income countries is a strategic goal in TB research, and the pipeline of diagnostic tools is rapidly growing: new ways of performing sputum smear microscopy and innovative technologies for molecular diagnosis have already been endorsed by WHO, or are under investigation [60]. To respond to the urgent need for simple and rapid diagnostic tools at the point of treatment in high-burden countries, a fully automated molecular test for *M. tuberculosis* detection and resistance to RIF testing was developed (Xpert®MTB/RIF) and has been endorsed by WHO in December 2010 [56]. Its capability to simultaneously detect mutations conferring resistance to RIF extends its usefulness beyond the diagnosis of TB (sensitivity 98.2 and 72.5% respectively for smear-positive and smear-negative samples; specificity 99.2%), also to first-line assessment of RIF resistance (99.1% sensitivity and 100% specificity) and prediction of multidrug resistance (99% sensitivity) [61]. Xpert®MTB/RIF system has the advantage to provide accurate results in less than 2 hours as it requires minimal biosafety supplies and training, so that patients can receive treatment from the same day on. According to WHO recommendations, Xpert®MTB/RIF, which is less sensitive than culture but more sensitive than microscopy [62], should be especially used as the initial diagnostic test in all individuals including migrants suspected of multidrug-resistant (MDR) TB or HIV-associated TB and in testing cerebrospinal fluid specimens from patients presumed to have TB meningitis; it may be used as a follow-on test to microscopy in settings where MDR and/or HIV is of lesser concern, especially in smear-negative specimens (conditional recommendation, recognizing major resource implications). With the introduction of Xpert®MTB/RIF, there has been an increase of the number of microbiologically confirmed TB in children [63], thus offering in low-income and middle-income countries, an opportunity for investigators to provide access to diagnosis for children beyond smear microscopy, and an increase of the number of pulmonary TB cases detected in HIV-positive patients when compared with microscopy [62]. Although with high specificity, Xpert®MTB/RIF has shown limited sensitivity for the detection of EPTB especially in HIV-positive individuals and among migrants in whom it can mimic cancer, bacterial and fungal infections [4, 64]. Other than Xpert®MTB/RIF test, new TB diagnostic tests may enhance diagnostic algorithms by offering rapid, point-of-care, or near-care detection of TB. One of these is the urine tests for lipoarabinomannan (LAM) and is detectable in the urine of all individuals with active TB [65]. Urine-based testing has advantages over sputum-based testing because urine is easy to collect and store, and lacks the infection control risks associated with sputum collection. The test is easy to perform, rapid (less than 30 minutes), and may be used at the point at which care is provided for TB or HIV. The urinary LAM assays currently available are unsuitable as general diagnostic or screening tests for TB, due to suboptimal sensitivity. The test was found to be cost-effective in sub-Saharan Africa when used for HIV-positive patients with CD4 counts of less than 100 per mm^3 [66], but lacks accuracy if used in patients with CD4 counts over 200 or in children. WHO recommends that LAM assay should be used for the diagnosis of TB in all HIV-positive persons with low CD4 counts or in those who are seriously ill,[4] and to assist in the diagnosis of TB in HIV-positive adult inpatients with signs or symptoms of TB (pulmonary and/or EPTB) who have a CD4 cell count less than or equal to 100 cells/L [4]. Other new generation NAAT kits have been released for research use [67], but further data are needed before their potential to assist TB control can be judged. Independent studies are required in settings representative of the intended use of the device.

6. Management and treatment of drug-resistant TB

So far TB treatment in migrant populations represents a challenge as it contributes considerably to illness and death especially in western countries. There are not only the economic but also the social costs. A number of social determinants, such as limited language, sociopsychological barriers, lack of employment, fear of expulsion, and access to health care facilities, often lead to a protracted diagnosis. Thus, TB treatment of these patients can be limited or inadequate and this is fundamental for conferring TB drug resistance.

6.1. MDR and XDR-TB management issues

The current standard of care of drug-susceptible MTB requires 6–9 months of combination therapy which includes a 2-month "intensive" phase of a four-drug cocktail containing RIF, INH, PZA, and EMB; followed by a longer "continuation" phase of RIF and INH to eradicate the remaining bacilli that have entered a dormant, slowly replicating the latent phase. Currently, standardized regimens require that patients' daily ingest up to four drugs under direct observation of a healthcare worker for a period of 6–9 months. In this setting, directly observed treatment (DOT) of TB reduces TB-related death, disability, and transmission; it is a highly cost-effective intervention, even in the lowest income countries [54]. Treatment of TB represents a therapeutic challenge because of not only the natural level high resistance of *M. tuberculosis* to antibiotics, but also because of the occurrence of new mutations that confer additional resistance as well as multidrug strains. The drug-resistant TB represents a constant threat to some groups of patients, including migrants, who do not take the medication once they start to feel better. Indeed, an increasing number of MDR-TB strains are isolated because of the poor compliance to treatment that characterizes migrants themselves. Nowadays, the insufficient treatment regimens, nonadherence, and poor availability of drugs are a major

[4]Respiratory rate >30/min, temperature >39°C, heart rate >120/min, severe difficulty to walk unaided.

cause of treatment failure, relapse of disease, and TB drug-resistance especially in migrants. Eastern European countries are among those with the highest rates of MDR-TB and have also the most drug-resistant (XDR) strains in the world[5] [15]. By the end of September 2009, at least one case of XDR-TB had been reported by each of the 25 countries in the European continent. The majority of European and other low prevalence countries, excluding some of the high priority countries in the WHO European Region (such as Latvia, Lithuania, Bulgaria, and Estonia), also reported higher prevalence of MDR-TB cases in migrants when compared to the native population [68]. The number of cases of XDR-TB diagnosed globally is rising as expected because of improved laboratory testing and reporting. The diagnosis of XDR-TB is equivalent today to a death sentence. Factors contributing to higher mortality rates in patients with XDR-TB include: resistance to six or more drugs, delayed diagnoses, prescribing ineffective drug therapies due to the lack of DST, and deprivation of programmatic access to effective SLD. During 2015, 105 countries reported cases of XDR-TB to the WHO [4]. However, the highest numbers were registered in 2014 and included India, Ukraine, South Africa, Belarus, and Kazakhstan [4]. In the United States, 15 cases of XDR-TB were reported to the CDC between 2009 and 2014 [4]. In Italy, the proportion of TB cases notified in foreigners increased from 22% in 1999 to 46% in 2008, paralleling the proportion of MDR-TB cases which consistently grew to 83% [13, 69]. A recent retrospective study conducted over the period 2008–2010 aimed to investigate drug-resistance proportions and drug-resistance profiles of *M. tuberculosis* strains circulating among immigrants and natives. It showed that the five countries mainly contributing to the TB resistance in foreigner groups in Italy were Romania (28.7%), Morocco (9.9%), Peru (5.8%), Pakistan (5.8%), and India (5.6%). Moreover, the MDR-TB prevalence in immigrants was consistent with that of their native countries (e.g., in 2009: Romania, 11.2%; Ukraine, 19%; Moldova, 44.3%). Differences in culture may impact significantly on TB prevention, diagnosis, and treatment in immigrants which, unlike the general population, are also at greater risk of having an infection with MDR-TB [14]. In general, patients who do not respond to previous TB therapy have an up to a 50-fold higher risk of having MDR- and XDR-TB. Other prominent risk factors include close contact to a patient with MDR-TB, migration, HIV infection, and young age. Moreover, as infection control policies are problematic in many developing countries, nosocomial transmission of MDR- and XDR-TB is 3–6 times higher in patients hospitalized for more than 14 days [70]. In particular, the risk increases in open hospital wards where advanced HIV-infected with low CD4 cell counts can facilitate the nosocomial spread of infection. The management of patients with MDR-TB, XDR-TB, or total resistant TB requires an appropriate and rapid diagnosis. After identification of high-risk groups, microbiological confirmation and appropriate treatment should be started [71, 72]. Confirmation of resistant-TB and identification of potentially effective drugs in an optimized combination treatment regimen should be done on the basis of antimicrobial DST. However, only 22% of countries worldwide routinely perform cultures and DST, and only 48% of the 46 countries in the WHO Africa region have ever undertaken a drug-resistance survey [4, 73]. Moreover, DST is often too expensive, especially in high-burden countries, and in many settings it is neglected because

[5]That is, MDR strains resistant to any FC and to at least one of three injectable SLD: KM, CM, AK.

of the lack of SLD [73, 74]. In general, treatment for MDR-TB can extend up to 2 years after microbiologic culture conversion and relies on more toxic, less efficacious second- or third-line agents, many of which are even more scarce than frontline drugs in affected areas [75].

6.2. Therapeutic concerns of MDR and XDR-TB in different population groups including migrants

Patients with MDR-TB strains should receive therapy based on individual DST including residual first-line (SM), EMB, PZA drugs, and SLD such as oxacin, KM, CM, ET, PAS, and CS. As with other antimicrobial agents, the use of SLD can generate resistant mutants. DST often shows poor reproducibility and lack of correlation with clinical response. The initial intensive phase of therapy should last 6–8 months and includes at least 4 months after culture conversion. Compared with the treatment of drug-susceptible TB, the treatment of MDR- and XDR-TB requires more drugs that are less well tolerated for a more prolonged duration. The available TB drugs against MDR/XDR-TB are included among a hierarchy of five groups, with first-line TB drugs listed in Group 1 and second-line drugs in Groups 2 through 5 [76]. Group 1 is composed of first-line TB drugs RIF, INH, PZA, and EMB; Group 2 contains the injectable agents embracing the bactericidal aminoglycosides (SM, AK, and KM) and CM, whereas Group 3 consists of FC including gatifloxacin and moxifloxacin. The remaining SLD ethionamide/prothionamide, CS, and PAS are inside Group 4 and are considered less potent and often less well tolerated by patients. Group 5 contains new antimicrobial agents, those with less clinical experience, and drugs with less proven efficacy in the management of drug-resistant TB such as clofazimine, developed in the 1950s to treat leprosy. Bedaquiline, delamanid, linezolid, clofazimine, meropenem, amoxicillin-clavulanate, and clarithromycin are included in this category. Although adherence to therapeutic programs is often impossible for immigrants as they are often lost in follow-up, at least five drugs (including an injectable agent) should be given for an "intensive phase" of up to 8 months. The specific drugs chosen depend on a patient's previous TB drug therapies and individual DST results. Thereafter, a "continuation phase" of least four oral drugs should be continued until a total minimum duration of 20 months. Prolonged therapy presents a range of practical challenges including prolonged hospitalization with conspicuous health care cost, toxicity (i.e., nephro- and ototoxicity with aminoglycoside drugs), and high loss to follow-up during continuation therapy. Finally, drug-resistant TB can represent in Africa a particular risk to individuals with HIV with high transmission of infection and high mortality [77]. Treatment success rates of MDR/XDR-TB vary between 36 and 79% [78, 79]. Surgery can have a positive adjunctive role with combination of antimicrobial drug therapy in the management of drug-resistant TB, but does not allow for shortening the duration of therapy [80].

Three groups of people deserve special attention in MDR/XDR TB management: children, pregnant women, and HIV-positive patients.

There are not enough data regarding optimal duration of MDR/XDR-TB treatment in children which may vary from case to case. Depending on the extent of the disease, the TB DST pattern and the immune status of the child, a total duration of treatment between 12 and 18 months following culture conversion could be acceptable, with the recommendation to continue the treatment only in particular cases to avoid relapse [30]. However, the clinical trials in children so far carried out are not enough to supporting this approach.

Regarding pregnancy, there is consensus that neither LTBI following contact of a patient with MDR/XDR-TB nor active MDR/XDR-TB requires cessation of pregnancy [81]. While safety of many drugs for the unborn child is unknown, treatment of pregnant females who develop MDR/XDR-TB or become pregnant during treatment can be successful without adverse events for the newborn, although aminoglycosides/polypeptides are not recommended for MDR/XDR-TB treatment during pregnancy [82]. Theoretically, breastfeeding should be recommended only in females who are not infectious. However, the known and theoretical benefits of continuing treatment seem to outweigh theoretical risks to the mother and fetus.

Being TB and HIV strictly related, HIV exacerbates TB and the phenomenon of MDR/XDR-TB is somehow increasing in these patients in whom HIV testing is not always evaluated especially in particular countries, thereby delaying the initiation of antiretroviral therapy (ART) which could significantly reduce mortality, relapse rates, and development of resistant strains [83]. This is especially true for immigrants in whom not only it is difficult the access HIV testing, but also ART testing. A large body of research has in fact shown that migrants are more likely to enter into the healthcare system late and are less likely to be retained at successive stages of the HIV treatment cascade.

MDR/XDR-TB has higher mortality rates especially in South Africa [83, 84] among MDR/XDR-TB and HIV coinfected cases with very low CD4 cell counts and limited access to ART. Timely diagnosis based on molecular assays is crucial to reduce the mortality associated with MDR/XDR-TB patients among HIV-infected persons. Owing to high case detection rates compared to smear microscopy, WHO recommends Xpert®MTB/RIF as a primary diagnostic test for TB in persons living with AIDS [4].

In conclusion, treatment for MDR/XDR-TB is far from optimal at present. In particular, treatment of MDR/XDR-TB in migrants living in high-income countries is associated with increased risk of therapy nonadherence, loss to follow-up, and in general, noncontinuity of anti-TB care that worsens drug-resistant TB. Migrants' slow progression through the TB or HIV treatment cascade can be attributed to feelings of confusion, inability to effectively communicate in the native language, and poor knowledge about administrative or logistical requirements of the healthcare system.

Novel therapeutic interventions with shorter treatment regimens with higher efficacy and better tolerability than those currently available are required. In addition, new drugs need to be developed and existing drugs for anti-TB properties should be reevaluated for their potential efficacy in the treatment of MDR/XDR-TB. In receiving high-income countries, the international community has responded with financial and scientific support, leading to new drugs [85] and regimens in advanced clinical development and an increasingly sophisticated understanding of resistance mechanisms and their application to all aspects of TB control and treatment. In the absence of a preventive vaccine, more effective diagnostic tools, and novel drugs, the control of MDR/XDR-TB will be extremely difficult. Moreover, the increasing rates of drug-resistant TB in Eastern EU, Asia, and sub-Saharan Africa is now threatening the gains made by TB control programs worldwide.

7. Conclusions and social issues

Although the WHO Report 2015 [4] with its "STOP TB" strategy has the goal to eliminate TB as a public health problem (defined as <1 case per 1 million population per year) by 2050, TB shows no signs of disappearing in the near future despite declining incidence in most high-income countries. TB is still one of the top three infectious killing diseases in the world, after HIV/AIDS that kills 3 million people each year, TB kills 2 million, and malaria kills 1 million [4]. In order to intensify the fights against this deadly disease, further efforts aimed to strength surveillance programs to accurately estimate the burden of all kinds of TB are of great significance. Considering the enormous number of migrants around the world [8] with its high rates in the USA and Europe (54 and 76 million, respectively), particularly in Germany, Russia, the UK, France, Spain, and Italy, other than Saudi Arabia, Canada, and Australia, the problem of TB is of foremost importance and deserves great attention in order to act promptly to find solutions.

Although migration in itself is not a definitive risk for TB, several factors can put migrants in vulnerable situations that push factors (desertification, famine/drought, political fear/persecution, poor medical care, loss of wealth, and natural disasters), and pull factors (search of job opportunities, better living conditions, better medical care, political and/or religious freedom and security) migrant people in and out of TB-endemic areas [86]. Social fragility of migrant populations, despite its heterogeneity, shows areas of health suffering in large part due to highly uncertain circumstances and integration policies in receiving countries, especially at the local level, difficulties in access to services, and to relational communicative problems. In fact, the slow or less rapid deterioration of the migrant health in the host country creates serious problems, both to the person who is sick, and to the community which is forced to support the social and economic costs that this entails. Therefore, understanding the changing socioenvironmental situation as well as population movements and their associated risks for TB infection is critical for control, containment, and elimination of this disease which still poses infection-control and public-health challenges in the twenty-first century. Providing services aimed to identify and treat TB in migrants, refugees, or asylum seekers who are at high TB risk is challenging and requires a multidisciplinary approach and a high rate of investment of resources, human, structural, and material [87]. In immigrants living in high-income countries there are crucial factors that play an important role in TB-drug adherence which include length of treatment course, complex regimens, medication side effects, poor access to health care services, poor communication with health care providers, lack of social support, negative perceptions, stigma, and discrimination. The lack of laboratory facilities in their country of origin made the laboratory diagnosis of infectious diseases, including TB, difficult in many parts of the African continent as well as in the majority of other poor and low resource countries, where the diagnosis continues to rely on century-old sputum microscopy. In recent years, a growing number of rapid and more sensitive tests for TB and drug-resistant TB, based on molecular methods, including Xpert®MTB/RIF, have become available to replace or parallel exist to conventional tests; however, current TB diagnostics are still suboptimal in their performance for childhood TB, smear-negative TB, EPTB, HIV-TB, and drug-resistant TB. Furthermore, there is no standard test for the identification of LTBI, which, if correctly identified in particular risk groups including migrants, could be appropriately treated in order to prevent the onset of TB. So far, neither test can reliably predict future disease among persons with positive tests, and strong positive tests do not suggest a higher risk.

Looking at the movement of people today, at world politics, and at the increasing gap between the rich and the poor, it is expected that the number of immigrants will increase and with it health risks of those on the move and, to a lesser extent, the risk of those in the receiving countries can also be anticipated. It is argued here that a substantial increase in funding for TB research is required. There is no vaccine with adequate effectiveness, and TB treatment regimens are protracted and have a risk of toxic effects. Moreover, fundamental understanding of the pathogenesis of this disease is inadequate. In order to achieve the ambitious targets of the End-TB strategy 2035 (95% reduction in TB deaths, compared with 2015), 90% reduction in TB incidence rate (less than 100 TB cases per million population, no affected families facing catastrophic costs due to TB), greater efforts are needed also regarding migrants interventions, such as support services to receive and treat migrants, improving their access to health facilities, preventing the development of drug resistance through high quality treatment of drug-susceptible TB, improving adherence to anti-TB treatment, and offering vaccination for TB especially to prevent TB meningitis in children in endemic areas. Control strategies need to be adapted to local realities after evaluation of data prevalence/incidence, feasibility, and cost effectiveness. TB transmission among immigrants and natives is still rare, although it could increase in case of limited TB control. Thus, interventions such as expansion of the free service package and education about TB diagnosis among community health personnel are urgently required for early LTBI or case detection among migrants, particularly those born in a country with a high incidence of disease or in those persons exposed to the contact with TB, like close relatives of infectious patients [87]. It is recommended that high-income countries and their institutions cooperate in the near future with high-burden countries [4]. One important goal inside the "Global Action Framework for Research towards TB Elimination," developed by WHO [4] for the period 2016–2025 will be in fact to translate the new technologies and innovative approaches into policies and practices and then adapt to particular country contexts as appropriate. This is only another rational approach that in future will help to reach some of the ambitious targets to control, perhaps stop TB, in the coming decades.

Abbreviations

RIF	Rifampicin
INH	Isoniazid
PZA	Pyrazinamide
EMB	Ethambutol
KM	Kanamycin
CM	Capreomycin

AK	Amikacin
CS	Cycloserine
PAS	P-aminosalicylic acid
FC	Fluoroquinolones
MDR-TB	Multi drug-resistant tuberculosis
XDR-TB	Extensive drug resistant-TB
SLD	Second-line drugs

Author details

Carlo Contini*, Martina Maritati, Marachiara di Nuzzo, Lorenzo Massoli, Sara Lomenzo and Anastasio Grilli

*Address all correspondence to: cnc@unife.it

Department of Medical Sciences, Section of Infectious Diseases and Dermatology, University of Ferrara, Ferrara, Italy

References

[1] Global Tuberculosis Report 2014. Geneva, Switzerland: World Health Organization 2014. Available from: http://apps.who.int/iris/bitstream/10665/137094/1/9789241564809_eng.pdf

[2] Frieden TR, Sterling TR, Munsiff SS, Watt CJ, Dye C. Tuberculosis. Lancet 2003, Sept 13; 362 (9387):887–99.

[3] Das PH, Horton R. Tuberculosis: time to accelerate progress. Lancet 2010, May 22; 375 (9728):1755-71755-1757.

[4] Global Tuerculosis Report 2015. Geneva, Switzerland. World Health Organization 2015 XXth Edition. Available from: http://apps.who.int/iris/bitstream/10665/191102/1/9789241565059_eng.pdf?ua=1. Accessed: October 2015.

[5] Pareek M, Greenaway C, Noori T, Munoz J, Zenner D. The impact of migration on tuberculosis epidemiology and control in high-income countries: a review. BMC Med. 2016; 14: 48.

[6] Dolin PJ, Raviglione MC, Kochi A. Global tuberculosis incidence and mortality during 1990–2000. Bull World Health Organ 1994; 72: 213–30.

[7] Dye C, Scheele S, Dolin P, Pathania V, Raviglione MC. Consensus statement. Global burden of tuberculosis: estimated incidence, prevalence, and mortality by country. WHO Global Surveillance and Monitoring Project. JAMA. 1999; 282: 677–86.

[8] Intenational Migration Report 2015. Available in http://www.un.org/en/development/desa/population/migration/publications/migrationreport/docs/MigrationReport2015_Highlights.pdf

[9] Zammarchi L, Bartalesi F, Bartoloni A. Tuberculosis in tropical areas and immigrants. Mediterr J Hematol Infect Dis. 2014; 6 (1): e2014043.

[10] Martinez VN Komatsu NK, De Figueredo SM, Waldman EA. Equity in health: tuberculosis in the Bolivian immigrant community of Sao Paulo, Brazil. Tropical Med Int Health. 2012; 17: 1417–24.

[11] Khyatti M, Trimbitas RD, Zouheir Y, Benani A, El Messaoudi MD, Hemminki K. Infectious diseases in North Africa and North African immigrants to Europe. Eur J Public Health. 2014; 24: 47–56.

[12] European Centre for Disease Prevention and Control/WHO Regional Office for Europe. (2012) Tuberculosis surveillance and monitoring in Europe 2012.

[13] Morandi M, Resi D, Morsillo F, Moro ML, D'Amato S, et al. La Tubercolosi in Italia Anno; 2008. pp. 1–24.

[14] Fattorini L, Mustazzolu A, Piccaro G, Pardini M, Filippini P, Giannoni F, et al. Drug-resistant tuberculosis among foreign-born persons in Italy. Italian Multicentre Study on Resistance to Antituberculosis Drugs Group. Eur Respir J. 2012; 40: 497–500.

[15] Nathanson E, Nunn P, Uplekar M, Floyd K, Jaramillo E, Lönnroth K, Weil D, Raviglione M. MDR tuberculosis—critical steps for prevention and control. N Engl J Med. 2010; 363: 1050–8.

[16] Ingrosso L, Vescio F, Giuliani M, Migliori GB, Fattorini L, Severoni S, Rezza G. Risk factors for tuberculosis in foreign-born people (FBP) in Italy: a systematic review and meta-analysis. PLoS One. 2014; 9(4): e94728. doi: 10.1371/journal.pone.0094728. eCollection 2014.

[17] Lobato MN, Hopewell PC. Mycobacterium tuberculosis infection after travel to or contact with visitors from countries with a high prevalence of tuberculosis. Am J Respir Crit Care Med. 1998; 158: 1871–5.

[18] Monge-Maillo B, Norman FF, Pérez-Molina JA, Navarro M, Díaz-Menéndez M, López-Vélez R. Travelers visiting friends and relatives (VFR) and imported infectious disease: travelers, immigrants or both? A comparative analysis. Travel Med Infect Dis. 2014; 12: 88–94. Epub 2013 Jul 29.

[19] White PJ, Abubakar I. Improving control of tuberculosis in low-burden countries: insights from mathematical modeling. Front Microbiol. 2016; 7: 394. eCollection 2016.

[20] Barniol J, Niemann S, Louis VR, Brodhun B, Dreweck C, Richter E, Becher H, Haas W, Junghanss T. Transmission dynamics of pulmonary tuberculosis between autochthonous and immigrant sub-populations. BMC Infect Dis. 2009; 9: 197.

[21] Heldal E, Kuyvenhoven JV, Wares F, Migliori GB, Ditiu L, Fernandez de la Hoz K, Garcia D. Diagnosis and treatment of tuberculosis in undocumented migrants in low- or intermediate-incidence countries. Int J Tuberc Lung Dis. 2008; 12: 878–88.

[22] Sridhar S, Pollock K, Lalvani A. Redefining latent tuberculosis. Future Microbiol. 2011; 6: 1021–35.

[23] Aldridge RW, Zenner D, White PJ, Muzyamba MC, Loutet M, Dhavan P, Mosca D, Hayward AC, Abubakar I. Prevalence of and risk factors for active tuberculosis in migrants screened before entry to the UK: a population-based cross-sectional study. Lancet Infect Dis. 2016; 16: 962–70. Epub 2016 Mar 21.

[24] Pareek M, Abubakar I, White PJ, Garnett GP, Lalvani A. Tuberculosis screening of migrants to low-burden nations: insights from evaluation of UK practice. Eur Respir J. 2011; 37: 1175–82. Epub 2010 Nov 11.

[25] Pareek M, Baussano I, Abubakar I, Dye C, Lalvani A. Evaluation of immigrant tuberculosis screening in industrialized countries. Emerg Infect Dis. 2012 Sep; 18: 1422–9.

[26] Sandgren A, Schepisi MS, Sotgiu G, Huitric E, Migliori GB, Manissero D, van der Werf MJ, Girardi E. Tuberculosis transmission between foreign- and native-born populations in the EU/EEA: a systematic review. Eur Respir J. 2014; 43: 1159–71. Epub 2013 Oct 10. Review.

[27] Schepisi MS, Gualano G, Piselli P, Mazza M, D'Angelo D, Fasciani F, et al. Active tuberculosis case finding interventions among immigrants, refugees and asylum seekers in Italy. Infect Dis Rep. 2016; 8: 6594. eCollection 2016 Jun.

[28] Tafuri S, Martinelli D, Melpignano L, de Palma M, Quarto M, Prato R, Germinario C. Tuberculosis screening in migrant reception centers: results of a 2009 Italian survey. Am J Infect Control. 2011; 39: 495–9. Epub 2011 May 14.

[29] European Centre for Disease Prevention and Control (ECDC) 2015. Available from: http://ecdc.europa.eu/en/publications/Publications/tuberculosis-surveillance-monitoring-Europe-2015.

[30] Alvarez GG, Clark M, Altpeter E, Douglas P, Jones J, Paty MC, Posey DL, Chemtob D. Pediatric tuberculosis immigration screening in high-immigration, low-incidence countries. Int J Tuberc Lung Dis. 2010; 14: 1530–7.

[31] Minodier P, Lamarrea V, Carleb M-E, Blaisa D, Ovetchkinea P, Tapiero B. Evaluation of a school-based program for diagnosis and treatment of latent tuberculosis infection in immigrant children. J Infect Public Health. 2010; 3: 67–75.

[32] Schraufnagel DE. Latent tuerculosis infection is a term that should go dormant and the significance of latent tuberculosis should be rethought. Ann Am Thor Soc. 2015; 13: 593–4.

[33] Lawn SD, Zumla AI. Tuberculosis. Lancet. 2011. Jul 2; 378 (9785): 57–72. Epub 2011 Mar 21.

[34] Hauck FR, Neese BH, Panchal AS, El-Amin W. Identification and management of latent tuberculosis infection. Am Fam Physician 2009; 79: 879–86.

[35] Rubinowicz A, Bartlett G, MacGibbon B, Greenaway C, Ronald L, Munoz M, Menzies D. Evaluating the role of primary care physicians in the treatment of latent tuberculosis: a population study. Int J Tuberc Lung Dis. 2014; 18: 1449–54.

[36] Kwan CK, Ernst JD. HIV and tuberculosis: a deadly human syndemic. Clin Microbiol Rev. 2011; 24: 351–76.

[37] Jeon CY, Murray MB. Diabetes mellitus increases the risk of active tuberculosis: a systematic review of 13 observational studies. PLoS Med 2008; 5: e152.

[38] Brown M, Miiro G, Nkurunziza P, Watera C, Quigley MA, Dunne DW, Whitworth JA, Elliott AM. Schistosoma mansoni, nematode infections, and progression to active tuberculosis among HIV-1-infected Ugandans. Am J Trop Med Hyg. 2006; 74: 819–25.

[39] Fares A. Racial differences in susceptibility to infection by mycobacterium tuberculosis. Ann Trop Med Publ Health. 2016; 5: 307–12.

[40] Franzetti F, Codecasa L, Matteelli A, Degli Esposti A, Bandera A, Lacchini C, Lombardi A, Pinsi G, Zanini F, El-Hamad I, Gori A. Genotyping analyses of tuberculosis transmission among immigrant residents in Italy. Clin Microbiol Infect. 2010 Aug; 16: 1149–54. Epub 2009 Oct 14.

[41] Garzelli C, Rindi L. Molecular epidemiological approaches to study the epidemiology of tuberculosis in low-incidence settings receiving immigrants. Infect Genet Evol 2012; 12: 610–8. Epub 2011 Oct 24.

[42] Lalvani A, Pareek M, Berrocal Almanza LC. Pre-entry screening for tuberculosis: the need for better evidence. Pathog Glob Health. 2015; 109: 44–5.

[43] Coker R, Bell A, Pitman R, Zellweger JP, Heldal E, Hayward A, Skulberg A, Bothamley G, Whitfield R, de Vries G, Watson JM. Tuberculosis screening in migrants in selected European countries shows wide disparities. Eur Respir J. 2006; 27: 801–7.

[44] Napoli C, Dente MG, Kärki T, Riccardo F, Rossi P, Declich S. Network for the control of cross-border health threats in the Mediterranean Basin and Black Sea. Screening for infectious diseases among newly arrived migrants: experiences and practices in non-EU countries of the Mediterranean Basin and Black Sea. Int J Environ Res Public Health. 2015; 12: 15550–8.

[45] Jiménez-Fuentes MA, Augé CM, Gómez MN, Peiró JS, de Souza Galvao ML, Maldonado J, Molina-Pinargote I, Orcau A, Cayla JA. Screening for active tuberculosis in high-risk groups. Int J Tuberc Lung Dis. 2014; 18: 1459–65.

[46] WHO: Global Tuberculosis Report 2012. Available from: http://apps.who.int/iris/bitstream/10665/44728/1/9789241564380_eng.pdf

[47] Centers for Disease Control and Prevention. Reported Tuberculosis in the United States, 2012.

[48] Taylor EM, Painter J, Posey DL, Zhou W, Shetty S. Latent tuberculosis infection among immigrant and refugee children arriving in the United States: 2010. J Immigr Minor Health. 2016; 18: 966–70.

[49] Amanatidou V, Syridou G, Mavrikou M, Tsolia MN. Latent tuberculosis infection in children: diagnostic approaches. Eur J Clin Microbiol Infect Dis. 2012; 31: 1285–94. Epub 2012 Jan 4.

[50] Pollock KM, Tam H, Grass L, Bowes S, Cooke GS, Pareek M, Montamat-Sicotte D, Kapembwa M, Taylor GP, Lalvani A. Comparison of screening strategies to improve the diagnosis of latent tuberculosis infection in the HIV-positive population: a cohort study. BMJ Open. 2012; 2: e000762.

[51] Haldar P, Thuraisingam H, Patel H, et al. Single-step QuantiFERON screening of adult contacts: a prospective cohort study of tuberculosis risk. Thorax. 2013; 68: 240–69.

[52] Lobue P, Menzies D. Treatment of latent tuberculosis infection: an update. Respirology. 2010; 15: 603–22.

[53] Mor Z, Kolb H, Lidji M, Migliori G, Leventhal A. Tuberculosis diagnostic delay and therapy outcomes of non-national migrants in Tel Aviv, 1998-2008. Euro Surveill. 2013; 18.

[54] WHO: Global Tuberculosis Report 2012. Available from: http://apps.who.int/iris/bitstream/10665/75938/1/9789241564502_eng.pdf

[55] Cavalli Z, Ader F, Valour F, Saison J, Boussel L, Dumitrescu O, Perpoint T, Chidiac C, May T, Ferry T; Lyon and TB Study Group. Clinical presentation, diagnosis, and bacterial epidemiology of peritoneal tuberculosis in two university hospitals in France. Infect Dis Ther. 2016; 5: 193–9. Epub 2016 Jun 13.

[56] WHO: Global Tuberculosis Report 2010. Available from: http://apps.who.int/iris/bitstream/10665/44425/1/9789241564069_eng.pdf

[57] European Centre for Disease Prevention and Control (ECDC) 2013. Available from: http://ecdc.europa.eu/en/publications/_layouts/forms/Publication_DispForm.aspx?List=4f55ad51-4aed-4d32-b960-af70113dbb90&ID=989

[58] Getahun H, Harrington M, O'Brien R, Nunn P. Diagnosis of smear-negative pulmonary tuberculosis in people with HIV infection or AIDS in resource-constrained settings: informing urgent policy changes. Lancet. 2007 Jun 16; 369 (9578): 2042–9.

[59] Tebruegge M, Ritz N, Koetz K, Noguera-Julian A, Seddon JA, Welch SB, Tsolia M, Kampmann B. Availability and use of molecular microbiological and immunological tests for the diagnosis of tuberculosis in europe. PLoS One. 2014 Jun 12; 9: e99129. eCollection 2014.

[60] Tapley A, Switz N, Reber C, Davis JL, Miller C, Matovu JB, Worodria W, Huang L, Fletcher DA, Cattamanchi A. Mobile digital fluorescence microscopy for diagnosis of tuberculosis. J Clin Microbiol. 2013; 51: 1774–8. Epub 2013 Apr 3.

[61] Boehme CC, Nabeta P, Hillemann D, Nicol MP, Shenai S, Krapp F, et al. Rapid molecular detection of tuberculosis and rifampin resistance. N Engl J Med. 2010; 363 (11): 1005–15. Epub 2010 Sep 1.

[62] Lawn SD, Mwaba P, Bates M, Piatek A, Alexander H, Marais BJ, et al. Advances in tuberculosis diagnostics: the Xpert MTB/RIF assay and future prospects for a point-of-care test. Lancet Infect Dis. 2013; 13: 349–61.

[63] Wang XW, Pappoe F, Huang Y, Cheng XW, Xu DF, Wang H, Xu YH. Xpert MTB/RIF assay for pulmonary tuberculosis and rifampicin resistance in children: a meta-analysis. Clin Lab. 2015; 61: 1775–85.

[64] Penz E, Boffa J, Roberts DJ, Fisher D, Cooper R, Ronksley PE, James MT. Diagnostic accuracy of the Xpert® MTB/RIF assay for extra-pulmonary tuberculosis: a meta-analysis. Int J Tuberc Lung Dis. 2015; 19: 278–84, i–iii.

[65] Peter J, Green C, Hoelscher M, Mwaba P, Zumla A, Dheda K. Urine for the diagnosis of tuberculosis: current approaches, clinical applicability, and new developments. Curr Opin Pulm Med. 2010; 16: 262–70.

[66] Shah M, Dowdy D, Joloba M, Ssengooba W, Manabe YC, Ellner J, et al. Cost-effectiveness of novel algorithms for rapid diagnosis of tuberculosis in HIV-infected individuals in Uganda. AIDS. 2013; 27: 2883–92.

[67] Fang R, Li X, Hu L, You Q, Li J, Wu J, et al. Cross-priming amplification for rapid detection of mycobacterium tuberculosis in sputum specimens. J Clin Microbiol. 2009; 47: 845–7.

[68] WHO. Global Tuberculosis Report 2007. Available from: who_report_2007_global_tb_control.pdf

[69] Contini C, Maritati M, Cultrera R, Di Nuzzo M. Infections in migrants: global and local epidemiological issues. Annali Online dell'Università di Ferrara. 2015; 10: 191–233. ISSN 2038-1034

[70] Andrews JR, Shah NS, Weissman D, Moll AP, Friedland G, Gandhi NR. Predictors of multidrug- and extensively drug-resistant tuberculosis in a high HIV prevalence community. PLoS One. 2010; 29; 5:e15735.

[71] Kalokhe AS, Shafiq M, Lee JC, Metchock B, Posey JE, Ray SM, Anderson A, Wang YF, Nguyen ML. Discordance in mycobacterium tuberculosis rifampin susceptibility. Emerg Infect Dis. 2012; 18: 537–9.

[72] Saleri N, Badoum G, Ouedraogo M, Dembele SM, Nacanabo R, Bonkoungou V, Cirillo D, Pinsi G, Matteelli A. Extensively drug-resistant tuberculosis, Burkina Faso. Emerg Infect Dis. 2010; 16: 840–2.

[73] McNerney R, Maeurer M, Abubakar I, Marais B, McHugh TD, Ford N, et al. Tuberculosis diagnostics and biomarkers: needs, challenges, recent advances, and opportunities. J Infect Dis. 2012; 205 Suppl 2: S147–58. Epub 2012 Apr.

[74] Sia IG, Wieland ML. Current concepts in the management of tuberculosis. Mayo Clin Proc. 2011; 86: 348–61.

[75] Zumla A, Chakaya J, Centis R, D'Ambrosio L, Mwaba P, Bates M, et al. Tuberculosis treatment and management—an update on treatment regimens, trials, new drugs, and adjunct therapies. Lancet Respir Med. 2015; 3: 220–34. Epub 2015 Mar 9.

[76] WHO. Global Tuberculosis Report 2013. Available from: http://apps.who.int/iris/bitstream/10665/91355/1/9789241564656_eng.pdf

[77] Cox HS, McDermid C, Azevedo V, Muller O, Coetzee D, Simpson J, et al. Epidemic levels of drug resistant tuberculosis (MDR and XDR-TB) in a high HIV prevalence setting in Khayelitsha, South Africa. PLoS One. 2010; 5(11): e13901.

[78] Falzon D, Gandhi N, Migliori GB, et al. Resistance to fluoroquinolones and second-line injectable drugs: impact on multidrug-resistant TB outcomes. Eur Respir J. 2013; 42: 156–68.

[79] Orenstein EW, Basu S, Shah NS, et al. Treatment outcomes among patients with multidrug-resistant tuberculosis: systematic review and meta-analysis. Lancet Infect Dis. 2009; 9: 153–61.

[80] Calligaro GL, Moodley L, Symons G, Dheda K. The medical and surgical treatment of drug-resistant tuberculosis. J Thorac Dis. 2014; 6(3): 186–95.

[81] Rohilla M, Joshi B, Jain V, Kalra J, Prasad GR. Multidrug-resistant tuberculosis during pregnancy: two case reports and review of the literature. Case Rep Obstet Gynecol. 2016; 2016: 1536281. Epub 2016 Feb 24.

[82] Lange C, Abubakar I, Alffenaar IWC, Bothamley G, Caminero JA, Carvalho ACC, et al. Management of patients with multidrug-resistant/extensively drug-resistant tuberculosis in Europe: a TBNET consensus statement. Eur Respir J. 2014; 44 (1): 23–63.

[83] United Nations Programme on HIV/AIDS (UNAIDS). Available from: http://www.unaids.org/en/resources/campaigns/20121120_globalreport2012

[84] Gandhi NR, Shah NS, Andrews JR, et al. HIV coinfection in multidrug- and extensively drug-resistant tuberculosis results in high early mortality. Am J Respir Crit Care Med. 2010; 181: 80–86.

[85] Hoagland DT, Liu J, Lee RB, Lee RE. New agents for the treatment of drug-resistant mycobacterium tuberculosis. Adv Drug Deliv Rev. 2016 May 2; pii: S0169-409X(16) 30136-3.

[86] Bidwell P, Laxmikanth P, Blacklock C, Hayward G, Willcox M, Peersman W, Moosa S, Mant D. Security and skills: the two key issues in health worker migration. Glob Health Action. 2014 Jul 28; 7: 24194. eCollection 2014.

[87] Raviglione M, Sulis G. Tuberculosis 2015: burden, challenges and strategy for control and elimination. Infect Dis Rep. 2016 Jun 24; 8 (2): 657087.

2

The World Health Organization Recommended TB Diagnostic Tools

Lynn S. Zijenah

Abstract

Tuberculosis (TB) is one of the top 10 causes of death worldwide. TB has further been exacerbated by the HIV/AIDS pandemic, the emergence of multidrug-resistant (MDR) TB and extensively drug-resistant TB. In 2015, approximately 1.4 million people and 400,000 who were HIV-negative and HIV-positive, respectively, died of TB. There were 10.4 million new cases with active TB of which 2.4 million were HIV co-infected and 480,000 new cases with MDR-TB. Conclusions: TB is a multifaceted disease and there is no one size fits all test for its diagnosis. In the 22 high TB burden countries (HTBBC), which harbour 80% of global TB, sputum smear microscopy with its low detection rate remains the most commonly used diagnostic test for pulmonary TB. Culture, the gold standard for TB diagnosis, the molecular-based tests for both rapid diagnosis and detection of drug resistant TB because of the requirement for specialized laboratories and trained personnel as well as other costs is not routinely used in most HTBBC. An accurate, affordable, point-of-care TB test, with no requirement for electricity, specialized laboratory, easily performed by healthcare personnel is what is urgently needed for TB control.

Keywords: sputum smear microscopy, TB-LAMP, LAM-LF, culture, MTB/RIF assay, line-probe assays

1. Introduction

Tuberculosis (TB), one of the top 10 major causes of death globally is a major public health priority. Of the 10.4 million people diagnosed with active TB in 2015, the majority occurred in people living in low- and middle-income countries. The TB epidemic has further been exacerbated by the HIV/AIDS pandemic and the emergence of multidrug-resistant (MDR) and extensively drug-resistant (XDR) TB. Of the estimated 1.8 million people who died in 2015, 1.4

million were HIV negative and 400,000 were HIV positive. In the same period, 480,000 cases of MDR TB and a further 100,000 that were estimated to be rifampicin-resistant [1].

TB mainly affects the lungs (pulmonary TB), however, it can affects other parts of the body such as the spine or brain (extrapulmonary TB). Although TB is a preventable and curable disease, failure to detect the disease early is one of the major bottlenecks to TB control. TB diagnostic tests with low sensitivity that were developed more than a century ago are still in use today. The detection case rates in the 22 high burden countries which harbor 80% of global TB burden is low (~50%) and even lower among the HIV-infected. [2]. From the 10.4 million people who developed TB in 2015, 4.3 million cases were not diagnosed or notified and only one quarter of MDR TB cases (132,000) were detected and reported. The reasons for the low detection and underreporting of TB are multifactorial and include limited or delayed access to appropriate diagnosis and care, large private sectors not reporting cases, and the lack of access to appropriate diagnostic tools due to geographic and/or financial barriers [3–5].

The WHO Strategic and Technical Advisory Group for Tuberculosis (STAG-TB) provides objective, ongoing technical and strategic advice to the WHO regarding TB diagnosis, care and control (http://www.who.int/tb/advisory_bodies/stag/en/index.html). The group which is comprised of 22 experts representing ministries of health, national TB control programs, academic and research institutions, civil society organizations, communities and patients affected by TB, and professional associations provides the WHO Director General with independent evaluations of the strategic, scientific, and technical aspects of WHO's area of work in TB. The group also reviews progress and challenges in TB-related core functions such as policies, strategies, and standards and make recommendations on committees and working groups. The STAG-TB reviews policy drafts and supporting documentation and may endorse the policy recommendation with or without revisions, request additional information and re-review the evidence in subsequent years, or reject the recommendation.

Below, we describe the WHO recommended TB diagnostic tools, the advantages and disadvantages as well as challenges in the implementation of the tools.

2. World Health Organization (WHO) approved TB diagnostic tools

2.1. Sputum smear microscopy for the diagnosis of pulmonary TB

Direct microscopic examination of sputum for acid-fast bacilli (AFB), the sputum smear microscopy (SSM) remains the most commonly used diagnostic test for pulmonary TB particularly in countries with a high rate of TB infection [6].

The test is conducted by placing a thin layer of the sputum (smear) on a glass slide. A series of special stains are then applied to the smear, and the stained slide is examined under a microscope for signs of the TB bacteria [7]. It is a simple inexpensive test which does not require sophisticated laboratory infrastructure or extensive training of laboratory personnel and the results are available within hours. Although its sensitivity is only about 50–60%, its high specificity (99–100%) ensures that only those who are positive receive the anti-TB treatment [8]. The detection rate is even lower in countries with a high prevalence of both pulmonary TB and HIV infection, as many patients with HIV and TB co-infection have very low levels of TB bacteria and are unable to produce good quality sputum leading to false negative results [9].

SSM has other limitations in addition to its low sensitivity. False positive results may occur in individuals that have been infected with NTB. False negative results particularly happen with children, older people and HIV-infected patients. Furthermore, SSM cannot be used to diagnose extrapulmonary TB. Many HIV-infected patients tend to have high rates of extrapulmonary TB compared to HIV negative individuals which probably contributes to the lower sensitivity of FM in this group of patients [9].

In the earlier years, a conventional light microscope for examining the AFB Ziehl-Neelsen (ZN) stains was recommended for SSM in low-income and middle-income countries where most of the world's TB cases occur [10, 11]. In high-income countries, AFB auramine O or auramine-rhodamine stains are examined by fluorescence microscopy (FM) which has a higher sensitivity than conventional ZN light microscopy. In these countries, FM is the most commonly used method for diagnosis of pulmonary TB [12].

In FM, the smear is illuminated with a quartz halogen or high pressure mercury vapor lamp, allowing a much larger area of the smear to be seen and resulting in more rapid examination of the specimen. The major advantage of FM is that it uses a lower power objective lens compared to conventional microscopy thus reducing the time of assessing the same area of a slide [13]. The major disadvantage of using FM is the expensive mercury vapor lamp which lasts a very short time. The lamp also takes a while to warm up, burn high amounts of electricity, and electricity supply problems can significantly shorten its life span [14]. The use of light emitting diodes (LEDs) which switch on extremely quickly, have an extremely long life, and do not explode can address some of these problems [14].

In 2006, a systematic review of 45 studies comparing conventional SSM with FM reported that FM has a higher sensitivity than the standard light microscopy but similar specificity with standard light microscopy [15]. In HIV positive patients, there was insufficient data to determine the value of FM.

Following a systematic review in September 2009, of a meta-analysis of published and unpublished data, the WHO assessed the evidence for the efficacy of LED microscopy. Subsequently in 2011 the WHO issued a policy statement recommending that conventional FM should be replaced by LED microscopy [16].

The advantages of LED microscopes are: they are less expensive, require less power and are able to run on batteries, the bulbs have a very long half-life and do not pose the risk of releasing potentially toxic products if broken.

In 2011, the WHO revised its earlier recommendations of using three sputum specimens collected on different days to same day microscopy using two sputum specimens collected at the same time, on the same day based on a systematic review of 37 eligible studies [17, 18]. However, the WHO recommended its use only in settings with a well-established laboratory network and a fully functional external quality assurance program for SSM including on-site evaluation and follow-up training for problem laboratories.

The revised recommendation has reduced the number of patient visits to the clinic, leading to a reduction in the numbers of TB positive cases that are lost to follow up, reduced laboratory workload as well as decreased time for diagnosis and initiation of anti-TB treatment with non-significant decrease in diagnostic yield [19].

2.2. Loop-mediated isothermal amplification (TB-LAMP) for diagnosis of pulmonary TB

A commercial molecular assay Loopamp MTBC Detection Kit was developed by Eiken Chemical Company Ltd. (Tokyo, Japan) for the detection of MTBC (TB-LAMP) [20].

The assay is based on loop-mediated isothermal amplification. It is a manual assay that requires less than 1 h to perform and the result can be read with the naked eye under ultra violet (UV) light. The assay consists of three steps, sample preparation (10–20 min), amplification (40 min), and visual detection of fluorescence light from the reaction tube using UV light (0.5–1 min) (**Figure 1**). Sputum is added to a heating tube containing the extraction solution which is then mixed by inverting, the heating tube is placed into the heating block to lyse and inactivate mycobacteria. The heating tube is then removed from the heating block and allowed to cool. The heating tube is then attached to an adsorbent tube and mixed by shaking until all the powder has been completely mixed with the solution. An injection cap is placed onto the adsorbent tube and screwed tightly to pierce the seal. The nozzle is then inserted into a reaction tube and drops of solution are transferred to the reaction tube. Amplification is carried out by loading the reaction tubes into the heating block and the reaction started. The amplification is stopped automatically after 40 min. For visual detection of fluorescent light, the reaction tubes are transferred into a fluorescence detector and the results recorded [21, 22].

The TB-LAMP assay has several features that makes it attractive as a diagnostics platform for resource-poor settings: it is fast (40 min), isothermal (requiring only a heat block), robust to inhibitors and reaction conditions that usually adversely affect polymerase chain reaction (PCR) methods, and it generates a result that can be detected with the naked eye. The major disadvantage of TB-LAMP is that it cannot detect drug resistance and is therefore only suitable for testing of patients at low risk of MDR TB [22].

In January 2016, WHO Guideline Development Group (GDG) conducted a systematic review and meta-analysis of 24 studies conducted after 01 January 2012 to evaluate the use of TB-LAMP on sputum samples from adults with signs and symptoms consistent with pulmonary TB that were conducted in settings with an intermediate or high burden of TB. Only 13

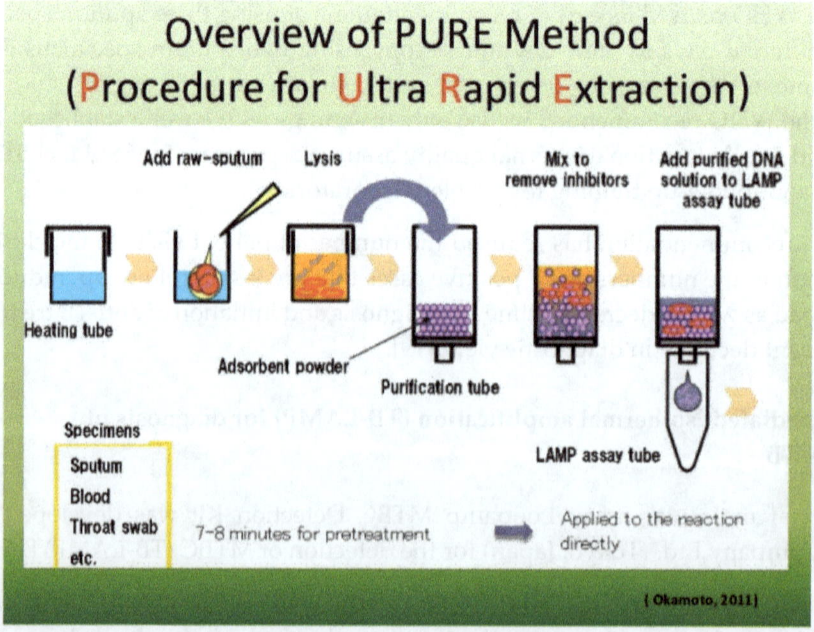

Figure 1. Overview of Pure method (procedure for ultra-rapid extraction [21]).

of the 24 studies met the eligibility criteria for inclusion in the systematic review. The pooled sensitivity of TB-LAMP was higher than that of SSM (78% vs. 63%). The pooled specificity of TB-LAMP was lower than that of SSM, 98% vs. 100%. In the HIV-infected patients, the pooled sensitivity of TB-LAMP was similar to that of SSM; 64% vs. 62% for SSM while specificity was the same, 99% for TB-LAMP and 99% for SSM. In the analysis of TB-LAMP for detection of pulmonary TB in adult patients who were SSM negative, TB-LAMP showed a 42% incremental yield [23].

In August 2016, WHO issued a policy recommendation on the TB-LAMP MTBC assay. TB-LAMP may be used as a replacement test for SSM to diagnose pulmonary TB in adults with signs and symptoms consistent with TB and TB-LAMP may be used as a follow-on test in adults with signs and symptoms consistent with pulmonary TB, especially when further testing of sputum smear-negative specimens is necessary. These recommendations apply to settings where conventional SSM can be performed, TB-LAMP should not replace the use of rapid molecular tests that detect TB and resistance to RIF, especially among populations at risk of MDR TB. Due to the limited evidence, it is unclear whether TB-LAMP has additional diagnostic value over SSM for testing persons living with HIV who have signs and symptoms consistent with TB. These recommendations are extrapolated to using TB-LAMP in children, based on the generalization of data from adults, while acknowledging the difficulties of collecting sputum specimens from children. TB-LAMP should not replace the Xpert MTB/RIF assay because the Xpert MTB/RIF assay can detect resistance to RIF whilst the former cannot [23].

2.3. Gene Xpert MTB/RIF assay

The Xpert MTB/RIF assay (Cepheid, Sunnyvale, CA, USA), is an automated semi-quantitative nested real-time PCR for the rapid detection of MTBC DNA and RIF resistance simultaneously, directly from unprocessed sputum within 2 h [24]. The assay has been extensively evaluated in various geographical settings and the diagnostic accuracy is good [25–31]. In a meta-analysis, the pooled sensitivity and pooled specificity of MTB/RIF were 88 and 95% respectively when used as an initial test for TB diagnosis. The pooled sensitivity was 80% in the HIV-infected patients. The pooled sensitivity and pooled specificity for detection of RIF resistance were 94 and 98% respectively. Thus, it was concluded that the MTB/RIF assay is sensitive and specific as an initial test for diagnosis of TB, TB associated HIV and MDR TB [32].

The assay is very simple to run and can be performed by nurses with very little training [33]. Briefly, the assay is carried out by adding the sample reagent in a volume twice that of the untreated sputum and the mixture incubated for 15 min. Two millimeters of the processed sputum is then transferred to the MTB/RIF assay catridge and then inserted into the Gene Xpert instrument, subsequent steps in the assay are completely automated and selfcontained. The advantages of the assay are its higher sensitivity when compared to SSM and shorter period (2 h) of obtaining the result when compared with culture which although it gives a definite diagnosis, it takes weeks. Furthermore the assay identifies RIF resistance within hours compared to the weeks taken to get any drug resistance result when using culture-based methods [34].

In 2011, WHO issued a policy statement recommending the use of the assay as a diagnostic tool for all people living with HIV who have signs and symptoms of TB, for people with unknown HIV status presenting with strong clinical evidence of HIV infection, for people who are seriously ill and suspected of having TB regardless of HIV status and those at risk of MDR TB [35].

Although it has been muted as a new test which represents a major milestone for global TB diagnosis and care and new hope for the millions of people who are at the highest risk of TB and drug-resistant disease, it has some disadvantages [36]. The disadvantages include the short shelf life of the cartridges (only 18 months), very stable electricity supply is required, the instrument needs to be recalibrated annually, and the cost of the test and the temperature ceiling is critical [37]. To address some of these challenges, a new machine, the Xpert Omni which is intended for point of care (POC) testing for TB and RIF resistance, using the same cartridges as those used in the current Xpert machine is currently under development. It is expected that it will be smaller, lighter and less expensive than the current Xpert machine and will also come with a built-in 4 h battery [38].

A next generation cartridge called the GeneXpert Ultra (Ultra) was launched on 24 March 2017, World TB Day [39]. Its sensitivity is higher than that of MTB/RIF with the greatest sensitivity gains being recorded among SSM negative-culture positive patients, and HIV infected-TB patients. It however, has a lower specificity than the MTB/RIF assay. The performance of the Ultra was assessed in 2016 in a multicentre non-inferiority study at 10 sites in 8 low- and middle-income countries. The performance of the Ultra assay was evaluated by the WHO Technical Experts Group in January 2016, which concluded that the Ultra test performed better than the MTB/RIF assay in TB diagnosis of children, HIV-infected patients and patients with extra pulmonary TB, who more often than not are difficult to diagnose, however, there is a need for more research to be conducted to improve the specificity of the new test [40].

The usefulness of the MTB/RIF has generated a lot of controversy. Some people consider the test to be extremely useful, as well as cost effective, and should be used in as many places as soon as possible while other people consider it not to be really suitable and practical at the present time for major use in low- and middle-income countries [41–43]. A clinical trial conducted in four African countries in 2013 comparing the use of the Xpert to SSM concluded that using the Xpert meant that more patients had a same day diagnosis and same day treatment initiation, but the benefits did not translate into lower TB morbidity [33].

In spite the negatives concerning the usefulness of the MTB/RIF in so far as the outcomes of its use are concerned, its introduction since 2010 has revolutionized TB diagnostics as a POC test offering rapid TB diagnosis and simultaneous detection of RIF resistance. More than 23 million Xpert machines had been procured in 130 countries and MDR TB diagnosis more than tripled by 2016 [44, 45].

2.4. Lipoarabinomannan urine strip test for TB diagnosis in HIV-infected patients

A POC lateral flow urine Lipoarabinomannan strip test (LF-LAM) developed by Alere Determine™ TB LAM Ag, Waltham, MA, USA for TB diagnosis is based on the detection of mycobacterial lipoarabinomannan (LAM) antigen in urine. Briefly 60 μL of freshly collected urine is applied to the test strip, incubated at room temperature for 25 min and the result recorded as negative if there was no presence of any band or recorded as positive and band graded using the manufacturer's reference card with bands of graded intensity. The LF-LAM test has been evaluated for accuracy of TB diagnosis in HIV-infected patients in various geographical settings [46–53] albeit with widely varying sensitivity (13–93%) and specificity (87–99%) [53]. The general consensus then was that the assay is most suitable for HIV-infected patients with CD4 counts < 200 cells/μL [54]. The variability in the performance characteristics of LF-LAM led the end users of the assay to request the WHO for guidance on the appropriate use of the assay.

In 2015, the WHO commissioned a systematic review of the use of LF-LAM assay for the diagnosis and screening of active TB in people living with HIV. The quantitative meta-analysis included 16 studies. Following the meta-analysis, the WHO recommended that the LF-LAM test may be used to assist in the diagnosis of TB in HIV positive adult in patients with signs and symptoms of TB (pulmonary and/or extra pulmonary) who have a CD4 cell count less than or equal to 100 cells/μL, or HIV positive patients who are seriously ill regardless of CD4 count or with unknown CD4 count [55]. This recommendation also applies to HIV positive children with signs and symptoms of TB (pulmonary and/or extra pulmonary) based on the generalization of data from adults while acknowledging very limited data and concern regarding low specificity of the LF-LAM assay in children [55].

The advantages of LAM include use of urine which is easily and rapidly obtained even from very ill patients compared to sputum, it is an easy to use POC test which can also be performed by trained nurses making it an ideal POC test. Its major disadvantage is that its use is restricted to a subgroup of HIV-infected TB suspects with low CD4+ T lymphocytes. The reasons for higher sensitivity and specificity in this group of patients are not fully understood. However, it is hypothesized that HIV patients with advanced immunosuppression may have a disseminated TB infection that is very difficult to rapidly diagnose with current tools. The patients may have a higher bacterial load associated with widespread infection and, therefore, antigen load, the greater likelihood of genitourinary tract TB and greater glomerular permeability to allow increased antigen levels in urine [55].

2.5. Culture for TB diagnosis and drug resistance testing

Culture remains the gold standard for TB diagnosis and drug-resistant testing. Ideally culture examinations should be done on all diagnostic specimens, regardless of AFB smear or nucleic acid amplification results. Positive cultures for MTB confirm the diagnosis of TB disease; however, in the absence of a positive culture, particularly in RLCs, TB disease may also be diagnosed on the basis of clinical signs and symptoms alone. Two types of broth culture systems; liquid and solid media are commercially available. The commercial liquid culture systems and molecular line-probe assays have been endorsed by the WHO as gold standards for rapid detection of MDR TB [56, 57].

The drug resistance of clinical isolates as determined by conventional methods (e.g., broth-based and agar proportion) is due to the presence of mutations in specific MTB genes [58]. These mutations often are single base pair changes in the DNA sequence of the bacteria. There are a variety of commercial assays and laboratory tests that can detect mutations associated with drug resistance. The assays are done on patient specimens or isolates from patient specimens. The liquid based systems such as BACTEC, MGIT, VersaTREK and MBBACT allow detection of most mycobacterial growth in 4–14 days compared to 3–6 weeks for solid media [59]. However these tests require specialized laboratories and skills that are often unavailable in the regions, particularly RLS, where most cases of TB and MDR TB occur [59].

As an interim solution while capacity for genotypic or automated liquid culture and drug sensitivity testing (DST) is being developed, in 2011, the WHO recommended non-commercial culture and DST methods for screening patients at risk for MDR TB namely (i) microscopic observation of drug susceptibility (MODS): a micro colony direct method in liquid culture, based on inoculation of specimens into drug-free and drug-containing media, followed by microscopic examination of early growth, (ii) colorimetric redox indicator (CRA): a direct or indirect method based on the ability of MTB to reduce nitrate, which is detected by a color reaction and (iii) nitrate reductase assay (NRI) methods: indirect methods based on the reduction of a colored indicator added to liquid culture medium on a microtitre plate after exposure of MTB strains to anti-TB drugs *in vitro*. These tests can only be used in reference laboratories and under strict laboratory protocols. The major disadvantage of these tests is that none can detect XDR TB and thus cannot replace the conventional culture and DST tests [60].

2.6. Molecular line-probe assays for diagnosis of TB and detection of drug resistance

The emergence of MDR TB and XDR TB threatens to reverse the gains that have been made in global control of TB. Rapid tests for detection of resistance to anti-TB treatment are urgently required for timeous and appropriate treatment which would lead to decreased morbidity and mortality as well as curbing new infections.

The standard first line drugs for anti-TB treatment include RIF and INH. In patients with MDR TB, drugs belonging to fluoroquinolines (FLQ) and second line injectable drugs (SLID) are used. The FLQ drugs include ofloxacin, levoflacin, moxifloxacin and gatifloxacin while the SLID include kanamycin (KAN), amikacin (AMK) and capreomycin (CAP) [61]. Patients with XDR TB are resistant to RIF, INH, plus any FLQ and at least one of the three SLIDs thus making them resistant to both first line and second line anti-TB drugs [61].

Turnaround time (TAT) for DST results using the conventional solid based methods ranges from 8 to 12 weeks [62] thus contributing to new infections as those infected continue to transmit drug-resistant TB. On 26 March 2007, the WHO recommended the use of liquid culture and DST in low- and medium-income countries [58] following evidence provided by the Foundation for Innovative New Diagnostics (FIND). Although the liquid media based tests such as BACTEC® (BD Diagnostics, Sparks, MD, USA), MGIT® (BD Diagnostics) and BacT/ALERT® (bioMe'rieux SA, Marcy l'Etoile, France) have a shorter TAT, they are more expensive, require specialized laboratories and trained laboratory personnel [63].

Nucleic acid amplification molecular methods offer several advantages over the conventional culture-based methods which include rapid diagnosis and standardized testing.

In 2005 a meta-analysis of one of the two commercially line-probe assays (LiPAs) that were available then; the INNO-LiPA Rif.TB (Innogenetics, Ghent Belgium) [64] was conducted.

The INNO-LiPA Rif.TB (LiPA) test simultaneously detects MTBC and a mutation in the *rpoB* gene associated with RIF resistance. The test involves extraction of DNA from cultures or directly from clinical specimens, amplification of the RIF resistance-determining region of the *rpoB* gene using PCR, hybridization of the biotinylated PCR products with immobilized probes and determination of results by color-metric development [64].

The meta-analysis to evaluate the accuracy of LiPA for RIF resistance detection comprised of 15 studies which comprised 11 studies that used culture isolates, 1 study that used clinical isolates and 3 studies that used both [64]. The sensitivity and specificity were greater than 95 and 100% respectively in 12 of the 14 studies that used culture isolates in the LiPA test. In the 4 studies that used clinical isolates in the LiPA test, sensitivity ranged between 80 and 100% whilst specificity was 100%. The authors concluded that although LiPA is a highly sensitive and specific test for detection of RIF resistance in culture isolates because of the lower sensitivity when used directly on clinical specimens, more evidence is required before the test can be used to detect MDR TB among populations at risk in clinical practice [64].

In 2008 a meta-analysis of the second LiPA commercially available in the early 2000, the Genotype MTBDR (Hain Life Sciences, Gmbh, Nehren Germany) was performed [65]. The Genotype MTBDR (MTBDR) test detects the mutations in the *rpo*B and *kat*G genes associated with RIF and isoniazid (INH) resistance respectively. The meta-analysis included 10 published articles contributing 14 comparisons and 15 comparisons for detection of RIF and INH respectively. The pooled sensitivity and specificity for RIF resistance across all the subgroups was 91.1 and 98.7% respectively. The pooled specificity for detection of INH resistance was 99.5%, but the sensitivity was variable and inconsistent, 84.3% (95% CI:76.6–89.8). Ling et al.

concluded that MTBDR assay also referred to as MTBDR*sl* Version 1 (now referred to simply as Hain version 1) has excellent accuracy for RIF resistance detection. Although specificity for detection of INH resistance was excellent, the sensitivity was modest and variable [65].

In 2008, following the two meta analyses to assess the diagnostic accuracy of LiPA and MTBDR assays, the WHO recommended the use of these LiPAs for MTBC and RIF resistance detection in sputum smear-positive specimens (direct testing) and in cultured isolates of MTBC (indirect testing) [66]. Since then, newer versions of the two LPAs have been developed and a third one, Nipro NTM + MDRTB detection kit 2 (Tokyo, Japan) which detects MTBC, RIF and INH resistance has been introduced.

The FIND evaluated the Nipro and the Hain version 2 LPAs and compared them with Hain version 1 in 2015. The study reported that these three LPAs showed equivalence for detecting TB and resistance to RIF and INH [67].

An updated systematic review of the accuracy of the three LiPAs (Hain version 1, Hain version 2 and Nipro) for detecting MTBC and resistance to RIF and INH was commissioned by the WHO in 2015. The review included 74 studies comprising 94 unique datasets of which 83 datasets evaluated Hain version 1, 5 evaluated Hain version 2, and 6 evaluated the Nipro assay. Subsequently, the WHO in 2016, issued a Policy update on the use of molecular LPAs for the detection of resistance to INH and RIF [68]. The mutation probes used for detection of RIF resistance *(rpoB)*, high level INH resistance (*katG*), and low-level isoniazid resistance (*inhA*) are the same for the three assays with the exception of the *katG* S315N mutation, which is included in the Nipro assay but not in Hain version 1 or version 2 [68].

Hain version 1 was developed to genotype resistance to FLQ via gryA, SLID resistance (SLID including KAN, AMK and CAP) via rrs and ethambutol (EMB) resistance via embB. Hain version 2 also targets gyrA but includes assays for gyrB mutations that are also associated with FLQ resistance. Furthermore, the assay incorporates further SLID resistance genotypes via the eis promoter region. The embB resistance component is not used in the Hain version 2.0 [69].

Subsequent to the meta-analysis, the WHO recommended that the commercial molecular LiPAs may be used as the initial test instead of phenotypic culture-based DST to detect RIF and INH in persons (children and adults) with a sputum smear-positive specimen (direct testing) or a cultured isolate of MTBC (indirect testing). However, the accuracy of detecting resistance to RIF and INH differs leading to an overall reduced accuracy of MDR TB diagnosis. LiPAs are not recommended to replace conventional culture-based DST, which may still be necessary to determine resistance to other anti-TB agents and to monitor the emergence of additional drug resistance. Furthermore, when the LiPA result does not detect INH resistance, conventional culture-based DST for INH may still be used to evaluate patients particularly for populations with a high pre-test probability of resistance to INH [68].

2.7. TB skin test for diagnosis of latent TB infection

Latent tuberculosis infection (LTBI) is defined as a state of persistent immune response to stimulation by *Mycobacterium tuberculosis* (MTB) antigens without evidence of clinically manifested active TB. LTBI will lead to active TB disease in approximately 5–10% of these individuals during their lifetimes; [70], the risk is higher in younger children [71], the immunocompromised or immunosuppressed [72, 73], and in people from countries with a high incidence of TB (≥40 cases per 100,000) [74].

Diagnosis of LTBI is important as those found positive may be initiated on prophylactic treatment, thus preventing development of active TB and indirectly preventing transmission for those found to have disease and commenced on anti-TB treatment.

The TB Skin test (TST) is one of the oldest diagnostic tests developed in the 19th century but which is still being widely used [75]. The standard recommended test is the Mantoux test, which is administered by intradermal injection of a 0.1 mL of liquid containing 5 tuberculin units (TU) of purified protein derivative (PPD) or 2 TU PPD RT23 (these are considered equivalent) into the top layers of skin of the forearm. The test is read 48–72 h after the injection [76]. Although widely used the test has several limitations; a positive reaction may be observed in both latent and active TB infection, therefore, it is unreliable in differentiating whether the person is currently having TB or had been infected in the past or at carrier stage; false positive reactions may occur which could be attributed to infection with non-tuberculosis mycobacteria (NTM), previous Bacillus Calmete Guerin (BCG) vaccination [77], incorrect method of TST administration, incorrect interpretation of reaction, incorrect bottle of antigen used; false negative reactions due to cutaneous anergy, recent TB infection (within 8–10 weeks of exposure), very old TB infection, very young age (less than 6 months old), recent live-virus vaccination (e.g., measles and smallpox), overwhelming TB disease, some viral illnesses (e.g., measles and chicken pox) [78, 79]. Thus, a confirmatory test such as sputum culture, is usually done to rule out an active TB infection.

HIV-infected patients may have a compromised ability to respond to the TST because of cutaneous anergy [80, 81]. Tuberculin skin testing assesses the ability to mount a delayed type hypersensitivity (DTH) cell mediated immune response to PPD. Since in HIV infection, there is a gradual decrease in CD4+ T lymphocytes, as HIV disease progresses, the HIV-infected patients tend to have an impaired DTH response, which plausibly may cause a false negative TST result.

The TST, however can be used for differential diagnosis of TB from sarcoidosis, another granulomatous disease with similarities to TB. Whilst TST has a high sensitivity for sarcoidosis, it has been reported to have a poor specificity for TB. In the general population, a negative TST is a specific test for sarcoidosis, in contrast, a positive TST in a sarcoidosis patient is a specific test for indicating TB. Thus a thorough TB workup should be done in a sarcoidosis suspect patient [82].

In 2015, the WHO strongly recommended the TST for diagnosis of latent TB in high- and upper medium-income countries with low TB burden (estimated TB incidence less than 100 per 100,000), in the HIV-infected patients, adult and child contacts of pulmonary TB cases, patients initiating anti-tumor necrosis factor treatment, patients receiving dialysis, patients preparing for organ or haematologic transplantation, and patients with silicosis [83].

2.8. Interferon gamma release assays for diagnosis of latent TB infection

The Interferon gamma release assays (IGRAs) measure, using an enzyme-linked immunosorbent assay (ELISA) or an enzyme-linked immunospot (ELISPOT) the release of Interferon-γ (IFN-γ) from T lymphocytes following stimulation of the cells with MTB-specific antigens

There are two commercially available IGRAs: the QuantiFERON® TB Gold (Cellestis Ltd., Carnegie, Victoria, Australia) and the T-SPOT® TB IGRAs (Oxford Immunotec, Oxford, United Kingdom).

In the first-generation QuantiFERON-TB assay, whole-blood is stimulated with PPD and ELISA used to measure the concentration of IFN-γ released by the T lymphocytes [84]. The enhanced form of the assay, the QuantiFERON-TB Gold uses the MTB-specific antigens: early-secreted antigenic target 6-kDa protein (ESAT-6) and culture filtrate protein 10 (CFP-10) instead of PPD [84]. In the newer version of the assay, QuantiFERON-TB Gold In-Tube, heparinized venous blood is added to the tube coated with the MTB-specific antigens; ESAT-6, CFP-10, and TB 7.7 [84].

In the T SPOT-TB assay, peripheral blood mononuclear cells are stimulated with ESAT6 and CFP10 and the released IFN-γ detected using an ELISPOT assay [85].

These assays are not routinely used in Resource-Limited Settings (RLS) because they are expensive, require expensive equipment and advanced technical expertise.

In 2015, the WHO recommended the use of IGRAs for the diagnosis and treatment of LTBI in people living with HIV, adult and child contacts of pulmonary TB cases, patients initiating anti-tumor necrosis factor treatment, patients receiving dialysis, patients preparing for organ or haematologic transplantation, and patients with silicosis, prisoners, healthcare workers, immigrants from high TB burden countries, homeless persons and illicit drug users and in high-income and upper middle-income countries with estimated TB incidence less than 100 per 100,000 [76].

The advantages of the IGRAs include only a single patient visit to conduct the TB test, the results can be available within 24 h, and prior BCG vaccination does not cause a false positive result. The disadvantages include; the requirement to process the collected blood specimen fairly rapidly (within 8–16 h following blood collection), laboratory facilities are required, and the test is only for latent TB. Furthermore, the IGRAs may not be as accurate in people who are HIV-infected [72].

2.9. Chest radiography

Chest X-rays (CXRs) are not considered as specific diagnostic tests for TB. However, because of the low sensitivity of SSM in TB diagnosis of HIV-infected patients, in 2007, the WHO recommended use of CXRs in HIV-infected patients who are SSM negative [86]. The chest X-ray plays an important role in the diagnosis of TB among people living with HIV and can also be an important entry point to diagnosing non-tubercular chest diseases, which are common among people living with HIV. CXR presentations of TB in HIV-infected patients are now well characterized and CXR play a significant role in shortening delays in diagnosis and should be performed early in the course of investigation of a tuberculosis suspect [86]. Indeed in a randomized controlled trial of Xpert MTB/RIF versus SSM conducted in four countries in southern Africa, the majority of the HIV-infected patients in the SSM arm who were smear-negative were commenced on anti-TB treatment based on radiological findings with or without clinical symptoms, whilst awaiting results from culture [33].

In 2016, the WHO published a factsheet and issued new recommendations and guidance on the use of chest radiography for TB detection in National TB care [87, 88]. CXR may play an essential role as a sensitive tool in diagnosis of childhood pulmonary and extra-pulmonary TB and in excluding active TB prior to treatment of LTBI. Since CXR on their own cannot establish a TB definite diagnosis, in an algorithm of TB screening that involves TB symptoms screening, CXR can also be used as a sensitive tool for screening for active TB, this may improve the pre-test probability of the subsequent diagnostic test and lead to a reduction in the number of people who need to undergo further diagnostic evaluation [89]. CXR is also used in TB prevalence surveys as it is considered the most sensitive screening tool for identifying those survey participants with a high probability of having TB. An abnormal CXR and or positive symptom screen is then followed by bacteriological confirmation [90].

The limitations in the wider use of chest X-rays, include non-availability at peripheral health facilities and the difficulty of interpreting results, even by trained physicians.

3. Conclusion

The upsurge of one the oldest known infectious diseases, TB, coupled with the HIV/AIDS pandemic, emergence of MDR TB and XDR TB has led to unprecedented efforts in developing new TB diagnostic tools which can detect TB and resistance to first line and second line anti-TB drugs more rapidly. Whilst SSM remains the most used tool in diagnosis of pulmonary TB in the majority of countries that harbor the highest burden of TB, new molecular-based amplification techniques, LiPAs which provide results faster have been developed. However, these tests are not available to the majority of the countries with the highest TB burden mainly because of costs, requirement of specialized laboratory and trained personnel with the exception of the Xpert MTB/RIF assay which can be performed by any healthcare giver after minimum training.

The urgent need for development of a true POC TB test with operational simplicity similar to the rapid HIV antibody POC test, which is accurate, easy to use, does not require a laboratory, laboratory trained personnel, nor electricity and is affordable cannot be overemphasized if the Global Strategy and Targets for Tuberculosis Prevention, Care and Control goal of eliminating TB as a public health threat by 2030 is to be achieved.

Acknowledgements

This publication, TESA II RegNet2015-1051 is part of the EDCTP2 Programme, which is supported under Horizon 2020, the European Union's Framework Programme for Research and Innovation.

Author details

Lynn S. Zijenah

Address all correspondence to: lzijenah@gmail.com

Department of Immunology, University of Zimbabwe College of Health Sciences, Harare, Zimbabwe

References

[1] WHO. Global Tuberculosis Report 2016. Geneva, Switzerland: WHO Press; 2016. www.who.int/tb/publications/global_report/en/ [Accessed: 20 August 2017]

[2] Peter JG, Theron G, Pooran A, Thomas J, Pascoe M, Dheda K. Comparison of two methods for acquisition of sputum samples for diagnosis of suspected tuberculosis in smear-negative or sputum scarce people: A randomised controlled trial. The Lancet Respiratory Medicine. 2013;**1**:471-478

[3] Subbaraman R, Nathavitharana RR, Satyanarayana S, et al. The tuberculosis cascade of care in India's public sector: A systematic review and meta-analysis. PLoS Medicine. 2016;**13**:e1002149

[4] Cazabon D, Alsdurf H, Satyanarayana S, et al. Quality of tuberculosis care in high burden countries: The urgent need to address gaps in the care cascade. International Journal of Infectious Diseases. 2017;**56**:111-116

[5] Wells WA, Uplekar M, Pai M. Achieving systemic and scalable private sector engagement in tuberculosis care and prevention in Asia. PLoS Medicine. 2015;**12**:e1001842

[6] Parsons LM, Somoskövi Á, Gutierrez C, et al. Laboratory diagnosis of tuberculosis in resource-poor countries: Challenges and opportunities. Clinical Microbiology Reviews. 2011;**24**:314-350

[7] Sputum Gram stain—Overview. University of Maryland Medical Center www.umm.edu/ency/article/. [Accessed: 05 September 2017]

[8] Siddiqi K, Lambert ML, Walley J. Clinical diagnosis of smear-negative pulmonary tuberculosis in low-income countries: The current evidence. The Lancet Infectious Diseases. 2003;**3**:288-296

[9] Getahun H, Harrington M, O'Brien R, Nunn P. Diagnosis of smear negative pulmonary tuberculosis in people with HIV infection or AIDS in resource-constrained settings: Informing urgent policy changes. Lancet. 2007;**369**:2042-2049

[10] Harries AD, Maher D, Nunn P. An approach to the problems of diagnosing and treating adult smear-negative pulmonary tuberculosis in high-HIV-prevalence settings in sub-Saharan Africa. Bulletin of the World Health Organization. 1998;**76**:651-662

[11] Foulds J, O'Brien R. New tools for the diagnosis of tuberculosis: The perspective of developing countries. The International Journal of Tuberculosis and Lung Disease. 1998;**2**: 778-783

[12] Shinnick TM, Iademarco MF, Ridderhof JC. National plan for reliable tuberculosis laboratory services using a systems approach. Recommendations from CDC and the association of public health laboratories task force on tuberculosis laboratory services. The Morbidity and Mortality Weekly Report. 2005;**54**(RR-6):1-12

[13] Toman K. What are the advantages and disadvantages of fluorescence microscopy? In: Frieden T, editor. Toman's Tuberculosis: Case Detection, Treatment, and Monitoring-Questions and Answers. 2nd ed. Geneva: World Health Organization; 2004. pp. 31-34

[14] Steingart KR, Henry M, Ng V, et al. Fluorescence versus conventional sputum smear microscopy for tuberculosis: A systematic review. The Lancet Infectious Diseases. 2006;**6**: 570-581

[15] TB diagnosis: Improving the yield with fluorescence microscopy. 2007. www.aidsmap.com/TB-diagnosis-Improving-the-yield-with-fluorescence-microscopy/. [Accessed: 05 September 2017]

[16] Fluorescent light-emitting diode (LED) microscopy for diagnosis of tuberculosis. WHO; 2011. http://www.who.int/tb/publications/2011/led_microscopy_diagnosis_9789241501613/en/ [Accessed: 05 September 2017]

[17] WHO. Same-day Diagnosis of Tuberculosis by Microscopy. Geneva: World Health Organization; 2011

[18] Mase SR, Ramsay A, Ng V, et al. Yield of serial sputum specimen examinations in the diagnosis of pulmonary tuberculosis: A systematic review. The International Journal of Tuberculosis and Lung Disease. 2007;**11**:485-495

[19] Cuevas LE, Yassin MA, Al-Sonboli N, et al. A multi-country non-inferiority cluster randomized trial of frontloaded smear microscopy for the diagnosis of pulmonary tuberculosis. PLoS Medicine. 2011;**8**:e1000443

[20] Boehme CC, Nabeta P, Henostroza G, et al. Operational feasibility of using loop-mediated isothermal amplification for diagnosis of pulmonary tuberculosis in microscopy centers of developing countries. Journal of Clinical Microbiology. 2007;**45**:1936-1940

[21] Mitarai S, Okumura M, Toyota E, et al. Evaluation of a simple loop-mediated isothermal amplification test kit for the diagnosis of tuberculosis. The International Journal of Tuberculosis and Lung Disease. 2011;**15**:1211-1217

[22] Ou X, Li Q, Xia H, Pang Y, Wang S, et al. Diagnostic accuracy of the PURE-LAMP test for pulmonary tuberculosis at the county-level Laboratory in China. PLoS One. 2014;**9**:e94544

[23] The Use of Loop-mediated Isothermal Amplification (TB-LAMP) for the Diagnosis of Pulmonary Tuberculosis: Policy Guidance. Geneva: World Health Organization; 2016

[24] Boehme CC, Nabeta P, Hillemann D, et al. Rapid molecular detection of tuberculosis and rifampicin resistance. The New England Journal of Medicine. 2010;**363**:1005-1015

[25] Lawn SD, Nicol MP. Xpert® MTB/RIF assay: Development, evaluation and implementation of a new rapid molecular diagnostic for tuberculosis and rifampicin resistance. Future Microbiology. 2011;**6**:1067-1082

[26] Boehme CC, Nicol MP, Nabeta P, et al. Feasibility, diagnostic accuracy, and effectiveness of decentralised use of the Xpert MTB/RIF test for diagnosis of tuberculosis and multidrug resistance: A multicentre implementation study. Lancet. 2011;**377**:1495-1505

[27] Zeka AN, Tasbakan S, Cavusoglu C. Evaluation of the GeneXpert MTB/RIF assay for the rapid diagnosis of tuberculosis and detection of rifampicin resistance in pulmonary and extrapulmonary specimens. Journal of Clinical Microbiology. 2011;**49**:4138-4141

[28] Hillemann D, Rusch-Gerdes S, Boehme C, Richter E. Rapid molecular detection of extrapulmonary tuberculosis by the automated GeneXpert MTB/RIF system. Journal of Clinical Microbiology. 2011;**49**:1202-1205

[29] Ligthelm LJ, Nicol MP, Hoek KGP, et al. Xpert MTB/RIF for rapid diagnosis of tuberculous lymphadenitis from needle-aspiration biopsy specimens. Journal of Clinical Microbiology. 2011;**49**:3967-3970

[30] Tortoli E, Russo C, Piersimoni C, et al. Clinical validation of Xpert MTB/RIF for the diagnosis of extrapulmonary tuberculosis. The European Respiratory Journal. 2012;**40**:442-447

[31] Theron G, Peter J, van Zyl-Smit R, et al. Evaluation of the Xpert MTB/RIF assay for the diagnosis of pulmonary tuberculosis in a high HIV prevalence setting. American Journal of Respiratory and Critical Care Medicine. 2011;**184**:132-140

[32] Steingart KR, Sohn H, Schiller I, et al. Xpert MTB/RIF assay for pulmonary tuberculosis and rifampicin resistance in adults. Cochrane Database of Systematic Reviews. 2013;**1**:1-131

[33] Theron G, Zijenah L, Chanda D, et al. Feasibility, accuracy, and clinical effect of point-of-care Xpert MTB/RIF testing for tuberculosis in primary-care-setting in Africa: A multicentre, randomised, controlled trial. Lancet. 2014;**383**:424-435

[34] Zijenah LS, Bandason T, Gwambiwa B, et al. Integration of point-of-care Xpert MTB/RIF and smear microscopy for TB diagnosis with point-of-care HIV tests, CD4 counts and treatment at a primary health care clinic in Harare, Zimbabwe. South African Respiratory Journal. 2014;**20**:104-111

[35] WHO. Automated Real-time Nucleic Acid Amplification Technology for Rapid and Simultaneous Detection of Tuberculosis and Rifampicin Resistance: Xpert MTB/RIF System: Policy Statement. Geneva, Switzerland: World Health Organization; 2011. http://www.who.int/tb/features_archive/xpert_rapid_tb_test/en/. [Accessed: 02 September 2017]

[36] Batz H. Towards Lab Free Tuberculosis Diagnosis. August: Access Campaign Medecins Sans Frontieres; 2011 www.msfaccess.org/ Accessed 05 September 2017

[37] Trébucq A, Enarson DA, Chiang CY, et al. Xpert MTB/RIF for national tuberculosis programmes in low income countries: When, where and how? The International Journal of Tuberculosis and Lung Disease. 2011;**15**:1567-1572

[38] Denkinger CM, Nicolau I, Ramsay A, Chedore P, Pai M. Are peripheral microscopy centres ready for next-generation molecular tuberculosis diagnostics? The European Respiratory Journal. 2013;**42**:544-547

[39] 2017 launch of new TB test Ultra backed by WHO recommendation. www.cepheid.com/us/about-us/news-events/press-releases/ [Accessed: 05 September 2017]

[40] WHO Meeting Report of a Technical Expert Consultation: Non-inferiority analysis of Xpert MTB/RIF Ultra compared to Xpert MTB/RIF. http://apps.who.int/iris/handle/10665/254792 [Accessed: 05 September 2017]

[41] Singh JA, Anant B. The ethics of national tuberculosis programmes in low income countries not rolling out Xpert MTB/RIF. The International Journal of Tuberculosis and Lung Disease. 2011;**15**:1563-1563

[42] Hanrahan CF, Selibas K, Deery CB, et al. Time to treatment and patient outcomes among TB suspects screened by a single point-of-care Xpert MTB/RIF at a primary care clinic in Johannesburg, South Africa. PLoS One. 2011;**8**:e66421

[43] Evans C. GeneXpert—A game changer for tuberculosis control? PLoS Medicine. 2011;**8**:e1001064

[44] World Health Organization website. WHO Monitoring of Xpert MTB/RIF Roll-Out. http://www.who.int/tb/areas-of-work/laboratory/status_xpert_rollout_dec_2016.pdf. [Accessed: 05 September 2017]

[45] Albert H, Nathavitharana RR, Isaacs C, Pai M, Denkinger CM, Boehme C. Development, roll-out and impact of Xpert MTB/RIF for tuberculosis: What lessons have we learnt and how can we do better? The European Respiratory Journal. 2016;**48**:516-525

[46] Peter J, Theron G, van Zyl-Smit R, Haripersad A, Mottay L, Kraus S, et al. Diagnostic accuracy of a urine lipoarabinomannan strip test for TB detection in HIV-hospitalised patients. The European Respiratory Journal. 2012;**40**:1211-1220

[47] Lawn SD, Kerhoff AD, Vogt M, Wood R. Diagnostic accuracy of a low-cost, urine antigen, point-of-care screening assay for HIV-associated pulmonary tuberculosis before antiretroviral therapy: A descriptive study. The Lancet Infectious Diseases. 2012;**12**:201-209

[48] Balcha TT, Winqvist N, Sturegard E, et al. Detection of lipoarabinomannan in urine for detection of active tuberculosis among HIV-positive adults in Ethiopian health centres. Tropical Medicine & International Health. 2014;**19**:734-742

[49] Drain PK, Losina E, Coleman SM, et al. Diagnostic accuracy of a point-of-care urine test for tuberculosis screening among newly-diagnosed HIV-infected adults: A prospective, clinic-based study. BMC Infectious Diseases. 2014;**14**:110

[50] Manabe YC, Nonyane BAS, Nakyingi L, et al. Point-of-care lateral flow assays for tuberculosis and cryptococcal antigenuria predict death in HIV infected adults in Uganda. PLoS One. 2014;**9**:e101459

[51] Shah M, Ssengooba W, Armstrong D, et al. Comparative performance of urinary lipoarabinomannan assays and Xpert MTB/RIF in HIV-infected individuals with suspected tuberculosis in Uganda. AIDS. 2014;**28**:1307-1314

[52] Nakiyingi L, Moodley VM, Manabe YC, et al. Diagnostic accuracy of a rapid urine lipoarabinomannan test for tuberculosis in HIV-infected adults. Journal of Acquired Immune Deficiency Syndromes. 2014;**66**:270-279

[53] Zienah LS, Kadzirange G, Bandason T, et al. Comparative performance characteristics of the urine lipoarabinomannan strip test and sputum smear microscopy in hospitalized HIV-infected patients with suspected tuberculosis in Harare, Zimbabwe. BMC Infectious Diseases. 2016;**16**:20

[54] Minion J, Leung E, Talbot E, Dhedha K, Pai M. Diagnosing tuberculosis with urine lipoarabinomannan systematic review and meta-analysis. The European Respiratory Journal. 2011;**38**:1398-1405

[55] WHO. The use of lateral flow urine lipoarabinomannan assay (LF-LAM) for the diagnosis and screening of active tuberculosis in people living with HIV severely HIV-infected patients with no available CD4 counts

[56] WHO. WHO policy statement. Molecular line probe assays for rapid screening of patients at risk of multidrug-resistant tuberculosis. 2008. http://www.who.int/tb/features_archive/policy_statement.pdf [Accessed: 02 September 2017]

[57] WHO. Use of liquid TB culture and DST in low and medium income settings. http://www.who.int/tb/laboratory/use_of_liquid_tb_culture_summary_report.pdf?ua=1 [Accessed: 05 September 2017]

[58] Chaudhary M, Gupta S, Khare S, Lal S. Diagnosis of tuberculosis in an era of HIV pandemic: A review of current status and future prospects. Indian Journal of Medical Microbiology. 2010;**28**:281-289

[59] Wilson ML. Recent advances in the laboratory detection of mycobacterium tuberculosis complex and drug resistance. Clinical Infectious Diseases. 2011;**52**:1350-1355

[60] World Health Organization. Noncommercial culture and drug-susceptibility testing methods for screening patients at risk for multidrug-resistant tuberculosis: policy statement; 2011

[61] Theron G, Peter J, Richardson M, Warren R, Dheda K, Steingart KR. GenoType® MTBDR#sl assay for resistance to second-line anti-tuberculosis drugs. Cochrane Database of Systematic Reviews. 2016;**9**:CD010705

[62] Dinnes J, Deeks J, Kunst H, Gibson A, Cummins E, Waugh N, et al. A systematic review of rapid diagnostic tests for the detection of tuberculosis infection. Health Technology Assessment. 2007;**11**:1-196

[63] Cruciani M, Scarparo C, Malena M, Bosco O, Serpelloni G, Mengoli C. Meta-analysis of BACTEC MGIT 960 and BACTEC 460 TB, with or without solid media, for detection of mycobacteria. Journal of Clinical Microbiology. 2004;**42**:2321-2325

[64] Morgan M, Kalantri S, Flores L, Pai M. A commercial line probe assay for the rapid detection of rifampicin resistance in mycobacterium tuberculosis: A systematic review and meta-analysis. BMC Infectious Diseases. 2005;**5**:62

[65] Ling DI, Zwerling AA, Pai M. GenoType MTBDR assays for the diagnosis of multidrug-resistant tuberculosis: A meta-analysis. The European Respiratory Journal. 2008; **32**:1165-1174

[66] Rossau R, Traore H, De Beenhouwer H, et al. Evaluation of the INNO-LiPA Rif.TB assay, a reverse hybridization assay for the simultaneous detection of mycobacterium tuberculosis complex and its resistance to rifampin. Antimicrobial Agents and Chemotherapy. 1997;**41**:2093-2098

[67] Report for WHO: non-inferiority evaluation of Nipro NTM+MDRTB and Hain GenoType MTBDRplus V2 line probe assays. Geneva: FIND; 2015. http://www.finddx.org/wp-content/uploads/2016/04/LPA-report_noninferiority-study_oct2015.pdf [Accessed: 04 September 2017]

[68] World Health Organization, WHO. The Use of Molecular Line Probe Assays for the Detection of Resistance to Second-Line Anti-Tuberculosis Drugs. Geneva: World Health Organization; 2016, 2016. http://www.who.int/tb/WHOPolicyStatementSLLPA.pdf Accessed: 05 September 2017

[69] Hain Life Sciences. Rapid Diagnosis of Tuberculosis Brochure. http://hain-lifescience.de/uploadfiles/file/produkte/mikrobiologie/mykobakterien/tbeng.pdf. [Accessed: 23 December 2015]

[70] Diel R, Loddenkemper R, Nienhaus A. Predictive value of interferon-γ release assays and tuberculin skin testing for progression from latent TB infection to disease state: A meta-analysis. Chest. 2012;**142**:63-75

[71] Kasprowicz VO, Churchyard G, Lawn SD, Squire SB, Lalvani A. Diagnosing latent tuberculosis in high-risk individuals: Rising to the challenge in high-burden areas. The Journal of Infectious Diseases. 2011;**204**(Suppl 4):S1168-S1178

[72] Santin M, Munoz L, Rigau D. Interferon-γ release assays for the diagnosis of tuberculosis and tuberculosis infection in HIV-infected adults: A systematic review and meta-analysis. PLoS One. 2012;**7**(3):e32482

[73] Chkhartishvili N, Kempker RR, Dvali N, et al. Poor agreement between interferon-gamma release assays and the tuberculin skin test among HIV-infected individuals in the country of Georgia. BMC Infectious Diseases. 2013;**13**:513

[74] Public Health England. World Health Organization (WHO) estimates of tuberculosis incidence by rate, 2012 (sorted by rate). 2014. https://www.gov.uk/government/publications/tuberculosis-tb-by-country-rates-per-100000-people. [Accessed: 03 September 2017]

[75] Menzies D. Tuberculin skin testing. In: Reichman LB, Hershfield ES, editors. Tuberculosis: A Comprehensive International Approach. New York: Marcel Dekker; 2000. pp. 279-322

[76] Nayak S, Acharjya B. Mantoux test and its interpretation. Indian Dermatology Online Journal. 2012;**3**:2-6

[77] Chaturvedi N, Cockcroft A. Tuberculosis screening among health service employees: Who needs chest X-rays? Occupational Medicine (London). 1992;**42**:179-182

[78] American Thoracic Society. Diagnostic standards and classification of tuberculosis in adults and children. American Journal of Respiratory and Critical Care Medicine. 2000;**161**: 1376-1395

[79] American Thoracic Society/Centers for Disease Control. Targeted tuberculin testing and treatment of latent tuberculosis infection. American Journal of Respiratory and Critical Care Medicine. 2000;**161**:S221-S247

[80] Markowitz N, Hansen NI, Wilcosky TC, et al. Tuberculin and anergy testing in HIV-seropositive and HIV-seronegative persons. Annals of Internal Medicine. 1993;**119**:185-193

[81] Graham NMH, Nelson KE, Solomon L, et al. Prevalence of tuberculin positivity and skin test anergy in HIV-1 seropositive and -seronegative intravenous drug users. Journal of the American Medical Association. 1992;**267**:369-373

[82] Smith-Rohrberg D, Sharma SK. Tuberculin skin test among pulmonary sarcoidosis patients with and without tuberculosis: Its utility for the screening of the two conditions in tuberculosis-endemic regions. Sarcoidosis, Vasculitis, and Diffuse Lung Diseases. 2006;**23**:130-134

[83] WHO. Guidelines on the Management of Latent Tuberculosis Infection. Geneva: World Health Organization; 2015. http://www.who.int/tb/publications/ltbi_document_page/en/

[84] Cellestis. Quantiferon-TB1 Gold. 2009. www.cellestis.com/. [Accessed: 05 September 2017]

[85] Oxford Immunotec. T.Spot-TB1. 2009. www.oxfordimmunotec.com/ [Accessed: 05 September, 2017] http://www.who.int/tb/publications/2011/mdr_tb_diagnostics_978924 1501620/en/ [Accessed: 01 September 2017]

[86] Improving the diagnosis and treatment of smear-negative pulmonary and extrapulmonary tuberculosis among adults and adolescents. Recommendations for HIV-prevalent and resource-constrained settings. World Health Organization; 2007 (WHO/HTM/ TB/2007.379); http://www.who.int/tb/publications/tb-diagnosishiv-recommendations/ en/ [Accessed: 5 September 2017]

[87] Summary of Current WHO Recommendations and Guidance on Programmatic Approaches. Geneva: World Health Organization; 2016

[88] World Health Organization. Radiography in Tuberculosis Detection. Summary of Current WHO Recommendations and Guidance on Programmatic Approaches. Geneva: World Health Organization; 2016

[89] TB World Health Organization. Systematic Screening for Active Tuberculosis: Principles and Recommendations. Geneva: World Health Organization; 2013 (WHO/HTM/TB/ 2013.04; http://apps.who.int/iris/bitstream/10665/84971/1/9789241548601_eng.pdf?ua=1) [Accessed: 05 September 2017]

[90] World Health Organization. Tuberculosis Prevalence Surveys: A Handbook. Geneva: World Health Organization; 2011 (WHO/HTM/TB/2010.17; http://www.who.int/tb/advisory_bodies/impact_measurement_taskforce/resources_documents/thelimebook/en/) [Accessed: 5 September 2017]

3

Modern Tools for Diagnosis in Tuberculous Ascites

Andra-Iulia Suceveanu, Despina Todescu, Laura Mazilu, Filippos Goniotakis Manousos, Roxana Hulea, Felix Voinea, Eugen Dumitru and Adrian Paul Suceveanu

Abstract

Tuberculosis (TB) is a highly contagious bacterial infection caused by *Mycobacterium tuberculosis* (MTB), affecting about 1/3rd of the world population and being responsible for lot of deaths worldwide, despite the progress achieved in the diagnosis and treatment fields. TB can affect the peritoneum, the TB ascites being a concern for physicians, especially when dealing with immunocompromised patients. The clinical presentation of TB ascites is challenging, due to nonspecific symptoms that make confusion with other diseases and the late results of cultures from ascites. The late diagnosis leads to a delayed treatment and high mortality. This manuscript describes recent tools used for early diagnosis in TB ascites. Molecular methods based on mycobacterial nucleic acid amplification tests (NAATs), polymerase chain reaction (PCR) detecting minimal amounts of bacterial DNA, or interferongamma release assays (IGRA) and biochemical methods such as the serum-ascites albumin gradient (SAAG) <1.1 g/dL, ratio between lactic dehydrogenase (LDH) in ascites fluid/serum total protein (TP) ratio of 0.5 and fluid ascites/serum LDH ratio of 0.6, and adenosine deaminase activity (ADA) > 40 UI/ml were recently considered more accurate diagnostic procedures. These methods allow a rapid and accurate differential diagnosis of ascites fluid, making possible the early treatment with appropriate drugs.

Keywords: peritoneal tuberculosis, ascites, diagnosis, molecular tests, biochemical tests

1. Introduction

Tuberculosis (TB) is a dangerous infection affecting about one third of the world population despite the availability of affordable and effective chemotherapy, remaining one of the major causes of death from a single infectious agent worldwide. The most affected organ is the lung. It is preventable through Bacillus of Calmette and Guérin (BCG) vaccination and curable with antituberculous drugs.

Tuberculosis is a serious and highly contagious bacterial infection which in humans is usually caused by bacteria called *Mycobacterium tuberculosis* (MTB), a member of the *Mycobacteriaceae* family. This complex also includes *M. bovis* and *M. africanum*. *M. bovis* is more frequently found in cattle and other animals, but it's also responsible for some cases in humans. *M. africanum* is more common in West African countries. Mycobacterial infection is spread through the air from one person to another and causes active disease or latent infection [1].

The absolute number of incident cases has been decreasing since the early 2000s. The lowest incidence rate is found in high-income countries including the United States of America, Canada, New Zealand, Western Europe, and Australia. The largest number of incident cases is found in low- and middle-income countries. In 2015, 61% of the new cases occurred in Asia, followed by 26% new cases in Africa (**Figure 1**) [2].

The HIV infection is the prevalent risk factor for the development of TB because HIV alters the pathogenesis of TB by producing a progressive decline in cell-mediated immunity and raises the chances of extrapulmonary involvement [3, 4].

Tuberculosis is a disease which typically involves the respiratory system, being characterized by the growth of tubercles in tissues, but it can affect any other organ, in which case it's called extrapulmonary tuberculosis (EPTB) and usually results from hematogenous dissemination, being particularly present in immunocompromised patients. In some cases the infection directly extends from an adjacent organ. The most common sites of extrapulmonary tuberculosis are the lymph nodes, abdomen, bones and joints, pleura, spinal cord, and brain [5, 6].

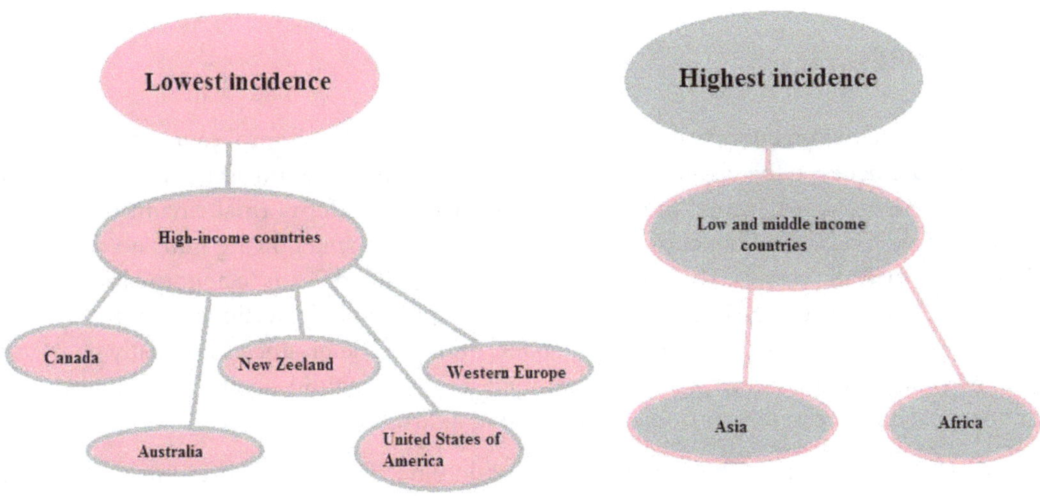

Figure 1. Worldwide incidence of TB infections.

Abdominal tuberculosis is a common form of extrapulmonary tuberculosis. The infection involving *M. tuberculosis* or *M. bovis* could be the result of a primary infection or the reactivation of a latent focus in immunocompromised patients. The spread of abdominal tuberculosis can be hematogenous or can result from direct contact with primary focus or ingestion of sputum containing bacilli from the active pulmonary focus. This form of EPTB affects the peritoneum, the gut, the abdominal lymph nodes, and sometimes, less frequently, the parenchymatous organs in the abdomen like the spleen, liver, and pancreas leading to severe complications. There are three types of abdominal tuberculosis: ascitic, obstructive, and glandular. Diagnosis can be achieved through different methods: ultrasound of the abdomen, CT/MRI scans, biopsies of the suspected organ, endoscopy, and various function tests.

Peritoneal tuberculosis is an uncommon site of extrapulmonary infection caused by *M. tuberculosis*. Patients susceptible of developing EPTB are those with malignant diseases, HIV infection, diabetes, and cirrhosis or patients treated with antitumor necrosis factor (TNF) agents or peritoneal dialysis. Peritoneal TB is divided into three types: the wet ascitic type, the fixed fibrotic type, and the dry plastic type. The wet ascitic type is more common and is associated with large amounts of free or loculated fluid in the abdomen. The high attenuation of the ascites in abdominal ultrasound is thought to be due to high protein and cellular content. Associated peritoneal enhancement is usually present.

Infection occurs frequently following reactivation of latent tuberculous in the peritoneum from hematogenous spread from a primary lung focus. It can also occur via hematogenous spread from active pulmonary or miliary TB. Not so often, the organisms enter the peritoneal cavity transmurally, from an infected small intestine or contiguously from tuberculous salpingitis. Over time, the visceral and parietal peritoneum becomes studded with tubercles [7–9].

2. Definition

Ascites is defined as an abnormal accumulation of fluid in the peritoneal cavity, the presence of serous fluid between the visceral and parietal peritoneum. The word ascites is derived from the ancient Greek word "*askos*" meaning a bag or a sack. Under normal circumstances, the amount of peritoneal fluid depends on a balance between plasma flowing into and out of the blood and lymphatic vessels. This balance, once being disrupted, leads to abnormal accumulation of fluid [10]. Ascites can be a consequence or a complication of infections, malignancy, and many severe diseases: cardiac, endocrine, hepatic, or renal. The prognosis is usually poor, but it depends on the underlying causes. Laboratory tests of ascitic fluid, clinical, paraclinical, and pathological data are required for the differential diagnosis.

Tuberculous ascites, one of the clinical signs of abdominal TB, implies accumulation of fluid in the abdomen, a swollen abdomen, and slightly raised tubercles of 1–2 mm all over the peritoneum. In EPTB, ascites develops secondary to "exudation" of proteinaceous fluid from the tubercles, similar to the mechanism leading to ascites in patients with peritoneal carcinomatosis, and it's often misdiagnosed in elderly patients. Most patients with tuberculous peritonitis have ascites at the time of diagnosis, while the rest present the advanced phase, the dry or fibroadhesive form of the disease [11, 12].

3. Clinical manifestations

Tuberculous peritonitis is a subacute disease, and its symptoms evolve over a period of several weeks or months.

The insidious onset of this condition and the fact that the diagnosis is rarely suspected explains why patients have symptoms for more than 4 months before the diagnosis is established. Tuberculous peritonitis should be considered in any patient presenting with several weeks of abdominal pain, fever, and weight loss. Systemic and constitutional manifestations are common. Symptoms may be mild, with fatigue, abdominal pain, and tenderness, or severe enough to mimic acute abdomen [13]. Other clinical manifestations could be:

- Constipation/diarrhea
- Nocturnal hyperhidrosis
- Low-grade fever
- Anorexia
- Malaise

The clinical presentation of TB ascites is challenging, since it is nonspecific and can be confused with a plethora of other infectious or noninfectious diseases, leading to a delayed diagnosis and treatment which are major factors that contribute to the high mortality of TB.

Another situation that contributes to a delayed diagnosis is the presence of multiple comorbidities such as HIV/AIDS, cirrhosis, uremia, or other chronic conditions. Additional illness results in atypical presentation of TB ascites which render the symptoms more difficult to identify and distinguish. Moreover, in elderly patients, clinical manifestation is minimal with abdominal discomfort, constipation, or fatigue, symptoms that most people tend to ignore as minor or non-perilous (**Figure 2**) [14, 15].

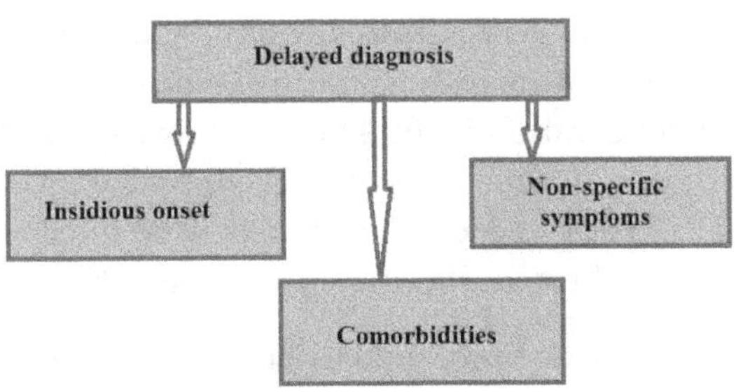

Figure 2. Factors associated with delayed diagnosis.

4. Diagnosis

Due to the fact that the nature of this disease is insidious, the diagnosis represents a challenge for clinicians. With the ever-increasing demographic shifts, more cases are now detected in areas where TB was a rarity until present. Unless a high degree of suspicion is maintained, the diagnosis can easily be missed or delayed [12].

Diagnostic techniques and procedures include:

- Clinical observation
- Imaging techniques: ultrasound, CT/MRI
- Laboratory tests
- Ascites fluid microbiologic and biochemical analysis

Generally, diagnosis is based on clinical suspicion, imaging of tuberculous infected zone, and detection of *M. tuberculosis* in ascitic fluid using acid-fast bacillus staining or culturing. The sensitivity of standard diagnostic methods such as Ziehl-Neelsen staining of smears and Lowenstein-Jensen culture done from ascitic fluid is very low for the diagnosis of abdominal TB. Ziehl-Neelsen staining of the ascitic fluid for mycobacterial detection is positive in only about 3% of the cases with proven TB peritonitis. Detection of mycobacteria requires the presence of more than 5000 bacilli/mL of specimen. In comparison, for positive culture, the presence of at least 10 organisms is considered to be sufficient. For a successful detection, culture methods based on a combination of liquid or biphasic media, together with solid media, are necessary [16, 17].

Nucleic acid amplification tests (NAATs) are molecular diagnostic methods based on amplification of mycobacterial nucleic acid. These are rapid methods that provide results within a day, and they are more specific and sensitive than Acid-Fast Bacillus Smear (AFB) smear. Albeit NAATs were originally designed for respiratory specimens, they can also be used on specimens from other TB sites like ascitic fluid samples, but this technique is still under evaluation.

Ascites of TB peritonitis obtained through ultrasound-guided paracentesis is an exudative type, and macroscopically its appearance is chylous and cloudy or turbid. Biochemically, the serum-ascites albumin gradient (SAAG) is now considered a more sensitive and specific measure than the ascitic total protein concentration which has been used for many years, in differentiating the ascites due to portal hypertension from ascites due to other pathophysiological mechanisms, such as tuberculous ascites which has a SAAG <1.1 g/dL and total proteins >3–4 g% [18, 19]. Combining LDH with total protein analysis has been explored for ascitic fluid. The cutoff values for three parameters in the ascitic fluid for differentiation between hepatic and non-hepatic ascites are as follows: LDH of 400 Sigma units, fluid/serum total protein (TP) ratio of 0.5, and fluid/serum LDH ratio of 0.6. The presence of any two of these three findings is usually associated with TB; the absence of all three indicates a hepatic cause [20].

Glucose concentration in the ascitic fluid, under normal conditions, is similar to that in the serum. Ascitic glucose concentration decreases due to consumption by bacteria, white blood cells, or cancer cells in the fluid in TB peritonitis. Ascitic glucose concentration is lower than normal in TB ascites, which makes it an indicator in differentiating tuberculosis from other diseases, such as cirrhosis. The ascitic/blood glucose ratio is a useful test in differentiating TB peritonitis from other causes of ascites [18].

Ascitic fluid adenosine deaminase activity (ADA) is considered a more sensitive and specific method used for early diagnosis of TB ascites. Even if the full physiological role of ADA is not yet completely understood, it is known that ADA values are notably higher (>40 U/L) in patients with TB ascites [21–23].

Non-biochemical tests of ascitic fluid, including cell counts, bacterial culture, and polymerase chain reaction (PCR), have an important role in diagnosing the cause of ascites.

The total cell count in tuberculous ascites is 150–4000/μL, and the cytologic examination shows over 70–80% lymphocytes and more than 250 leucocytes/mm^3 (**Table 1**).

The sensitivity of direct microscopic smear detection of acid-fast bacilli in the ascitic fluid (0–6%) and ascitic fluid mycobacterial culture (20–35%) is low, and because of the delay in obtaining the results of mycobacterial cultures of ascitic fluid, the mortality is high, and the value of these tests in the differential diagnosis of ascites is limited.

Recently, a new approach to the fast diagnosis of bacterial infections emerged, including tuberculosis. The advanced molecular techniques provided a new method represented by PCR which can detect minimal amounts of bacterial DNA and improves the rates of bacterial identification from 4 to 6 weeks for microbiological cultures to 24 hours. In diagnosing TB effusions, PCR appears to be an ideal tool, with 94% sensitivity and 88% specificity, becoming a rapid and reliable method for identification of infectious ascites [24].

The tuberculin skin testing (TST or purified protein derivative (PPD) skin test) is controversial, despite the high specificity of this test which is between 95 and 99%. Skin testing is currently used only for detection of latent infection because of its low sensitivity and low positive predictive value. At the moment, there are no recommendations for using this test to diagnose active

Type	**Exudative**
Appearance	Chylous and cloudy/turbid
Total cell count	150–4000/μL
Leucocytes	>250/mm^3
Lymphocytes	>70–80%
Total proteins	>3–4 g%
ADA	>40 U/L
LDH	>400 SU
Glucose	<6 mg/dL
SAAG	<1.1 g/dL

Table 1. Characteristics of tuberculous ascites.

disease like tuberculous peritonitis. At best, tuberculin skin testing can only offer auxiliary information. Several studies have reported positivity rates ranging between 24 and 100% with no significant difference between high and low endemicity areas. Currently, the recommendations about the cut point for the induration differ depending on the risk scale. For patients at low risk, the cut point is at 15 mm; in cases of moderate risk, the cut point is 10 mm, and for those at high risk, the cut point is 5 mm. Generally, about 50% of the patients would have false-negative reactions to this test, suggesting the fact that it has many potential sources of error. In conclusion, anergy testing may yield confusing information and is no longer recommended for diagnosis [25].

A great scientific advance has been the development of an IFN-c-based test with an 89% sensitivity, which is a quantitative in vitro assay evaluating the cell-mediated immune response to *M. tuberculosis* and has excellent agreement with tuberculin skin testing. The principle of this test is that previously sensitized T lymphocytes release IFN-c in response to stimulation by purified protein derivative (PPD).

In the past few years, the tuberculin skin test has been replaced by T-cell-based interferon-gamma release assay (IGRA) which is more sensitive and more specific. IGRA is an in vitro test used in all circumstances in which the TST is currently used, including evaluation of immigrants, surveillance programs, or contact investigations [26]. There are three commercially available IFN-γ tests: QuantiFERON-TB Gold assay (QFN-Gold), QuantiFERON-TB Gold *In-Tube* assay (QFN-G-IT), and T-SPOT.TB assay. They are rapid immunodiagnostic tests that can detect interferon-γ (IFN-γ) produced by lymphocytes in response to *Mycobacterium tuberculosis* (MTB). T-SPOT.TB test is a blood IFN-γ assay that measures the number of IFN-γ-producing T cells by identifying IFN-γ release when stimulated by MTB-specific antigens, including early secretory antigenic target 6 and culture filtrate protein 10, using enzyme-linked immunospot assay. QuantiFERON-TB Gold test is the predecessor of QuantiFERON-TB Gold In-Tube test, and they both measure production of IFN-γ in culture supernatant using enzyme-linked immunosorbent assay (ELISA). This measurement is possible by circulating T cells in whole blood being challenged with *M. tuberculosis*-specific antigens. The advantage of blood IGRA tests over tuberculin skin tests is the fact that IGRAs do not cross-react with the Bacillus of Calmette and Guérin (BCG) vaccine antigens, but suboptimal results can be possible in diagnosing EPTB because they aren't able to distinguish latent infection from active disease [27]. According to some researches, *M. tuberculosis* antigen-specific T cells may accumulate at infection sites; therefore, investigating body fluid IGRAs may increase the accuracy of EPTB diagnosis [28, 29].

Imaging techniques used for detection of TB ascites are ultrasound and computed tomography. These methods also increase the accuracy of several procedures like paracentesis or peritoneal biopsies, providing a safer and affordable replacement to diagnostic laparoscopy [30].

Ultrasound is the most sensitive and reliable method of detecting ascites, guiding paracentesis and monitoring the effects of therapy. It can detect even small volumes of fluid (as little as 100 ml of fluid could be detected). Ascites is usually seen as an anechoic space. In TB ascites, particulate matter within the ascitic fluid or fine, mobile strands, representing echogenic debris, can be detected. Less commonly, the ultrasound can reveal calcifications in the walls of encysted ascitic fluid [12].

On computed tomography the ascitic fluid has high attenuation values, between 20 and 45 HU, and the peritoneum is symmetrically thickened and nodular. Frequently, an early sign of abdominal TB is a thickened mesentery (>15 mm) with mesenteric lymph nodes.

Many studies concluded that ultrasonography and computed tomography are complementary to each other in detecting TB ascites, as they provide different details. CT focuses on the peritoneum and omental and mesentery involvement, and the ultrasound shows fine, mobile septations (**Figure 3**) [31].

However, the only certain way to diagnose TB ascites is the histological examination. Various methods that include excision, laparoscopy, needle biopsy and ultrasound-guided biopsies, endoscopy, computed tomography (CT), or endoscopic ultrasound are used to establish the

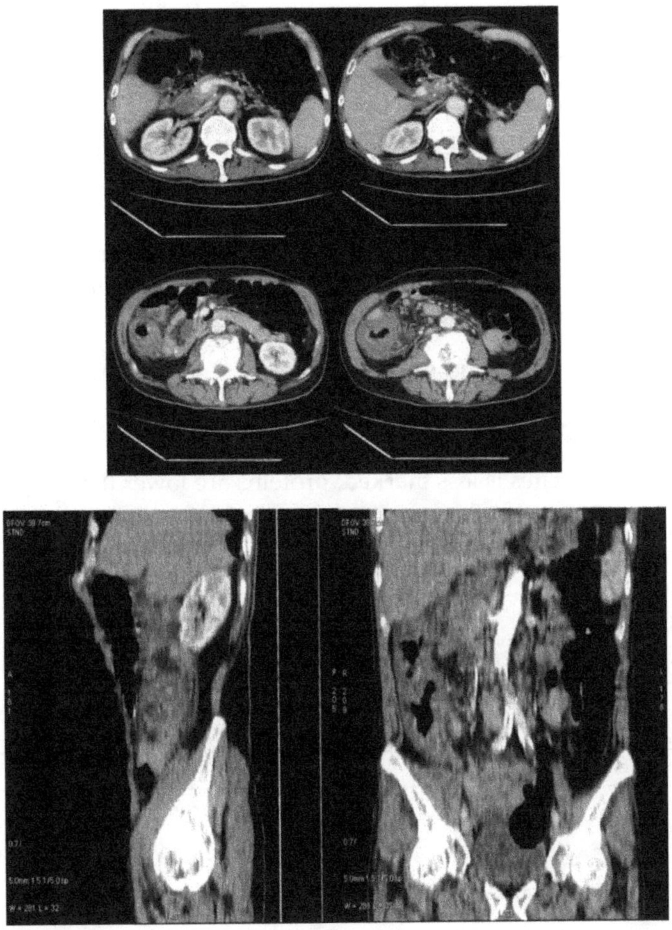

Figure 3. Circumferential parietal thickness, with an edematous appearance of the appendix, cecum, ascending colon, and up to the hepatic flexura, associating stripe thickening of adjacent fat. Multiple adenopathies containing calcifications and central necrosis. Fluid accumulation in the peritoneal cavity associating symmetrical, iodophilic thickening of parietal peritoneum. Osteolytic areas with an adjacent osteosclerotic reaction in L2, L3, and L4 vertebrae. Parafluid accumulation in L2–L3 and L3–L4 intervertebral spaces that reaches the anterior epidural space and the roots of L2 and L3 nerves, extending to L3–L4 adjacent smooth tissues, with no visible border toward the right psoas muscle.

diagnosis. The presence of granulomas is typical for TB ascites [32]. The relative sensitivities of different procedures and the potential therapeutic benefits should be considered in making the choice of diagnostic approach. In superficial TB lymphadenitis, fine needle aspiration (FNA) biopsy of affected lymph nodes is the gold-standard diagnostic technique. Excision biopsy has the highest sensitivity, whereas FNA is less invasive and may be useful. If FNA examination results are doubtful, excision biopsy may be needed. Laparoscopy with target peritoneal biopsy is the current first-line investigation in the diagnosis of peritoneal TB [33, 34]. Several studies revealed a diagnostic accuracy of 84–96% for TB peritonitis.

Generally, tissue biopsy is superior to fluid aspiration in providing positive culture results. The diagnosis is more accurate when the biopsy results and polymerase chain reaction assays are combined with culture results [35].

5. Differential diagnosis

The main differential diagnosis is peritoneal carcinomatosis, which can be difficult to distinguish, especially in older patients. The nodules of carcinomatosis are larger, usually more than 3 mm, more vascular, and more irregular than the tuberculous ones which rarely surpass 1–2 mm. Carcinomatosis is seen as an irregular peritoneal thickening with nodular implants, while TB peritonitis is suggested by the presence of a smooth peritoneum with symmetrical thickening, ascites, and enlarged lymph nodes of low attenuation [31].

Other less likely considerations include:

- Ascites in liver diseases: the liver is enlarged and irregular; proteins are lower than 4 g%.
- Nephrotic syndrome: ascites is less marked; proteins are lower than 4 g%.
- Nutritional edema (hypoproteinemia) has many other signs of protein deficiency; proteins are also lower than 4 g%.
- Starch peritonitis, sarcoidosis, and Crohn's disease may resemble the laparoscopic features of TB peritonitis, but the presence of caseating granuloma establishes the diagnosis (**Table 2**) [36, 37].

The most important differential diagnosis	Less likely considerations
	Ascites in liver disease
	Nephrotic syndrome
Peritoneal carcinomatosis	Hypoproteinemia
	Sarcoidosis
	Starch peritonitis
	Crohn's disease

Table 2. Differential diagnosis.

There are a few signs that additionally suggest the diagnosis of TB peritonitis: normal serum levels of CA 19–9 and carcinoembryonic antigen (CEA), elevated serum levels of CA 125, fever, and lymphocyte-predominant benign ascites, but only biopsies yield the final diagnosis [38, 39].

6. Treatment

Treatment is initiated not only in patients with confirmed diagnosis but also in patients with strong suspicion of TB, because a delay in treatment initiation can lead to significant mortality. TB treatment initiation includes also individuals with ascites associated with fever, weight loss, imaging signs of TB, personal history of TB, or contact with a tuberculosis case.

Despite the fact that most guidelines on the treatment of tuberculosis suggest that 6 months of treatment is sufficient for extrapulmonary tuberculosis (except for the case of bone tuberculosis or tuberculous meningitis), most physicians treating peritoneal tuberculosis use antituberculous therapy for 9 to 12 months [40, 41].

Drug treatment is the most important modality and follows standard regimens and principles. There are currently five drugs that are considered first-line medications: isoniazid, rifampicin, pyrazinamide, streptomycin, and ethambutol. Second-line drugs are only used in case of resistance to first-line therapy (extensively drug-resistant tuberculosis or multidrug-resistant tuberculosis), and they are represented by aminoglycosides, fluoroquinolones, polypeptides, cycloserine, thioamides, and terizidone. There is also a third-line therapy with uncertain or unproven efficacy including rifabutin, macrolides, linezolid, thioacetazone, thioridazine, arginine, bedaquiline, and vitamin D [42]. Drug-resistant disease varies substantially in different areas of the world and may occur in cases of poor patient management, nonadherence to prescribed regimen, or as a result of malabsorption of the antituberculous drugs.

The treatment of TB peritonitis in patients with HIV is usually the same, but because HIV-infected patients are often taking multiple drugs, some of which may interact with antituberculous ones; it is strongly recommended to consult the experts in HIV-related TB.

The "complete response" to antituberculous treatment means complete resolution of symptoms and ascites within 6 months; in most cases, laboratory tests return to normal values within 3 months. Persistence of ascites means "no response" [43, 44].

7. Conclusions

Peritoneal tuberculosis is still common in areas of the world where TB is prevalent and its incidence ratio is likely to increase as a consequence of population migrations.

Ascites can be a complication of an aggregate of diseases, which carries an unfavorable prognosis that depends on the causes, the moment of diagnosis, and the start of the treatment.

Establishing the diagnosis of TB ascites requires a high index of suspicion because of its insidious development. In any patient with several weeks of abdominal pain, weight loss, fever, and lymphocytic dominant ascites with SAAG < 1.1 g/L, as well as in patients with ascites belonging to special population groups, such as indigenous or older people, or patients with ascites as the primary symptom, ascitic TB peritonitis should be considered in differential diagnosis. This syndrome behaves clinically like many abdominal diseases that are often ignored, leading to a significant impact on morbidity and mortality due to a delayed diagnosis and treatment. Older laboratory tests lack sensitivity and specificity in establishing the diagnosis. Histological examination, considered the gold-standard diagnosis method, is an invasive procedure with high risk of complications. More accurate methods such as molecular tests based on mycobacterial nucleic acid amplification tests (NAATs), PCR techniques used to detect bacterial DNA, or interferon-gamma release assays (IGRA) and biochemical methods such as the serum-ascites albumin gradient (SAAG), ratio between LDH in ascites fluid/ serum total protein (TP) ratio and fluid ascites/serum LDH ratio, adenosine deaminase activity (ADA), and imagistic techniques were recently considered for an efficient positive diagnosis of TB ascites, making possible the early treatment with appropriate tuberculostatic drugs.

Author details

Andra-Iulia Suceveanu*, Despina Todescu, Laura Mazilu, Filippos Goniotakis Manousos, Roxana Hulea, Felix Voinea, Eugen Dumitru and Adrian Paul Suceveanu

*Address all correspondence to: andrasuceveanu@yahoo.com

Faculty of Medicine, Ovidius University, Constanta, Romania

References

[1] Dye C, Lönnroth K, Jaramillo E, et al. Trends in tuberculosis incidence and their determinants in 134 countries. Bulletin of the World Health Organization. 2009;87:683

[2] Walter ND, Jasmer RM, Grinsdale J, et al. Reaching the limits of tuberculosis prevention among foreign-born individuals: A tuberculosis-control program perspective. Clinical Infectious Diseases. 2008;46:103. DOI: 10.1086/523733

[3] Canadian Thoracic Society and The Public Health Agency of Canada and Licensors. Canadian Tuberculosis Standards. 7th ed. Ottawa: Public Health Agency of Canada; 2013. pp. 247-273

[4] Schluger NW, Rom WN. The host immune response to tuberculosis. American Journal of Respiratory and Critical Care Medicine. 1998;157:679-691

[5] Mehta JB, Dutt A, Harvill L, Mathews KM. Epidemiology of extrapulmonary tuberculosis. A comparative analysis with pre-AIDS era. Chest. 1991;99:1134

[6] Gherasim L. Non-surgical diseases of the peritoneum - Ascites. Internal Medicine. Vol. 3. Ed. Medicala; 1998. pp. 1159-1176

[7] Lazarus A, Thilagar B. Abdominal Tuberculosis. Disease-a-Month. 2007;53(1):32-38

[8] Dineen P, Homan WP, Grafe WR. Tuberculous peritonitis: 43 years experience in diagnosis and treatment. Annals of Surgery. 1976;184:717-722

[9] Sanai FM, Bzeizi KI. Systematic review: Tuberculous peritonitis—presenting features, diagnostic strategies and treatment. Alimentary Pharmacology and Therapeutics. 2005;22(8): 685-700

[10] Lin-Lin H, Harry Hua-Xiang X, Sen-Lin Z. Ascitic Fluid Analysis in the Differential Diagnosis of Ascites: Focus on Cirrhotic Ascites. Available from: https://www.ncbi.nlm.nih.gov/pmc/articles/PMC4521252

[11] Chow KM, Chow VC, Hung LC, Wong SM, Szeto CC. Tuberculous peritonitis-associated mortality is high among patients waiting for the results of mycobacterial cultures of ascitic fluid samples. Clinical Infectious Diseases. 2002;35:409-413

[12] Jain R, Sawhney S, Bhargava DK, Berry M. Diagnosis of abdominal tuberculosis: Sonographic findings in patients with early disease. American Journal of Roentgenology. 1995;165:1391-1395

[13] Bernhard JS, Bhatia G, Knauer CM. Gastrointestinal tuberculosis: An eighteen-patient experience and review. Journal of Clinical Gastroenterology. 2000;30:397-402

[14] Al Karawi MA, Mohamed AE, Yasawy MI, et al. Protean manifestations of gastrointestinal tuberculosis: Report on 130 patients. Journal of Clinical Gastroenterology. 1995;20: 225-232

[15] Gonnella JS, Hudson EK. Clinical patterns of tuberculous peritonitis. Archives of Internal Medicine. 1966;117:164-169

[16] Yeager HJ Jr, Lacy J, Smith L, LeMaistre C. Quantitative studies of mycobacterial populations in sputum and saliva. The American Review of Respiratory Disease. 1967;95: 998-1004

[17] Gupta S, Kumari S, Banwalikar JN, Gupta SK. Diagnostic utility of the estimation of mycobacterial antigen A60 specific immunoglobulins IgM, IgA and IgG in the sera of cases of adult human tuberculosis. Tubercle and Lung Disease. 1995;76:418-424

[18] Tarn AC, Lapworth R. Biochemical analysis of ascitic (peritoneal) fluid: What should we measure? Annals of Clinical Biochemistry. 2010;47:397-407

[19] Mansour-Ghanaei F, Shafaghi A, Bagherzadeh AH, Fallah MS. Low gradient ascites: A seven year course review. World Journal of Gastroenterology. 2005;11:2337-2339

[20] Sevinc A, Sari R, Fadillioglu E. The utility of lactate dehydrogenase isoenzyme pattern in the diagnostic evaluation of malignant and nonmalignant ascites. Journal of the National Medical Association. 2005;97:79-84

[21] Riquelme A, Calvo M, Salech F, et al. Value of adenosine deaminase (ADA) in ascitic fluid for the diagnosis of tuberculous peritonitis: A meta-analysis. Journal of Clinical Gastroenterology. 2006;40(8):705-710

[22] Segura RM, Pascual C, Ocana I, et al. Adenosine deaminase in body fluids: A useful diagnostic tool in tuberculosis. Clinical Biochemistry. 1989;22:141-148

[23] Blake J, Berman P. The use of adenosine deaminase assays in the diagnosis of tuberculosis. South African Medical Journal. 1982;62:19-23

[24] Schwake L, von Herbay A, Junghanss T, Stremmel W, Mueller M. Peritoneal tuberculosis with negative polymerase chain reaction results: Report of two cases. Scandinavian Journal of Gastroenterology. 2003;38:221-224

[25] Arend SM, van Meijgaarden KE, de Boer K, de Palou EC, van Soolingen D, Ottenhoff TH, van Dissel JT. Tuberculin skin testing and in vitro T cell responses to ESAT-6 and culture filtrate protein 10 after infection with *Mycobacterium marinum* or *M. kansasii*. The Journal of Infectious Diseases. 2002;186:1797-1807

[26] Pai M, Zwerling A, Menzies D. Systematic review: T cell-based assays for the diagnosis of latent tuberculosis infection: An update. Annals of Internal Medicine. 2008;149:177-184

[27] Wagner D, Hörster R, Lange B, Lange C. Evaluation of T-cell interferon-gamma-release assays for the diagnosis of latent and active tuberculosis. Deutsche Medizinische Wochenschrift. 2008;133:354-357

[28] Sharma SK, Tahir M, Mohan A, Smith-Rohrberg D, Mishra HK, Pandey RM. Diagnostic accuracy of ascitic fluid IFN-gamma and adenosine deaminase assays in the diagnosis of tuberculous ascites. Journal of Interferon & Cytokine Research. 2006;26:484-488

[29] Greco S, Girardi E, Masciangelo R, Capoccetta GB, Saltini C. Adenosine deaminase and interferon measurements for the diagnosis of tuberculous pleurisy: A meta-analysis. The International Journal of Tuberculosis and Lung Disease. 2003;7:777-786

[30] Burrill J, Williams CJ, Bain G, et al. Tuberculosis: A radiologic review. Radiographics. 2007;27(5):1255-1273

[31] Ha HK, Jung JI, Lee MS, et al. CT differentiation of tuberculous peritonitis and peritoneal carcinomatosis. AJR American Journal of Roentgenology. 1996;167:743-748

[32] Mimica M. The usefulness and limitations of laparoscopy in the diagnosis of tuberculous peritonitis. Endoscopy. 1992;24:588-591

[33] Barry RE, Brown P, Read AE. Physicians use of laparoscopy. British Medical Journal. 1978;2:1276-1278

[34] Chu CM, Lin SM, Peng SM, et al. The role of laparoscopy in the evaluation of ascites of unknown origin. Gastrointestinal Endoscopy. 1994;40:285-289

[35] Bhargava DK, Shriniwas, Chopra P, et al. Peritoneal tuberculosis: Laparoscopic patterns and its diagnostic accuracy. The American Journal of Gastroenterology. 1992;87:109-112

[36] McHutchison JG. Differential diagnosis of ascites. Seminars in Liver Disease. 1997;17:191-202

[37] Alexandrakis MG, Moschandrea JA, Koulocheri SA, Kouroumalis E, Eliopoulos GD. Discrimination between malignant and nonmalignant ascites using serum and ascitic fluid proteins in a multivariate analysis model. Digestive Diseases and Sciences. 2000;45:500-508

[38] Louhimo J, Finne P, Alfthan H, Stenman UH, Haglund C. Combination of HCG beta, CA 19-9, and CEA with logistic regression improves accuracy in gastrointestinal malignancies. Anticancer Research. 2002;22:1759-1764

[39] Xiao W, Liu Y. Elevation of serum and ascites cancer antigen 125 levels in patients with liver cirrhosis. Journal of Gastroenterology and Hepatology. 2003;18:1315-1316

[40] Treatment Duration for Abdominal Tuberculosis. July, 2015. Available from: https://clinicaltrials.gov/ct2/show/NCT01124929 [Accessed 2 March 2016]

[41] World Health Organization. Guidelines on the Management of Latent Tuberculosis Infection. Geneva: WHO; 2015. Available from: http://www.who.int/tb/publications/ltbi_document_page/en/[Accessed 2 March 2016]

[42] Lonnroth K, Castro KG, Chakaya JM, Chauhan LS, Floyd K, Glaziou P, Raviglione MC. Tuberculosis control and elimination 2010-50: Cure, care, and social development. Lancet. 2010;375:1814-1829

[43] Lonnroth K, Uplekar M. Invest in breaking the barriers of public-private collaboration for improved tuberculosis care. Bulletin of the World Health Organization. 2005;83:558-559

[44] Mendez A, Raviglione MC, Laszlo A, Binkin N, Rieder HL, Bustreo F,Cohn DL, Lambregts-vanWeezenbeek CS, Kim SJ, Chaulet P, et al. Global surveillance for antituberculosis-drug resistance, 1994-1997. World Health Organization-International Union against Tuberculosis and Lung Disease Working Group on Anti-Tuberculosis Drug Resistance Surveillance. The New England Journal of Medicine. 1998;338:1641-1649

4

Breast and Cervix Uteri: Rare Locations for *Mycobacterium tuberculosis* Infections and Complications

Manuela Cristina Russu, Şerban Nastasia,
Daniela Degeratu and Ruxandra Viorica Stănculescu

Abstract

Breast and cervix uteri are rare locations for *Mycobacterium tuberculosis* (*MbT*) infection and *MbT* association to cervical cancer is more rare in European countries. This chapter analyses two cases of rare locations of tuberculosis (TB) in young Romanian women. The first patient presented a chronic primary TB breast abscess, non-pregnancy related with periods of apparent healing and repeated areolar fistula formation. In the second case, the unexpected discovery of secondary TB endocervical granulomatous inflammation with caseous necrosis on a radical hysterectomy specimen, performed after chemoradiotherapy for squamous non-keratinizing cell carcinoma is presented. Worldwide incidence, risk factors, hypothetic mechanisms of primary/secondary breast and cervix uteri *MbT* infection, the association to high-risk HPV, microbiological diagnosis difficulties, the differentials to pyogenic abscesses, other chronic granulomas and breast cancer treatment issues are presented in the reviewed literature, focusing on the peculiarities of these rare locations and complications. It is recalled an old concept of "therapeutic antitubercular" test when all other assessments steps are usefulness.

Keywords: tuberculosis, breast abscess, cervical caseous granuloma, carcinoma

1. Introduction

Tuberculosis (TB) is an old disease, known since 5000BC, and contemporary professional and scientific communities are challenged by the WHO's *"Global Tuberculosis Report 2017"* showing 6.3 million new cases of TB in 2016, with about 16% expected to die due to TB by 2020.

These data may be connected to the lack of an effective vaccine, and of sensitive and rapid diagnostic tests, to the appearance of multidrug resistant strains of *Mycobacterium tuberculosis* (*MbT*) [1, 2]. Low income, immunosuppressive disorders, worldwide travels and immigration are associated to TB globalization [3]. Breast and uterine cervix are rare locations for *MbT* even in TB endemic countries [1]. This chapter analyses two cases of rare locations of TB in young women from Romania, a middle-income country. The first case is a chronic, non-pregnancy-related primary breast abscess, with areolar fistula formation between periods of apparent healing. The second case is an association of secondary endocervical tuberculosis to a squamous cervical carcinoma in a young woman with a previous lung tuberculosis, without activation during/after specific cervical cancer therapy. In Europe, there are few papers in the form of case reports on breast or cervix uteri tuberculosis. Breast and cervix uteri tuberculosis are uncommon diseases with non-specific clinical, imagistic and or cytological/histological findings. Misdiagnosis or the diagnosis after many negative assessments for these rare TB locations are common, because biopsy specimens are paucibacillary, and other investigations such as microscopy and culture are frequently negative, as it is the PCR for *MbT*. *MbT* can simulate cervical carcinoma in premenopause and postmenopause [4, 5] due to abnormal vaginal bleeding at clinical presentation.

We intent to review and refresh the theories/hypothesis on the epidemiology, pathophysiology, diagnosis and therapeutic issues on these rare *MbT* locations and complications. In countries like Romania, where TB is non-endemic and the diagnosis for extra pulmonary tuberculosis is a surprise, the golden standard of microbiological evidence of *MbT* is rare, even with the new molecular techniques. It is reconsidered the "old concept of the therapeutic test" with antitubercular drugs, which was proved to be active in pulmonary tuberculosis.

2. Cases presentation

First case: A 31 years old Caucasian woman, higher studies and salaried, married, nuligesta, on combined oral contraceptives, no family or personal history of tuberculosis or known exposure to a person with tuberculosis, no mammary surgery, is presenting in December 2014 with nipple retraction and inversion, skin redness and thickening, over a breast inflammatory tumor of 2 x 1 cm size, in the internal upper quadrant of the right breast, freely mobile and a fistula at areola level, with no axillary or cervical lymphadenopathy, and normal left breast. The systemic examination is non-contributory, and no associated constitutional symptoms, as fever, no weight and appetite loss are registered.

The patient had three previous similar episodes, since 2007, with a fistula of the right breast abscess, sterile cultures for aerobic/anaerobic germs, and yeasts in the nipple purulent discharge.

Routine hematological and biochemical investigations, and serum prolactin levels are normal, HIV test is negative. Breast sonography reveals skin thickening, nipple retraction and dilated terminal ducts and ill-defined thick-walled cystic mass of 2.9 cm diameter.

The cytological examination after Giemsa stain from the fistula's purulent discharge shows a rich cellular smear, with many polymorphs background, lymphohistiocytic aggregates and Langhans type multinuclear giant cells, fibrin debris and rare epithelial cells, which conducted to the conclusion of a chronic breast inflammatory granuloma.

It is decided and incision-excision of the inflammatory mammary gland tissue was performed, with large drainage of the remaining cavity, samples collection for pathology/microbiology and no other unwanted events as shock or toxemia.

In January 2015, a new fistula occurred on the opposite on the opposite area of the right nipple, with discharge of purulent material, without fever or other general symptoms, as she never presented at each previous medical consultations (**Figure 1**).

The cultures for aerobic/anaerobic germs and yeasts are sterile, the pathological examination discovers rare epithelial cells of squamous type, lymphocytes, plasma cells, histiocytes, multinuclear giant cells of Langhans type and a multitude of blood vessels. The Ziehl Neelsen stain for acid-fast bacilli and PCR for *MbT* from sample collected at excision biopsy are negative (**Figure 2(A, B)**).

The chest X-ray examination is normal and the PPD skin test is 10 mm.

In March 2015, a 6 months antitubercular treatment (ATT) with three drugs was recommended: isoniazid, rifampicin and ethambutol with intensive therapy for the first 3 months is administered. The follow up from May 2015 (after 2 months of intensive therapy) shows remission of the fistulas, heal of the skin, the persistency of the nipple retraction and a 2 kg weight gain. The patient had a total 9 months ATT (**Figure 3**).

The final diagnosis is primary non-gestational breast tuberculosis abscess.

The second case: A 29 years merchandise by occupation, smoker of five cigarettes per day, non-alcoholic, married since 10 years is presenting for repeated postcoital abnormal vaginal bleeding and blood-stained discharge since 6 months. History: physiology: the menarche:

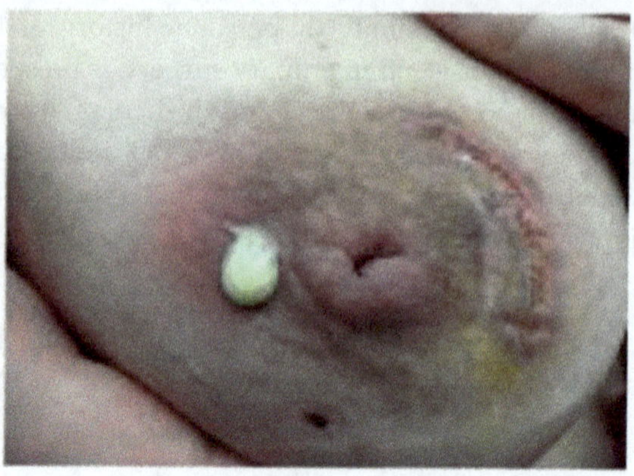

Figure 1. Photograph of the scar from slowly-healing post-incision/excision-drainage wound of the right breast, and the new fistula on the opposite part of the right areola and purulent discharge.

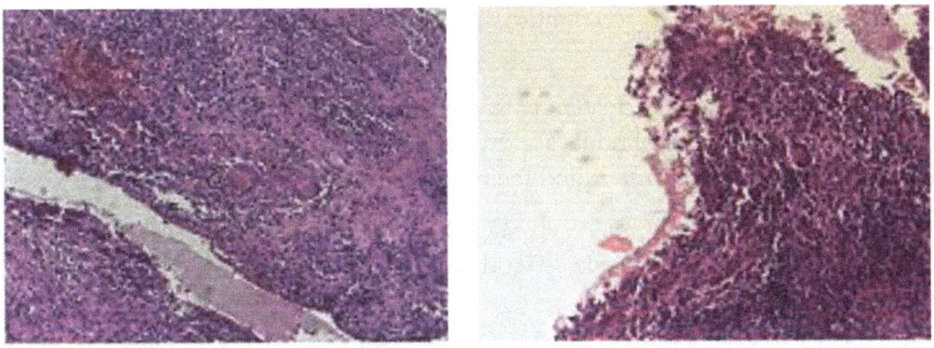

A B

Figure 2. Pathological images (**A.** Hematoxylin & Eosin, 40X; **B.** Hematoxylin & Eosin, 20X): Inflammatory granulomatous lesions: Rich chronic inflammatory infiltrate, with many histiocytes (with epithelioid aspect) and frequent multinuclear giant cells Langhans-type. Collection of Degeratu Daniela, "Dr I. Cantacuzino" Laboratory of Pathology.

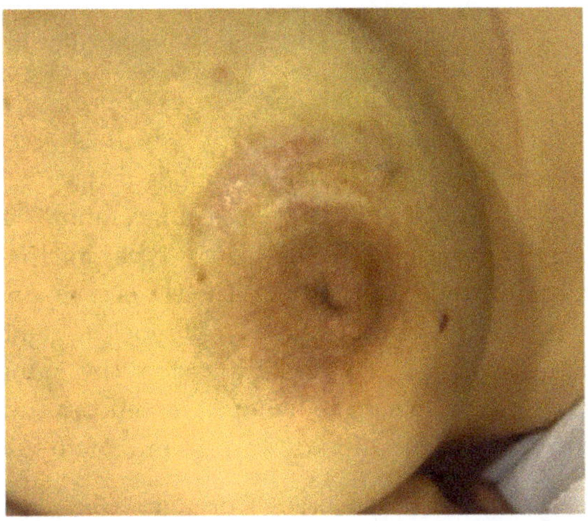

Figure 3. Photograph of the right breast after two months of intense active antitubercular treatment. Patient in recumbent position with healed wound, without sinuses of the areola, and inverted nipple.

14 years; 2 full-term spontaneous deliveries; 1 abortion; pathology: pulmonary tuberculosis (treated and considered healed in 2002); no surgical illness. LMP: August 20, 2008, immunological pregnancy and HIV tests: negative. General physical examination was essentially normal; abdominal examination revealed no mass, no ascites, no hepatosplenomegaly and no other abnormality.

Vaginal speculum examination: an irregular, cauliflower-like tumor of 4 cm in the largest size on the anterior cervical ridge, spontaneously bleeding, and on touch; normal vaginal walls and bilateral fornices.

Vaginal bimanual examination: anteverted uterus of normal shape, and volume, firm, mobile and no adnexal mass.

Per-rectal examination: smooth rectal mucosa, and freely mobile, no induration or nodularity of both parametrials.

Pap smear: epithelioid-like cell clusters with atypia. Colposcopic examination increased vascularity on the posterior cervical ridge, acetowhite on the anterior cervical ridge, with negative iodine stain with precise contour around the previously described cauliflower-like tumor.

Provisional diagnosis of carcinoma cervix stage I B was kept, and after preliminary investigations, patient was posted for multiple cervical biopsies—the tumor and from other four cardinal points in the vicinity.

The histopathological diagnosis came out to be squamous non-keratinizing cell carcinoma (**Figure 4**), and the specific tests for viral infection had revealed the presence of genotype 33 HPV.

Hematological test: low degree anemia (Hb: 11.0 mg/dL, Ht; 34%), leukocytosis and thrombocytosis.

Biochemical and coagulation tests: normal.

Chest radiography showed fibrous and fibro-nodular sequelae of pulmonary tuberculosis.

After 4 weeks of radiotherapy (tele-radiation and 2 cures of brachytherapy) plus chemotherapy (cisplatin), the patient is proposed for surgery, which is accepted and it is done a Wertheim's radical hysterectomy with bilateral pelvic node dissection. The post-surgery pathological examination showed a cervix with large areas of ulceration, polymorph inflammatory infiltrate and multinuclear giant cells of foreign body type, micro-calcifications and small islands of squamous non-keratinizing cancer cells. The endocervix presents a granulomatous inflammation with caseous necrosis and Langhans multinuclear giant cells. The vaginal part and the lateral part of the cervix have no neoplastic invasion. The endometrium is atrophic, the ovaries have albicans bodies, the tubes have hypoplastic mucosa,and the examination of 10 lymphnodes shows their reactive aspect, lipo-dystrophy and micro-calcifications.

PCR for *MbT* was performed on archived tissue (formalin-fixed paraffin embedded uterine tissue) following detection of cervical TB by pathology, was positive in the cervix. The patient

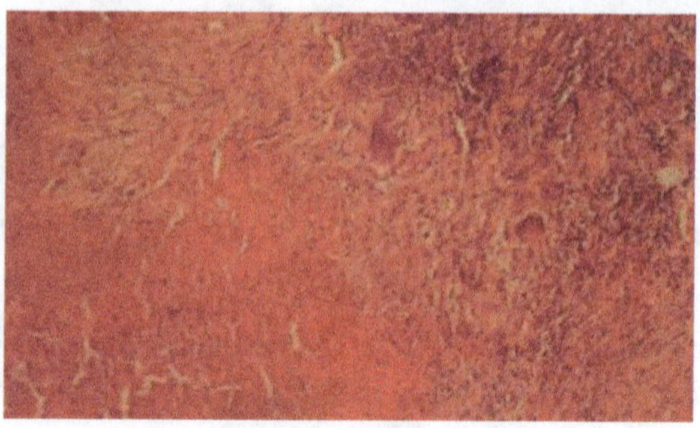

Figure 4. Two confluent epithelioid caseous granulomas with Langhans-type gint multinuclear cells and lymphocytic inflammatory infiltrate at the periphery, HE stain, 10 x. Collection of Degeratu Daniela, "Dr I. Cantacuzino" Laboratory of Pathology.

has a normal evolution post-radio, chemotherapy and post-surgery, without any reactivation of the pulmonary tuberculosis.

3. Epidemiology: risk factors

3.1. Epidemiology of breast tuberculosis

Breast TB was first described in a very young woman by Sir Astley Cooper in 1829 as "scrofulous swelling of the bosom", and the location of *MbT* in the cervix uteri was first described 2 years later by Renaud (1831). Extrapulmonary TB was reported in nearly 18% of cases in USA [6], and TB location in the breasts is extremely rare in Western populations from 0.025 to 0.1% of all surgically treated breast diseases. In the last 20 years, the Southern European countries such as Greece, Turkey, Italy and Spain reported rare such cases, and 0.64–3.59% of all mammary treatable conditions are in developing countries from Asia [7], where the overall incidence of histological confirmed breast TB is 0.4% per year [8]. In India, the incidence of breast TB is five times less common than carcinoma of the breast [8]. There are described fluctuations in the incidence of generally breast TB, with the highest incidence in Southern Turkey in 2007 [10], and in the last 8 years (**Table 1**) the reported cases with primary breast TB have an increasing incidence all over the world, as it is the Romanian case, which had the first episode in 2007. Mammary involvement is nearly equal in frequency in the right and left (40.0 vs. 44.0%) [10], bilateral disease is rare [11, 12], as it is the infra-mammary location of tuberculosis [13]. Breast tuberculosis is affecting women in the reproductive age,

Continent	Number of cases since the year 2000 (00)																
	00	01	02	03	04	05	06	07	08	09	10	11	12	13	14	15	16
Europe	1 It	0	0	1 Gr	0	1 T	1 T	1 Ch	0	3 T	0	0	0	0	0	1 R	0
Africa	0	1 Mo	1 Mo	0	0	0	0	0	0	0	0	0	1 Mo	0	0	0	0
Asia	8 In		1 In	0	0	0	35 In	0	1 In	0	2 In Tw	3 Ir In	8 In	2 In	8 Ir In	0	0
North America	0	0	0	0	0	0	0	0	0	0	0	0	1 Mx	0	0	0	1 US
South America	0	0	3 Br	0	0	1 Br	0	0	0	1 Br	0	0	0	1 Co	0	0	0
Australia New Zeeland	0	0	0	0	0	0	38	0	0	0	0	0	0	0	0	0	0

It, Italy; Gr, Greece; T, Turkey; Ch, China; R, Romania; Mo, Morocco; In, India; Tw, Taiwan; Ir, Iran; Br, Brasil; Mx, Mexico; Co, Columbia; US, United States of America.

Table 1. Annual worldwide published cases with primary breast tuberculosis (last 16 years medical literature - Google scholar, Medline, web of science).

21–30 years, predominantly, a case being reported during pregnancy [14], and rarely in prepubescent [15] and elderly postmenopausal women [16], the last category being more affected in the early twentieth century, and in the last years it is discovered in women and men [17, 18]. None of the recognized risk factors (multiparity, lactation, trauma, past history of suppurative mastitis, breast surgery/breast reconstruction [19, 20], silicon breast introduction or AIDS [21] was present in the Romanian reported case.

3.2. Epidemiology of cervix uteri tuberculosis

In developing countries like India, TB is a major socioeconomic burden, afflicting 14 million people mostly in the reproductive age group (15–45 years). Regarding the genital tract, fallopian tubes are involved in almost all the cases of pelvic tuberculosis, endometrium in 50–60% and ovaries in 20–30% [22]. Cervical tuberculosis accounts for 0.1–0.65% of all cases of the disease and 5–24% of genital tract [23].

4. Pathophysiology

4.1. Pathophysiology of breast tuberculosis

The breast was considered an organ that offers resistance to the survival and multiplication of the tubercle bacillus [24], like other organs such as spleen, skeletal muscle or cervix uteri, and this property is one of the reasons for the uncommon diagnosis of breast TB, and in countries like India it is supposed that the breast TB is confused to carcinoma [25], or to a pyogenic breast abscess [26], or to other diseases [27], tubercular mastitis being a "great masquerader" [28]. In contrast to this quality, when breast is infected with *MbT*, it was proved that BRCA 1/2 network is suppressed during infection suggesting that breast cell proliferation suppression is a feature of Koch bacilli survival [29].

Breast TB is described to be primary or isolated, and secondary. The primary breast TB is appreciated when the breast infection is the only manifestation of the disease, no demonstrable tuberculous focus exists elsewhere in the body [30], and the infection is through abrasions or through the openings of the ducts in the nipple. Primary breast TB is rare in comparison to secondary to lung or extrapulmonary, and the authors consider that the Romanian case is among primary breast tuberculosis. The secondary type is appreciated when a pre-existing lesion is located elsewhere in the body. Secondary *MbT* can spread by three routes such as hematogenous, lymphatic or directly from the primary location such as lung, pleura, ribs, mediastinum and articular lesions. It is supposed that the patient had acquired the *MbT* during a plain long distance travel, some previous years ago, when she claimed the first episode of breast inflammation; extensive travels seem to be responsible for tuberculosis globalization, statement common to others' physicians [3], which is an explanation for a primary men's breast tuberculosis, as it the case of a 44 years old Lithuanian man living in UK [18]. In countries where TB is endemic, young lactating women are more prone to develop breast tuberculosis, being described an incidence that can vary in the limits of 7–33% [31–33]. All types of *Mycobacterium spp.*, and other types of antigens or foreign bodies, as milk during pregnancy or lactational period, are met by a vigorous cell-mediated hypersensitivity reaction involving macrophages, epithelioid and giant cells, Th1 lymphocytes, and their cytokines, which are activated and are developing the granulomas [34].

In Romania, like in countries with endemic tuberculosis as India, Pakistan, China, Iran and Korea, tubercular infection is seen more frequent secondary to a tubercular focus such as lungs, pleura or lymph nodes, which very frequently actually may not be detected clinical or radiological [26]. The breast infection is acquired usually from lungs by many routes (hematogenous, lymphatic via tracheobronchial, paratracheal, mediastinal lymph trunks or internal mammary nodes), by spread from contiguous structures and by ductal infection [8]. *MbT* is affecting differently breast structures, according to route of contamination: the epithelium of the ducts (primary) or of the lobules (secondary) with loss of acinar structures; and the entire epithelial lining of the lobules is destroyed, caseating necrosis appearing in the center of the lesion, and the destructive mechanisms are progressing and involving the skin, which may ulcerate and create fistula/sinuses; in other cases, specially in elder women, the mechanisms of repair/restoration are developing excessive dense fibrous tissue.

4.2. Pathophysiology of cervix uteri tuberculosis: Hypothesis on the association to cervical cancer

Pelvic organs are infected from a primary focus, elsewhere in the body, most commonly from lungs, by hematogenous spread. The cervix may be infected, as a part of this process, by lymphatic dissemination from the infected tube, or by direct extension from the endometrium. It is discussed a cervical infection from the sexual partner/partners with tuberculous epididymitis, being discussed the increased risk when there are multiple sexual male partners, especially in China [35]. It is discussed a relative immunity of the cervix to *MbT* as it was shown previously for other organs, which is probably connected to the inability of the bacillus to penetrate the squamous epithelium *of portio* vaginalis, and to cervical mucus resistance, but in rare cases, cervical TB may be a primary infection, *MbT* being introduced by a partner with tuberculous epididymitis or other genitourinary disease [36], but the sexual partner of the reported patient was negative for pulmonary TB. It was suggested the role of the sputum used as a sexual lubricant [22].

In the nineteenth century, it was a controversy as whether tuberculosis and cancer can coexist in the same organ; Carl von Rokitansky (1855) was the first to propose the view that there is a definite antagonism between the two, meaning that tuberculosis and cancer cannot be present in the same organ, but after the influences of Votta J Paul work and through his own further experience, Rokitansky later changed his previous generally accepted view, and admitted that tuberculosis and carcinoma can coexist, but that this coexistence is rather rare. The Romanian report on this pathological association is done for its rarity in Europe, and to the best of authors' knowledge, in the last 45–50 years, two similar cases in Romania (Iaşi) by Luchian et al. [37] and one case in Poland [38] are described. The question is whether tuberculosis is before cancer, or the presence of the viral infection made possible the secondary location of the *MbT*. The pathological exams of the reported case did not revealed extensive granulomatous reaction, or cancer metastases in the endometrium, tubes, ovaries and lymph nodes. Since many years from the first description of the association of these two life-threatening pathologies, host response as the basic mechanism of specific defense against infection and tumor factors that enable such a response are also discussed since long time [39], being not completely known/understood, they may benefit from the host's previously compromised immunity: *MbT* and HPV can potentate each other.

The *MbT* is a facultative intracellular parasite that grows well in non-activated macrophages. When large numbers of these bacilli have grown intracellularly within such macrophages, a cytotoxic immune response, herein called tissue-damaging delayed-type hypersensitivity kills the macrophages, forming the caseous center of the tubercle, where the tubercle is surviving; such a delayed-type hypersensitivity was first described for the pulmonary tuberculosis [40], and this patient have suffered from pulmonary tuberculosis 7 years earlier. The progression of cervical dysplasias to invasive, lethal cervical cancers has been attributed to diverse factors such as immune, hormonal, and nutritional status, or co-infection with other sexually transmitted agents, supporting data being equivocal [41].

The contemporary professional societies are sure on primary immune defense system deficiency or incapacities to some infections, bacterial and viral, which were demonstrated in the systemic circulation and in some bodies locations – in the cervix uteri or in the breast. In North America [42], Western Europe [43, 44] and recently in China [45], it was proved the shifted balance between T helper 1 (Th1)-type and Th2-type cytokines in cervical dysplasia [42, 46], the involvement and increase of invariant natural killer T (iNKT) cells (which are in small number in condyloma acuminatum, in mild and moderate dysplasias [47]), and the cytokines production from cervical keratinotytes [48] the main targets of HPV infection as the stratified epithelium cells, and the main source of cytokines [49], as type I interferon (IFN)-γ, tumoral necrosis factor (TNF)-α, transforming growth factor (TGF)-α, interleukin-1 (Il-1), interleukin-6 (Il-6), interleukin −8 (Il-8) expressions are involved in immune system modulation (all of them being parts of innate immune system), in the evolution from persistent high-risk HPV-infected cells to the development of high-grade cervical intraepithelial neoplasia and cervical cancer, because the keratinocytes cannot destroy the fact high-risk HPV, and that may work also on *MbT* infection evolution, and complications. Parallel to these conditions, it is the individual cellular system of defense [50], involved in early phases of infection [51, 52]. Flow cytometry is revealing an increased level of CD3+ T, CD + 4 cells [53, 54] among both epithelium and stromal layers of the cervical tissues, contributing to the suppression of local immunity. In conjunction to these details is the presence of the population of monocytes/macrophages in the endocervix, with increasing number in cervical high-grade lesions with the parallel decrease in Langerhans cells, in contrary to what occurs in non-infected tissues [55]. All these facts contribute to the escape of HPV to tissue innate and acquired immune system, which is also influenced by the viral epitopes E6 and E7 [56], and evolution from less invasive to more advanced invasive cervical HPV-induced carcinoma is associated to a higher number of T and B lymphocytes, macrophages and induced nitric oxide synthase-expressing cells in the peritumoral stroma, so cell migration being proportional to the progression of the lesion [54]. Some studies show that these high number of inflammatory cells and compounds may open the way to bacterial infections, being additional mediators [57].

Insertional mutagenesis by HPV is another proposed tumor-promoting mechanism, but recent studies have not supported this hypothesis [58]. No common, recurring genetic alterations that cooperate with HPV to promote cervical cancer progression have been identified since Harald Zur Hausen first identified HPV as the causal transmissible agent of cervical cancer nearly 40 years ago [59]. To the pressing question to the biological basis of cervical cancer progression which is to be resolved since long time, the discover of the loss of a major tumor supressor *LkB1* [60, 61] or somatically acquired mutations in this tumor supressor *LKB1* [62], which is considered to be similar to p53. When *LKB1* deficiency/mutations, a primary cervical tumor confined to the cervix at the time of diagnosis has a bad prognosis: early metastasis and patient death, after the initial diagnosis despite aggressive therapy including radiation treatment. These abnormalities were first discovered in connection to Peutz-Jeghers Syndrome [63] and pulmonary cancer [64]. The *MbT* was proved to reduce host's immunity to high-risk HPV types for cervical cancer. The Chinese study "Shanxi Province Cervical Cancer Screening Study I" [36] showed an increasing magnitude of effect of *MbT* with increasing severity of disease in an isolated women population from rural China, as is demonstrated by the increasing odds ratios from 1.68 for HPV positivity to 1.75 for persistent HPV and then 2.08 for CIN3+. Associated to these findings, it was showed that TB and cervical inflammation were diagnosed in 1% of the women, and associated with 90% higher odds of oncogenic HPV infection and 113% higher odds of persistent HPV infection. The authors of the "Shanxi Province Cervical Cancer Screening Study I" are considering that their results are consistent with the novel hypothesis that TB may provide an immunological profile that is associated with an increased susceptibility to HPV infection. In conjunction to this hypothesis, we can speculate like that *MbT* is associated to the loss/mutations in *LKB1* tumor suppressor, because persistence of small islands of squamous non-keratinizing cancer cells after radiation and chemotherapies.

5. Diagnosis

Regarding the diagnosis, one must consider the clinical presentation, physical examination, laboratory results, specially the microbiological ones and imagistic tools, and after the difficulties of the Romanian first published case of breast tubercular abscess on must reconsider an old concept of diagnosis—the "therapeutic" test.

5.1. Clinical presentation: physical examinations

5.1.1. Clinical presentation of breast TB

Clinical presentation of breast TB is variable regarding symptoms/signs: swelling of the breast 48.1% [65]; painless hard lump in approximately 60% cases [66], or pain is revealed as the first complain of some patients [67, 68] or up to 18.5% of cases [65]; rarely are recorded multiple lumps, the lump being with irregular borders, sometimes with skin fixation or to the underlying muscle or even chest wall, clinical findings imposing differential to breast carcinoma [69], situation which is much more suggested by the presence of an isolated breast mass, sometimes skin fixated "peau d'orange" sign, and without an associated sinus tract; abscess, unique or multiples; skin thickening; and skin sinus/fistula/multiple discharge sinuses [70], nipple retraction or inversion, nipple hyperpigmentation or focal discoloration –when the disease is long time duration [69], breast shape and sizes change, axillary lymphadenopathy (axillary lymph nodes are found in one-third of cases with breast TB [33]. Constitutional symptoms as fever, weight loss, night sweats or a failing of general health are infrequently encountered [71, 72].

5.1.2. Clinical diagnosis of cervix uteri tuberculosis

Irregular vaginal and postcoital bleeding with different aspects could occur at the cervix speculum examination such as exophytic-cauliflower aspect, tumoral-granulomatous, ulcerative and polypoid endocervical [73]. In many countries, even where tuberculosis is endemic, the majority of cases remain asymptomatic, but infected, and are discovered incidentally or remain undiscovered [22, 74]. Cervical examination of cases with cervical tuberculosis is normal in 90% cases, and the rest presents non-specific macroscopic changes, ulcerative/hypertrophic nodular lesions like proliferative cauliflower growth or fistulas/sinuses, or friable papillary growth covering almost the entire ectocervix. All these aspects may simulate invasive cervical cancer, or a miliary appearance [75–77]. There are reported cases with entire genital tract involvement, with myometrial alterations [78, 79], and association with tuberculosis of vulva and vagina [80].

5.2. Laboratory assessment

Current hematological and biochemical analysis are minimally influenced in cases with these *MbT* locations. It is cited a high level of white blood cells, and of ESV [77].

5.2.1. Bacteriological diagnosis

The golden standard for TB diagnosis is to detect acid-fast bacilli (AFB) in the infected tissue, but it is well known how difficult is the Ziehl-Neelsen stain or the cultures for BK to become positive [67, 72, 81], because the necessity of a high number *MbT* in the smear (more than 10,000 bacilli/mL), and the slow growth of all mycobacterial species, including *MbT,* fact that partially explains the delay of TB diagnosis. It was recommended scanning with high-power oil immersion because these diagnosis difficulties, but the practice proved that scanning with a X 40 objective should suffice in most cases. There were proposed alternative stains to the conventional Ziehl-Neelsen stain, such as auramine/auramine-rhodamine using fluorescence technique [82], which in association to a higher power examination (x 600) may have better detection for *MbT* [83].

It is known that biopsy specimens that are cultured on Löwenstein-Jensen medium at room temperature yield pigmented mycobacterial colonies in 2–4 weeks. In the literature of bacteriology, it is very important the place for sampling, and leveling that may affect the sensitivity of a stain in the detection of rare organisms as *Mycobacterium spp.* or fungi. On the other side, for a better discovery for *MbT,* it is recommended to examine at least two blocks of biopsy instead of one [84]. In India, it is reported that are possible positive cultures of nipple discharge for *Staphylococcus aureus* associated with positivity for *MbT* [85].

Actually many infections are detected by immunological assays proving the host competence, but for TB this aim is still a future desire; a very recently study of North American Universities' Microbiology and Pathology Laboratories [86] have confirmed the limitations of serodiagnosis for active tuberculosis, including poor sensitivity and increased reactivity with *non-tuberculous mycobacterium*-positive patients.

5.2.1.1. *Bacteriological diagnosis of breast tuberculosis*

The molecular diagnosis from clinical specimens is the aim of modern diagnosis of *MbT,* since many years, and this may be accomplished by nuclear acid amplification (NAA). The used methods allow the detection of mycobacterial DNA or RNA directly from the specimens, before the culture results are available [87]. Food and Drug Administration had accepted since the year 2000, two types of NAA, which were initially used for pulmonary tuberculosis, and later in extrapulmonary cases. The NAA is usually recommended when the smear evaluation is negative for AFB, and when clinical suspicion is very high, or when TB is endemic, but there are controversies on the specificity, sensitivity of the methods regarding the origin of specimen from respiratory tract or other sites [88]. The recommended tests are the enhanced *MbT* Direct Test (E-MTD; Gen-Probe, San Diego, CA) and Amplicor *MbT* Test (Amplicor; Roche Diagnostic Systems, Inc., Branchburg, NJ), and associated to these tests there were many studies about each value, specially for differential to granulomatous mastitis [12, 83, 89] or for the value of polymerase chain reaction (PCR) for real time *MbT* to compare to formalin-fixed, paraffin-embedded histologic specimens [90].

The real-time PCR for *MbT* on paraffin-embedded tissue is available with a high specificity of 99%, but low sensitivity of 65% for breast tissue in contrast to other types of specimens such as cerebral spinal fluid, urine and bronchoalveolar lavage, where sensitivity of more than 90% is reported, with comparable specificity [91, 92].

In the Romanian case, the molecular test—PCR for *MbT* on paraffin-embedded breast tissue was negative, and there are some researches [83, 93, 94] sustaining that molecular tests are not always relevant for the diagnosis of TB in smear-negative specimens. It is appreciated that real-time PCR for *MbT* is useful if positive, and confirms the presence of *MbT,* but if negative does not rule out the possibility of an infection [83]. Breast TB is paucibacillary and consequently tests such as microscopy, culture and NAA tests such as PCR techniques do not have the same diagnostic utility as they do in pulmonary tuberculosis [95]. There are some explanations for the negativity of the described tests for BK identification. One old explanation [84] is that the microorganisms have been killed and/or removed by the inflammatory process. Other explanation for PCR negativity is the existence of *non-tuberculous* infections such as *Corynebacterium* spp. [96], or *non-tuberculous mycobacterium,* which are now more common than tuberculosis in Western countries, and therefore would not be detected by this assay.

5.2.1.2. *Bacteriological diagnosis in cervical tuberculosis*

The demonstration of the presence of *MbT* in the cervix uteri with the Ziehl-Neelsen staining was proved to be difficult in many reported cases all over the world, even in India and China

[97]. In the Romanian case, *MbT* presence in the endocervix was confirmed by PCR for *MbT* performed on archived tissue (formalin-fixed paraffin-embedded uterine tissue).

5.3. Cytological diagnosis

5.3.1. Cytological diagnosis of breast tuberculosis

Actually fine needle aspiration cytology (FNAC) is considered a minimally invasive diagnosis method for breast pathology [98], including TB, because is revealing chronic granulomatous inflammation with caseating necrosis, presence of Langhans giant cell, and lymphocytic aggregates [99–101], but some studies are showing that in one quarter of cases FNAC is negative for breast tuberculosis diagnosis [71], because tissue samples collected at FNAC are not usually adequate for evaluation, or because caseating necrosis can be absent on the specimen. The absence of necrosis on breast specimen from FNAC does not exclude tuberculosis, which is sustained by other histological abnormalities [102]. In these situations, the next step for the diagnosis of mammary TB is the pathologic evaluation of specimens collected at open surgical biopsy [71], as it was done in the Romanian case, after the evaluation of the smear from fistula discharge.

5.3.2. Cytological diagnosis of cervix uteri tuberculosis

The Pap smear, a non-invasive procedure, may help in the diagnosis by the discover of epithelioid and multinucleated histiocytic cells, described since many years ago and rediscuss actually [103–105], fact that prompts further investigation. The epithelioid cells are elongated cells with pale eosinophilic cytoplasm, indistinct cell borders having large oval/elongated nuclei with a delicate chromatin pattern in singles/clusters. Multinucleated histiocytic cells, typical of Langhan's cells type, have large number of delicate, often ovoid nuclei, some overlapping, arranged peripherally and often in horseshoe fashion. The presence of those multinucleated histiocytic giant cells may help to differentials to herpes virus infection—the cells have epithelial origin, but lower number of nuclei, and show characteristic crowding/molding without overlapping with eosinophilic inclusion in nuclei and cytoplasm, and also in post radiotherapy of postmenopausal women smears, where the cells have bad outline, and may contain some phagocytosed debris with radiation-induced changes [104]. In countries with endemic tuberculosis, it is appreciated that the Papanicolaou smear is helping very much the staff, the Ziehl-Neelsen stain of cervical smear, and fluorescent technique and culture are confirming later [105]. The Romanian woman was not postmenopausal, a viral infection with high-risk HPV was clearly demonstrated, by genotyping of the cervix after surgery, but these type of cells were absent in the smear.

5.4. Pathological diagnosis of *MbT* infection

5.4.1. Pathological diagnosis in breast MbT *infection*

There are known two pathological classifications of breast tuberculosis: an old one—McKeown and Wilkinson [106] cited by Bahoroon [107], and a recent one—Tewari and Shukla [7].

McKeown and Wilkinson [106] had classified breast tuberculosis into five pathological varieties: (1) nodular—the most common variety presenting as a localized mass, with extensive caseation, and little fibrosis; (2) diffuse or disseminated—second most common variety, involving the entire breast with multiple intercommunicating foci of tubercles within the breast, which caseate leading to ulceration and discharging sinuses; (3) sclerosing—extensive fibrosis rather than caseation is present, suppuration is rare, the entire breast is hard, the nipple is retracted/inverted, category which is often mistaken for breast carcinoma; (4) tuberculous mastitis obliterans, characterized by duct infection producing proliferation of the lining epithelium, and marked epithelial and periductal fibrosis; and occlusion of the ducts, with appearance of cystic spaces, and all these resemble "cystic mastitis" and (5) acute miliary tuberculous mastitis, which occurs as a part of generalized miliary tuberculosis. The last two entities have only historical importance, being rarely described in the recent medical literature.

The Indian pathologists [108] have introduced a new pathological classification of breast tuberculosis, with three categories: (1) nodulo-caseous tubercular mastitis; (2) disseminated/confluent tubercular mastitis and (3) tubercular breast abscess.

There are some controversial discussions about the "granulomatous mastitis", diagnosed during childbearing period, usually in parous women, in early 1930s, which are frequently misdiagnosed as tuberculosis or carcinoma [108], with negative culture for *MbT*, and with cytological and immunocytochemical findings definitely for differential diagnosis from breast tuberculosis at fine needle aspiration cytology [109] or at open surgery. The pathological changes induced by *MbT* in breast make the differences to other breast pathology, "idiopathic granulomatous mastitis", which is also a "masquerader" [25, 28]. Tuberculous mastitis is often considered a form of "granulomatous mastitis" secondary to breast *MbT* infection, and some authors reserve the term of "granulomatous mastitis" to "idiopathic granulomatous mastitis", a chronic breast inflammatory entity [110]. Granuloma is a defense mechanism against antigens, which stay in many organs without inactivation. The granulomatous lesions are classified into infectious, vasculitis, immunological, chemicals and neoplasia [35], or the recent classification is more simple: infectious and non-infectious granulomas, with the prove from new studies that pathogenic microorganism are suspected to be a cause of granuloma in non-inflammatory diseases [111].

The etiology of "granulomatous mastitis" is unclear, being postulated, and sometimes proved, the autoimmune factors [112], sarcoidosis, fat necrosis, undetected organisms (as blastomycosis, actinomycosis, cryptococcosis, histoplasmosis, filarial infection and corynebacterium), Wegener's granulomatosis, reaction to childbirth, and use of oral contraceptives, ductular ectasis [113] the last two factors are present in the reported case. "Granulomatous mastitis" was the first diagnosis in authors' mind at the beginning of investigations, and this is partially an explanation of the delay in diagnosis, and late specific antitubercular treatment, as in other cases from literature in the last years [12]. These breast pathologies – tuberculosis and "idiopathic" granulomatous mastitis are considered "masquerader" [28] or "imitator" [89].

There are described some pathological characteristics [107, 114, 115], which make the differentiation between the "idiopathic "granulomatous mastitis"—first described by Kessler and Wolloc [113], and breast TB. TB is affecting all breast structures (lobules, ducts, fat; some pathologists consider that ducts are specially affected), and the tubercular granulomas are associated to caseating necrosis which makes the name of "caseating granulomas", and the difference from "idiopathic "granulomatous mastitis [107, 116], which was named "lobular non caseous granuloma" (**Table 2**). The isolation of *MbT* in the central necrosis increases the sensitivity of the diagnosis.

There are mentioned some other types of "necrositing granulomas" in which infections-inflammation are frequently associated, and are proved with special stains (as Ziehl-Neelsen or Grocott Methamine Silver), and/or by cultures, and other granulomas with infection-inflammatory aspect, but without associated infections as eosinophylic necrosis or basophilic necrosis [83], as is Wegener's granulomatosis, and less commonly rheumatoid nodule, necrotizing sarcoid granulomatosis, infarct and lymphomatoid granulomatosis [83]. The granulomas with eosinophilic necrosis have regular rounded contour, the rim being formed of epithelioid histiocytes with multinucleated giant cells, and the center may have coagulative type of necrosis, which is like an infarct. The Wegener's granulomatosis is characterized by 'dirty' basophilic necrosis with irregular geographic necrosis; the necrosis is rimmed by palisading histiocytes and scattered multinucleated giant cells, with hyperchromatic nuclei and peripheral to the necrosis is the necrotizing vasculitis in vessels. The vessels display transmural fibrinoid necrosis, and the necrosis of the media with admixed necrotic neutrophils, which contributes to the diagnosis with true necrotizing vasculitis. The granuloma of the Romanian case has multiple normal vessels. The parenchymal necrosis of the necrotizing

Characteristic	"Idiopathic" granulomatous mastitis	Tubercular mastitis
Macroscopic characteristic		
Isolated or multiple breast masses	Common	Common
Multiple sinuses or fistulas	Absent	Present
Abscess	Common	Uncommon
Focal discoloration of areola	Absent	Present
Microscopic characteristic		
Structure affected	Mammary lobules from one breast, rarely bilateral	All mammary structures: ducts, lobules, fat, commonly bilateral
Type of lesion	Granulomas of the lobules	Granulomas of all mammary structures
Histological components of breast's granulomas	Epithelioid histiocytes, Langhans giant cells, lymphocytes, plasma cells, and occasionally eosinophils	Epithelioid histiocytes, Langhans giant cells, lymphocytes, rare plasma cells, and eosinophils
Foamy cells	Absent	Present
Caseating necrosis	Absent	Present
Fibrosis	Present	Present
Fat necrosis	Present	Present

Table 2. Macroscopic and microscopic characteristics of "idiopathic" granulomatous mastitis and tubercular mastitis (modified from Akcan et al. [114]; Baslaim et al. [115]; Bahoroon [107]; Lacambra et al. [109]).

sarcoid granulomatosis is variable, usually eosinophilic but can be irregular and basophilic, mimicking Wegener's granulomatosis.

The pathological characteristics of the "idiopathic" lobular non-caseating granulomas and of tuberculosis caseating granuloma of the breast are listed in **Table 2**, and it is considered [83] that no single histological feature may distinguish infectious necrotizing granulomas from other specific disorder as Wegener's granulomatosis or sarcoidosis, being necessary a combination of multiple pathological features to establish the specific diagnosis.

The first reported case of this chapter is a primary breast TB, with no personal history, or other focus on the systemic physical/radiological examinations for TB. The diagnosis of breast TB must follow the general principles: clinical and laboratory. The clinical presentation of breast TB is variable regarding symptoms/signs: swelling of the breast—48.1% [10]; painless hard lump—approximately 60% cases, or pain is revealed as the first complain of some patients [67, 68] or up to 18.5% of cases [10]; rarely are recorded multiple lumps, with irregular borders, sometimes with skin fixation or areola fixation, or to the underlying muscle or even chest wall, clinical findings imposing differential to breast carcinoma [69], situation which is much more suggested by the presence of an isolated breast mass, sometimes skin fixated-"peau d'orange" sign, and without an associated sinus tract; ulceration of areola [117], or of the skin covering the mammary gland [118]; abscess, unique or multiples [85]; skin thickening and skin sinus/fistula/multiple discharge sinuses [70], nipple retraction or inversion, nipple hyperpigmentation or focal discoloration—when the disease is long time duration [69], or distruction of nipple-areola region [19], breast shape and sizes are changed, axillary lymphadenopathy (axillary lymph nodes are found in one-third of cases with breast TB). Constitutional symptoms as fever, weight loss, night sweats or a failing of general health are infrequently encountered [71, 72].

5.4.2. Pathological diagnosis of cervical tuberculosis

The cervical tuberculosis diagnosis is commonly established by the Papanicolaou smear without any dysplasia, positivity for acid-fast bacilli, and the cervical biopsy (punch, loop excision biopsy) showing granulomatous inflammation with caseous necrosis, facts that were absent in the Romanian case. The presence of the viral infection is clearly proved by genotyping of the cervix after surgery. The endocervical curettage which has the possibility to diagnose associated endocervical tuberculosis was not done, because they believe that exocervical lesion was the only cause of abnormal bleeding. The pulmonary tuberculosis was 7 years previously registered, and the genital location was diagnosed in the endocervical glands, on the specimen collected at hysterectomy—after radiotherapy and chemotherapy. The presence of the endocervical tubercle bacillus was indirectly diagnosed by the pathologic examination the presence of caseous necrosis and Langhans multinuclear giant cells, and by PCR for *MbT*. The diagnosis of TB depends also upon the isolation of the *MbT* on microscopy, and culture, and by the PCR. Culture of *MbT* and acid-fast staining was not done, the cervical granulomas were noted at pathological examination after surgery, on a formalin-fixed specimen. The presence of characteristic, typical caseous granuloma was appreciated sufficient to make the diagnosis [77, 119], but many researchers consider that it is very important to distinguish between the granulomatous reaction and tuberculosis by more specific methods [120]. The presence of stroma caseous necrosis was sufficient for the positive diagnosis of cervical TB in the Romanian authors' opinion. The granuloma diagnosis is a microscopic diagnosis. The microscopy of the cervical specimen after radical hysterectomy reveals an aggregate of immune cells, appearing as epithelioid macrophages, and if a foreign body or a parasite is not observed inside the granuloma, stains for acid-fast bacilli, and fungi are ordered as mycobacteria and fungi (such as *Cryptococcus, Blastomyces, Coccidioides* and *Aspergillus* can be seen on hematoxyline-eosine, preferentially in the area of necrosis rather than the surrounding viable area) are frequently the cause of this type of inflammation [31]. In cases with samples fixed in formalin the detection of the infectious agent is recommended to be done by molecular analysis, PCR for *MbT* in the Romanian case [91, 118].

5.5. Imaging diagnosis of rare tuberculosis locations

5.5.1. Radiological imaging of breast tuberculosis

Radiological imaging of breast tuberculosis is appreciated not to be diagnostic, and the described mammographic images are in connection to three patterns of breast tuberculosis: nodular, disseminated and sclerosing patterns [121]. Some radiological characteristics are common for all patterns, like the change in shape, and outline of the breast mass—seen in the standard views, the reduction in size of the affected breast, skin thickening, nipple retraction and ill-defined breast mass [122]. In previous radiological studies, the skin bulge and sinus tract sign, which connects the breast density to a localized skin thickening or to the skin bulge are the radiological features strongly suggestive for tubercular breast abscess [66].

In the Romanian case, the mammography was not recommended, because authors thinking was dominated by a chronic inflammation with repeated episodes of recurrence, as a granulomatous mastitis or a plasma cell mastitis.

Some clinicians [123] recommend computed tomography scan, when are doubtful cases, for the differentiation of primary and secondary lesions, to evaluate accompanying pulmonary disease, if it is present or to detect the continuity of the breast lesions with the thoracic wall or pleura, and associated lesions of the lungs.

5.5.2. Ultrasonography for breast tuberculosis

In the literature, there are controversies about the value of ultrasonography for breast TB diagnosis. On one side, it is mentioned no specificity of the ultrasound examination [121]: the breasts' lesions may appear as heterogeneous, hypoechoic, irregularly or ill-bordered masses of different sizes, but usually small sizes, with internal echoes or thick-walled cystic lesions, some mass may present posterior acoustic enhancement, in association to the fistula formation, and the thickening of Cooper's ligaments and subcutaneous tissues, as it was revealed in the Romanian case. On the other side, it is mentioned an unique finding strongly suggestive for breast TB: the presence of a dense sinus tract connecting an ill-defined breast mass to localized skin thickening and bulge [14].

Regarding the vascularisation of the breast tubercular masses, the blood flow was not observed within the lesions, while increased circumferential vascularization was seen in the color Doppler ultrasound, and the spectral evaluation shows a low resistance monophasic flow pattern [121].

5.5.3. Magnetic resonance imaging (MRI) for breast/cervix uteri tuberculosis diagnosis

If on recommend MRI imaging for breast TB, it is possible to detect parenchymal asymmetry with enhancement, micro-abscesses, and peripherally enhanced masses. MRI may reveal lymphadenopathy along the pelvic walls, with an abnormal signal to the entire body of the uterus and sometimes when the entire uterus is infected by *MbT,* the endometrial cavity, myometrium, and junctional zone could not be differentiated and thus the radiological appearance was consistent with Asherman's syndrome [77].

5.6. Antitubercular therapeutic test for rare location tuberculosis diagnosis

There are cases with pulmonary and extrapulmonary TB with negative molecular test—PCR for *MbT* from clinical specimens or it is not possible to recommend and use the rapid very efficient modern molecular NAA for detection of mycobacterial DNA or RNA directly from the specimens as it was previously discussed. In countries with endemic TB, it is since long time discussed and recently it is recalled an empirical antitubercular therapy even in the absence of positive acid-fast bacilli, and without culture—positive results, or when it is the suspicion of TB or when the "idiopathic" granulomatous mastitis is found and it is not responding to metothrexate or corticosteroids [108, 117].

TB is considered to be actually under-diagnosed in Romania, and the Romanian health history had a similar management in cases which are mentioned before, and in these conditions, the final diagnosis of the case with primary recurrent non-gestational breast abscess was done after the antitibercular" therapeutic" test, which was efficient after the first two months. More details are in the subsection 8 on "Treatment".

6. Differential diagnosis

6.1. Differentials for breast tuberculosis

The breast tuberculosis can be confused with breast carcinoma, specially in elder women [27, 28, 69, 124], who present an isolated ill defined, irregular, occasionally hard breast lump without sinuses/fistula, but pain is present more frequently in the tuberculous lump than in carcinoma. Involvement of the nipple and areola is rare in tuberculosis, but fixation of the lump to the skin may be present as a part of the inflammatory process, which is present in both pathological entities A high index of suspicion needs to be maintained if a breast lump is associated with a sinus or indolent lump in an immigrant women if this is encountered in the western countries. The coexistence of tubercular axillary lymphadenitis with breast carcinoma can falsely over-stage the disease [125], and is reported an association of the metastasis of breast carcinoma and axillary tuberculous lymphadenitis [126]. In postmenopausal women is considered that the diagnosis of breast TB does not exclude a concomitent cancer [3], situation that was first reported by Pilliet and Piatot in (cited by [27]).

In cases with discharging sinuses associated to a breast lump it is necessary to make the differentiation from actinomycosis by the absence of sulfur granules in the discharge and by fungal culture [9].

For women from countries with endemic tuberculosis from Asia and Africa, or immigrated from that countries, the association of breast carcinoma and tuberculosis must be thought, specially when the data are confusing [3, 127, 128], as it is when on records tuberculosis of axillary lymph nodes with primary breast cancer [129], or axillary lymph nodes with granulomas and a breast carcinoma [72, 130].

Beside carcinoma there are other misdiagnosis risks as "idiopathic" granulomatous mastitis (**Table 2**, for pathological differential), or plasma cell mastitis (which may mimic histological the tuberculosis by the presence of foreign body giant cells, epithelioid cells which are arranged in tubercles, besides plasma cells, polymorphs, lymphocytes and few foamy macrophages, but is missing the caseation which makes the differential from tuberculosis- [131], lupus mastitis [132], eritema nodosus [133].

In the last years there are described recurrent breast abscess to be more frequent due to non-tuberculous mycobacterial infection [20, 134], cases with similar clinical presentation, with granulomas.

6.2. Differentials for cervix uteri tuberculosis

When women's complaints are present, and cervical examination shows cervical changes it is considered to think about both pathologies, separately or associated in countries with high risks for these pathologies. There are discussed other viral cervical infections as HIV, herpes virus simplex, other sexual transmitted (Treponema pallidum, Trichomonas vaginalis, Neisseria gonorrhea) or parasitic diseases as schistosomal, amoebic, brucella, tularaemia which may induce chronic cervical granulomas, sarcoidosis, and foreign body reaction [77], or more rare an epithelioid granulomas in Hodgkin's disease [39].

7. Complications of breast/cervix uteri tuberculosis

When not adequate treated, TB mastitis is followed by abscesses, which can penetrate the retromammary space [135], or to the ribs [136], formation of sinuses, and nipple retraction, and irreversible inversion, recurrences even with surgical drainage/excision, and breast mutilation [26].

In the case with the association of two severe immunosuppressive diseases as tuberculosis and cancer there are risks for reactivating the lung tuberculosis, for lung metastases from cervical cancer, and of high mortality in patients with coexistent disease [137, 138].

8. Treatment of breast/cervix uteri tuberculosis

Treatment may cure the disease with antitubercular drugs, and surgery is rarely required, being used in cases resistant to medical treatment. The specific antitubercular treatment was delayed in the Romanian case with breast abscess as is frequently mentioned in literature [24], because the difficulties of the positive and differential diagnosis, and because tuberculosis is under-diagnosis in contemporary Romania, but the attitude regarding tuberculosis was similar in the Romanian health history to that from tuberculosis endemic countries: to recommend empirical antitubercular therapy even in the absence of positive AFB, and without positive culture results, when it is a suspicion of TB or when the granuloma is found. In many cases, the decision for the antitubercular treatment is taken after the failure of corticoids and methotrexate therapy for "idiopathic" granulomatous mastitis [108, 117, 139].

Based on patient profile, clinical features and lack of response to usual antibiotic therapy, it is recommended a four-drug (isoniazid, rifampin, ethambutol and pyrazinamide) 6-month course of Directly Observed Therapy Short-Term (DOTS) - Category I [117], but the response to treatment is variable and not dramatic. There are reported excellent results with such management [101].

There are no specific available guidelines for chemotherapy of breast TB, and the therapy generally follows guidelines that are used for pulmonary TB. The regimen consists of a 2 month intensive phase (isoniazid, rifampicin, pyrazinamide and ethambutol), followed by a 4 month continuation phase (isoniazid and rifampin). It is recommended another regimen with extension of continuation therapy for a longer period to 7 months [9, 140–142] or more up to 12–18 months [140], because the wish to lower the relapse rate. There is also a regimen which combines first and second lines antitubercular drugs, including kanamycin, ofloxacin, ethionamide, para-amino salicylic acid (PAS), pyrazinamide and isoniazid, with the reason of the risk of multidrug resistant strains [143]. The breast lesions and tenderness are steadily improved after 2 months of intensive therapy the breast lesions and tenderness are steadily improved [83] (**Table 3**).

Treatment duration	Initial phase treatment (intensive therapy)	Continuation treatment
6 months*	2 months of: 300 mg isoniazid, 600 mg rifampin, 1500 mg pyrazinamide, 1000 mg ethambutol or streptomycin 1 g per day	4 months of isoniazid, rifampin
9 months**	2 months of: 300 mg isoniazid, 600 mg rifampin, 1500 mg pyrazinamide, 1000 mg ethambutol per day	7 months of isoniazid, rifampin

*Al-Marri et al. [122]; Jalali et al. [102]; Mirsaeidi et al. [6], Bahoroon [107]; Gon et al. [28]; Singal, et al. [13].
**Daali et al. [141]; Khanna et al. [9]; Kumar et al. [143].

Table 3. Breast antitubercular regimens.

In the Romanian primary recurrent non-gestational breast abscess was recalled as the old concept of the "antitubercular therapeutic" test, for the final diagnosis and it was proved to be efficient after the first 2 months, and the association of isoniazid and rifampin was continued with excellent results up to 9 months.

Surgery was imposed in the Romanian case because of abscess complications in the conditions of *MbT* late diagnosis. It was a minimal surgical intervention required for drainage and excision biopsy of abscesses' wall. Surgery is commonly reserved for selected cases, in particular situations, and in different manner:

- According to the presence of breast masses/lump and abscesses with fistula: simple or segmental mastectomy or quadrantectomy or drainage of abscess with large excision of the necrotic tissue of the breast and excision of the axillary lymph nodes when involved [25].
- Breast abscesses with negative bacteriological tests in order to diagnose by excision biopsy of the abscess wall and drainage of abscess with fistula [16, 21, 67].
- In cases refractory to medication [69].
- Residual lumps after antitubercular therapy, excision of sinus [9, 10].
- Mastectomy when is severe breast destruction [14].

A special mention is for the percutaneous treatment with drainage controlled by CT and specific antibiotic antitubercular drugs [123], especially when resistance to ATT is discovered [144], as it is done for pulmonary TB and for abdominal collections [145].

The ATT are usually recommended for cervix uteri tuberculosis for minimum 6 months [146], healing being proved by repeated biopsy. The chemo and radiotherapy, and the radical surgical intervention done in the Romanian case were imposed by the initial diagnosis of squamous non-keratinized cervical carcinoma stage IB, tubercular cervicitis being a postoperative surprise, and it was decided to avoid a new cure of AAT because the postoperative assessments for *MbT* lung or general reactivation were negative.

9. Conclusions

- Breast tuberculosis should be considered as a differential diagnosis of breast inflammatory disease or masses, all over the world, not only where tuberculosis is endemic.
- Tuberculosis must be suspected in recurrent breast inflammatory disease with negative current cultures, and negative tests as Ziehl-Neelsen stain, culture and PCR for *MbT*.
- The pathologic examination of the open biopsy in the reported case is suggesting the diagnosis of a granulomatous mastitis, and the multinuclear giant cells of Langhans type presence ensure the diagnosis of tubercular granulomatous mastitis even in the absence of the characteristic caseous necrosis.

- The final diagnosis of breast TB was established by specific antitubercular drugs, which represents a Tuberculosis Diagnosis Test, and may avoid or delay breast characteristic mutilations when treatment is not adequate.
- The cervix uteri tuberculosis presence and its association to ecto/endocervical cancer is to be suspected not only in developing countries with endemic tuberculosis and high rates of HPV/HIV infections, in patients with primary lung/other organs tuberculosis.

Author details

Manuela Cristina Russu[1*], Şerban Nastasia[2], Daniela Degeratu[3] and Ruxandra Viorica Stănculescu[4]

*Address all correspondence to: manuela_russu@yahoo.com

1 "Dr. I. Cantacuzino" Clinical Hospital, "Carol Davila" University of Medicine and Pharmacy, Bucharest, Romania

2 "Dr. I. Cantacuzino" Clinic of Obstetrics and Gynaecology, "Carol Davila" University of Medicine and Pharmacy, Bucharest, Romania

3 "Dr. I. Cantacuzino" Laboratory of Pathology, Bucharest, Romania

4 Department of Pathological Obstetrics, Emergency "St Pantelimon" Clinical Hospital, "Carol Davila" University of Medicine and Pharmacy, Bucharest, Romania

References

[1] World Health Organization. Global Tuberculosis Report 2017. Geneva, Switzerland: Licence CCBY-NC-SA0IGO. Available from: http://apps.who.int/iris

[2] Prezzemolo T, Guggino G, Pio La Manna M, Di Liberto D, Dieli F, Caccamo N. Functional signatures of human CD4 and CD8 T cell responses to *Mycobacterium tuberculosis*. Frontiers in Immunology. 2014;**5**:180

[3] Bouti K, Soualhi M, Marc K, Zahraoui R, Benamor J, Bourkadi E, Iraqi G. Postmenopausal breast tuberculosis – Report of 4 cases. Breast Care (Basel). 2012;**7**(5):411-413

[4] Micha JP, Brown JV 3rd, Birk C, Van Horn D, Retenmaier MA, Golstein BH. Tuberculosis mimicking cervical carcinoma-case report. European Journal of Obstetrics & Gynecology. 2007;**28**(4):316-318

[5] Agrawal S, Madan M, Leekha N, Raghunandan C. A rare case of cervical tuberculosis simulating carcinoma cervix. Cases Journal. 2009;**2**:161

[6] Mirsaeidi SM, Masjedi MR, Mansouri SD, Velayati AA. Tuberculosis of the breast: Report of 4 clinical cases and literature review. Eastern Mediterranean Health Journal. 2007;**13**(3):670-676

[7] Tewari M, Shukla HS. Breast tuberculosis: Diagnosis, clinical features, and management. The Indian Journal of Medical Research. 2005;**122**:103-110

[8] Al-Marri MR, Almosleh A, Almoslmani Y. Primary tuberculosis of the breast in Qatar: Ten year experience and review of the literature. The European Journal of Surgery. 2000; **166**:687-690

[9] Khanna R, Prasanna GV, Gupta P, Kumar M, Khanna S, Khanna AK. Mammary tuberculosis: Report on 52 cases. Postgraduate Medical Journal. 2002;**78**(921):422-424

[10] Tanrikulu AC, Abakay A, Abakay O, Kapan M. Breast tuberculosis in Southeast Turkey: Report of 27 cases. Breast Care (Basel). 2010;**5**(3):154-157

[11] Kant S, Dua R, Goel MM. Bilateral tubercular mastitis: A case report. Lung India. 2007; **24**:90-93

[12] Ruiz-Moreno JL, Peña-Santos G. Bilateral tuberculous mastitis nulliparous patient, initially treated as idiopathic granulomatous mastitis. Ginecología y Obstetricia de México. 2012;**80**(3):228-231

[13] Singal R, Bala J, Gupta S, Goyal S, Mahajan NC, Chawla A. Primary breast tuberculosis presenting as a lump: A rare modern disease. Annals of Medical and Health Sciences Research. 2013;**3**(1):110-112. DOI: 10.4103/2141-9248.109470

[14] Bani Hani KE, Yaghan RJ, Matalka IL, Mazahrich TS. Tuberculous mastitis: A disease not to be forgotten. The International Journal of Tuberculosis and Lung Disease. 2005; **9**(8):920-925

[15] Chellaoui M, Taleb A, Chat L, Achaabane E, Alami D, Najid A, Benamour-Ammar H. Tuberculosis of the breast: A case report. Journal de Radiologie. 2002;**83**(6 Pt 1):742-744

[16] Gupta R, Singal R, Gupta A, Singal S, Shahi S, Singal R. Primary tubercular abscess of the breast-an unusual entity. Journal of Medicine and Life. 2012;**5**:98-100

[17] Jaideep C, Kumar M, Khanna AK. Male breast tuberculosis. Postgraduate Medical Journal. 1997;**73**:428-429. DOI: 10.1136/pgmj.73.861.428

[18] Brown S, Thekkinkattil KD. Tuberculous cold abscess of breast: An unusual presentation in a male patient. Gland Surgery. 2016 Jun;**5**(3):361-365. DOI: 10.21037/gs.2016.01.02

[19] Rimmer J, Hamilton S, Gault D. Recurrent mycobacterial breast abscesses complicating reconstruction. British Journal of Plastic Surgery. 2004;**57**(7):676-678

[20] Atallah D, El Kassis N, Araj G, Nasr M, Nasnas R, Veziris N, Sarkis D. Mycobacterial infection of breast prosthesis–a conservative treatment: A case report. BMC Infectious Diseases. 2014;**14**:238

[21] Gupta PP, Gupta KB, Yadav RK, Agarwal D. Tuberculous mastitis. A review of seven consecutive cases. The Indian Journal of Tuberculosis. 2003;**50**:47-50

[22] Chowdhury NNR. Overview of tuberculosis of the female genital tract. Journal of the Indian Medical Association. 1996;**94**:345-361

[23] Carter JR. Unusual presentations of genital tract tuberculosis. International Journal of Gynaecology and Obstetrics. 1990;**33**:171-176

[24] Lin TL, Chi SY, Liu JW, Chou FF. Tuberculosis of the breast: 10 years' experience in one institution. The International Journal of Tuberculosis and Lung Disease. 2010;**14**(6): 758-763

[25] Daryanani A, Sundeep P, Rodrigues G, Kumar S, Kudva R. Tuberculosis mastitis masquerading as carcinoma breast. The internet. Journal of Tropical Medicine. 2002;**1**(2)

[26] Chowdri NA, Parray FQ, Dar RA, Malik AA, Mushtaque M, Malik RA. Tubercular mastitis – A rare presentation. International Journal of Surgery. 2010;**8**(5):398-400

[27] Morino GF, Rizzardi G, Gobbi F, Baldan M. Breast tuberculosis mimicking other diseases. Tropical Doctor. 2007;**37**(3):177-178

[28] Gon S, Bhattacharyya A, Majumdar B, Kundu S. Tubercular mastitis - a great masquerader. Turkish Journal of Pathology. 2013;**29**(1):61-63

[29] Kaewseekhao B, Naranbhai V, Rovtrakul S, Namwat W, Paemance A, Lulitanond V, Chaiprasert A, Faksri K. Comparative proteomics of activated THP-1 cells infected with *Mycobacterium tuberculosis* identifies putative clearance biomarkers for tuberculosis treatment. PLoS One. 2015;**10**(7):e0134168. Published online 2015 Jul 27. DOI: 10.1371/journal.pone.0134168

[30] Yanamandra U, Pathak N, Naithani N, Grover N, Nair V. Tuberculosis of breast: Unusual manifestation of tuberculosis. Journal of Infection and Chemotherapy. 2011; **18**(1):109-111. DOI: 10.1007/s10156-011-0296-0. Epub 2011 Aug 31

[31] Banerjee SN, Ananthakrishnan N, Mehta RB, et al. Tuberculous mastitis: A continuing problem. World Journal of Surgery. 1987;**11**:105-109. DOI: 10.1007/BF01658471

[32] Shinde SR, Chandawarkar RY, Deshmukh SP. Tuberculosis of the breast masquerading as carcinoma: A study of 100 patients. World Journal of Surgery. 1995;**19**:379-381. DOI: 10.1007/BF00299163

[33] Mehta G, Mittal A, Verma S. Breast tuberculosis-clinical spectrum and management. The Indian Journal of Surgery. 2010;**72**:433-437. DOI: 10.1007/s12262-010-0166-5

[34] James DG. A clinicopathological classification of granulomatous disorders. Postgraduate Medical Journal. 2000;**76**:457-465

[35] Zhao FH, Varanasi AP, Cunningham CA, Graubars DI, Hu SY, Chen F, Barrett CJ, Qiao YL, Forman MR. Tuberculosis and oncogenic HPV: Potential co-infections in women at high-risk of cervical cancer in rural China. Asian Pacific Journal of Cancer Prevention. 2011;**12**(6):1409-1415

[36] Richards MJ, Angus D. Possible sexual transmission of genitourinary tuberculosis. International Journal of Tuberculosis and Lung Disease (IJTLD). 1998;**2**:439

[37] Luchian N, Dobreanu N, Cordon Tărăbuţă G, Costăchescu G. Considerations on 2 cases of association between cancer and tuberculosis of the uterine cervix. Revista Medico-Chirurgicală a Societăţii de Medici şi Naturalişti din Iaşi. 1967;**71**:1025-1028

[38] Sabilinska B, Szufladowicz R. Tuberculosis of the cervix uteri after radiation therapy of uterine cervix cancer. Ginekologia Polska. 1971;**43**(1):85-87

[39] O'Connell MJ, Schimpff SC, Kirschner RH, Abt AB, Wiernik PH. Epithelioid granulomas in Hodgkin's disease. JAMA. 1975;**233**:886-889

[40] Dannenberg AM Jr. Roles of cytotoxic delayed-type hypersensitivity and macrophage-activating cell-mediated immunity in the pathogenesis of tuberculosis. Immunobiology. 1994;**191**(4-5):461-473

[41] Steben M, Duarte-Franco E. Human papillomavirus infection: Epidemiology and pathophysiology. Gynecologic Oncology. 2007;**107**:S2-S5

[42] Scott M, Nakagawa M, Moscicki A-B. Cell-mediated immune response to human papillomavirus infection. Clinical and Diagnostic Laboratory Immunology. 2001;**8**(2):209-220

[43] Stanley M. HPV-immune response to infection and vaccination. Infectious Agents and Cancer. 2010;**5**(1):19 http://www.infectagentscancer.com/content/5/1/19

[44] Bais AG, Beckmann I, Lindemans J, Ewing PC, Meijer CJLM, Snijders PJF, Helmerhorst TJM. A shift to a peripheral Th2-type cytokine pattern during the carcinogenesis of cervical cancer becomes manifest in CIN III lesions. Journal of Clinical Pathology. 2005;**58**:1096-1100

[45] Hu T, Yang P, Zhu H, Chen X, Xie X, Yang M, Liu S. Accumulation of invariant NKT cells with increased IFN-γ production in persistent high-risk HPV-infected high-grade cervical intraepithelial neoplasia. Diagnostic Pathology. 2015;**10**:20. DOI: 10.1186/s13000-015-0254-8

[46] Spellberg B, Edwards JE. Type1/type 2 immunity in infectious diseases. Clinical Infectious Diseases. 2001;**32**:76-102

[47] Satam MN, Suraiya JN, Nadkarni JJ. Natural killer and antibody-dependent cellular cytotoxicity in cervical carcinoma patient. Cancer Immunology, Immunotherapy. 1986; **23**:56-59

[48] Woodworth CD, Simpson S. Comparative lymphokine secretion by cultured normal human cervical keratinocytes, papillomavirus-immortalized, and carcinoma cell lines. The American Journal of Pathology. 1993;**142**:1544-1555

[49] Schröder JM. Cytokine networks in the skin. Journal of Investigative Dermatology. 1995; **105**:20S-24S

[50] Witkin SS, Giraldo P, Linhares I, Ledger WJ. Individual immunity and susceptibility to female genital tract infection. American Journal of Obstetrics and Gynecology. 2000;**183**: 252-256

[51] Banks L, Moreau F, Vousden K, et al. Expression of the human papillomavirus E7 oncogene during cell transformation is sufficient to induce susceptibility to lysis by activated macrophages. Journal of Immunology. 1991;**146**:2037-2042

[52] Barnard P, McMillan NA. The human papillomavirus E7 oncoprotein abrogates signaling mediated by interferon-alpha. Virology. 1999;**259**:305-313

[53] Hohn H, Pilch H, Gunzel S, Neukirch C, Hilmes C, Kaufmann A, Seliger B, Maeurer MJ. CD4+ tumor-infiltrating lymphocytes in cervical cancer recognize HLA-DR-restricted peptides provided by human papillomavirus-E7. Journal of Immunology. 1999;**163**:5715-5722

[54] Da Silva CS, Michelin MA, Etchehere RM, Adad SJ, Murta FC, et al. Local lymphocytes and nitric oxide synthase in the uterine cervical stroma of patients with grade III cervical intraepithelial neoplasia. Clinics (São Paulo, Brazil). 2010;**65**(6):575-581

[55] Parr MB, Parr EL. Mucosal immunity in the female and male reproductive tract. In: Ogra PL et al., editors. Handbook of Mucosal Immunology. San Diego: Academy Press; 1996. pp. 677-689

[56] Stanley M, Coleman N, Chamberst M. The Host Response to Lesions Induced by Human Papillomavirus. Vaccine against Virally Induced Cancers. Vol. 187. Wiley, Chichester: Ciba Foundation Symposium; 1994. pp. 21-44

[57] Ben-Baruch A. Inflammation-associated immune suppression in cancer: The roles played by cytokines, chemokines and additional mediators. Seminars in Cancer Biology. 2006;**16**:38-52

[58] Dall KL, Scarpini CG, Roberts I, Winder DM, Stanley MA, et al. Characterization of naturally occurring HPV16 integration sites isolated from cervical keratinocytes under noncompetitive conditions. Cancer Research. 2008;**68**:8249-8259

[59] Zur Hausen H. Condylomata acuminata and human genital cancer. Cancer Research. 1976;**36**:794

[60] Gurumurthy S, Hezel AF, Berger JH, Bosenberg MW, Bardeesy N. LKB1 deficiency sensitizes mice to carcinogen-induced tumorigenesis. Cancer Research. 2008;**68**:55-63

[61] Hezel AF, Bardeesy N. LKB1; linking cell structure and tumor suppression. Oncogene. 2008;**27**:6908-6919

[62] Wingo SN, Gallardo TD, Akbay EA, Liang M-C, Contreras CM, Castrillon D. Somatic LKB1 mutations P romote cervical cancer progression. PLoS One. 2009;**4**(4):e5137

[63] Esteller M, Avizienyte E, Corn PG, Lothe RA, Baylin SB, et al. Epigenetic inactivation of LKB1 in primary tumors associated with the Peutz-Jeghers syndrome. Oncogene. 2000; **19**:164-168

[64] Ji H, Ramsey MR, Hayes DN, Fan C, McNamara K, et al. LKB1 modulates lung cancer differentiation and metastasis. Nature. 2007;**448**:807-810

[65] Tanrikulu AC, Abakay A, Abakay O, Kapan M. Breast tuberculosis in Southeast Turkey: Report of 27 cases. Breast Care (Basel). 2010;**5**(3):154-157. Epub 2010 May 11

[66] Makanjuola D, Murshid K, Al Sulaimani S, Al Saleh M. Mammographic features of breast tuberculosis: The skin bulge and sinus tract sign. Clinical Radiology. 1996;**51**(5):354-358

[67] Harris SH, Khan MA, Khan R, Haque F, Sved A, Ansari MM. Mammary tuberculosis: Analysis of thirty-eight patients. ANZ Journal of Surgery. 2006;**76**(4):234-237. DOI: 10.1111/j.1445-2197.2006.03692

[68] Khodabakhshi B, Mehravar F. Breast tuberculosis in Northeast Iran: Review of 22 cases. BMC Womens Health. 2014;**14**:72

[69] Maroulis I, Spyropoulos C, Zolota V, Tzorakoleftherakic E. Mammary tuberculosis mimicking breast cancer: A case report. Journal of Medical Case Reports. 2008;**2**:34

[70] Singal R, Dalal AK, Dalal U, Attri AK. Primary tuberculosis of the breast presented as multiple discharge sinuses. The Indian Journal of Surgery. 2013;**75**:66-67

[71] Akçay MN, Saglam L, Polat P, Erdogan F, Albayrak Y, Povoski SP. Mammary tuberculosis – Importance of recognition and differentiation from that of a breast malignancy: Report of three cases and review of the literature. World J. Surgical Oncology. 2007;**5**:67

[72] Alzaara A, Dalal N. Co-existence of carcinoma in tuberculosis in one breast. World Journal of Surgical Oncology. 2008;**6**:29

[73] Singhal SR, Chaudhry P, Nanda S. Genital tuberculosis with predominant involvement of cervix: A case report. Clinical Reviews and Opinions. 2011;**3**(5):55-56

[74] Wadhwa N, Singh UR, Saith SA. Report of two unsuspected cases of cervical tuberculosis. Indian Journal of Pathology & Microbiology. 2005;**3**:390-392

[75] Jyotima A, Gupta JK. Female genital tuberculosis: A retrospective clinicopathologic study of 501 cases. Indian Journal of Pathology & Microbiology. 1993;**4**:389-397

[76] Chakraborthy P, Roy A, Bhattacharya S, Addhya S, Mukherjee S. Tuberculous cervicitis: A clinicopathological and bacteriological study. Journal of the Indian Medical Association. 1995;**5**:167-168

[77] Lamba H, Byrne M, Goldin R, Jenkins C. Tuberculosis of the cervix: Case presentation and a review of the literature. Sexually Transmitted Infections. 2002;**78**:62-63

[78] Sinha R, Gupta D, Tuli N. Genital tract tuberculosis with myometrial involvment. International Journal of Gynaecology and Obstetrics. 1997;**57**:191-192

[79] Sachan R, Patel ML, Gupta P, Verma AK. Genital tuberculosis with variable presentation: A series of three cases. MI Case Report. 2012:bcr2012006665. DOI: 10.1136/bcr-2012-006665

[80] Akhlaghi F, Hamedi AB. Postmenopausal tuberculosis of the cervix, vagina and vulva. International Journal of Gynecology & Obstetrics. 2004;**3** Online publication

[81] Morsad F, Ghazli M, Boumzgou K, et al. Mammary tuberculosis: A series of 14 cases. Journal de Gynecologie, Obstetrique et Biologie de la Reproduction (Paris). 2001;**30**:331-337

[82] Woodard BH, Rosenberg SI, Farham R, et al. Incidence and nature of primary granulomatous inflammation in surgically removed material. The American Journal of Surgical Pathology. 1982;**6**:119-129

[83] Aubry MC. Necrotizing granulomatous inflammation: What does it mean if your special stains are negative? Modern Pathology. 2012;**25**(Suppl 1):S31-S38

[84] Ulbright TM, Katzenstein AA. Solitary necrotizing granulomas on the lung. The American Journal of Surgical Pathology. 1980;**4**:13-28

[85] Tauro LF, Martis JS, George C, Kamath A, Lobo G, Hegde BR. Tuberculous mastitis presenting as breast abscess. Oman Medical Journal. 2011;**26**:53-55

[86] She CR, Litwin MC. Performance of a tuberculosis serologic assay in various patient populations. American Journal of Clinical Pathology. 2015;**144**:240-246

[87] Soini H, Musser JM. Molecular diagnosis of mycobacteria. Clinical Chemistry. 2001;**47**: 809-814

[88] Wiener RS, Della-Latta P, Schluger NW. Effect of nucleic acid amplification for *Mycobacterium tuberculosis* on clinical decision making in suspected extrapulmonary tuberculosis. Chest. 2005;**128**:102-107

[89] Ruiter AM, Vegting IL, Nanayakkara PW. Idiopathic granulomatous mastitis: A great imitator? MBJ Case Report. 2010;**03**:28-44

[90] Park DY, Kim JY, Choi KU, Lee JS, Lee CH, Sol MY, Suh KS. Comparison of polymerase chain reaction with histopathologic features for diagnosis of tuberculosis in formalin-fixed, paraffin-embedded histologic specimens. Archives of Pathology & Laboratory Medicine. 2003;**127**(3):326-330

[91] Buckwalter SP, Wengenack NL. Detection of mycobacteria in paraffin-embedded tissue using lightcycler PCR. American Society for Microbiology. 104th General Meeting; New Orleans, LA; 23-27 May, 2004

[92] Nyendak MR, Lewinsohn DA, Lewinsohn DM. New diagnostic methods for tuberculosis. Current Opinion in Infectious Diseases. 2009;**22**:174-182

[93] Katoch VM. Newer diagnostic techniques for tuberculosis. The Indian Journal of Medical Research. 2004;**120**:418-428

[94] Veziris V. Bacteriological diagnosis of tuberculosis. La Revue du Praticien. 2012;**62**(4): 490-492

[95] Pai M, Riley LW, Colford JM Jr. Interferon-gamma assays in the immunodiagnosis of tuberculosis: A systematic review. The Lancet Infectious Diseases. 2004;**4**:761

[96] Taylor GB, Paviour SD, Musaad S, Jones WO, Holland DJ. A clinicopathological review of 34 cases of inflammatory breast disease showing an association between corynebacteria infection and granulomatous mastitis. Pathology. 2003;**35**:109-119

[97] Saichandran S, Vijayan S, Thirunavukkarasu AB, Sankuppa FS, Singh DA. Rare case of cervical tuberculosis which simulated carcinoma of the cervix. Journal of Clinical and Diagnostic Research. Jun 2013;7(6):1189-1190

[98] Yu YH, Wei W, Liu JL. Diagnostic value of fine-needle aspiration biopsy for breast mass: A systematic review and meta-analysis. BMC Cancer. 2012;**12**:41

[99] Thompson SK, Donzelli J, Jensen JA, Pachucki C, Eng AM, Reyes VC. Breast and cutaneous mycobacteriosis: Diagnosis by fine-needle aspiration biopsy. Diagnostic Cytopathology. 1997;**17**(1):45-49

[100] Kakkar S, Kapila K, Singh MK, Verma K. Tuberculosis of the breast. A cytomorphologic study. Acta Cytologica. 2000;**44**:292-296

[101] Mehrota R. Fine needle aspiration diagnosis of tuberculous mastitis. Indian Journal of Pathology & Microbiology. 2004;**47**(3):377-380

[102] Jalali U, Rasul S, Khan A, Baig N, Khan A, Akhter R. Tuberculous mastitis. Journal of the College of Physicians and Surgeons–Pakistan. 2005;**15**:234-237

[103] Misch KA, Alison S, Deirdre T, O'Sullivan JC, Onuigbo W. Tuberculosis of the cervix: Cytology as an aid to diagnosis. Journal of Clinical Pathology. 1976;**29**:313-316

[104] Samantaray S, Parida G, Rout N, Giri SK, Kar R. Cytologic detection of tuberculous cervicitis. Acta Cytologica. 2009;(5):594-596

[105] Kalyani R, Sheela S, Rajini M. Cytological diagnosis of tuberculous cervicitis: A case report with review of literature. Journal of Cytology. 2012 Jan;**29**(1):86-88

[106] McKeown KC, Wilkinson KW. Tuberculosis of the breast. The British Journal of Surgery. 1952;**39**:420-429

[107] Bahoroon S. Tuberculosis of the breast. Annals of Thoracic Medicine. 2008;**3**(3):110-114

[108] Sriram KB, Moffatt D, Stapledon R. Tuberculosis infection of the breast mistaken for granulomatous mastitis: A case report. Cases Journal. 2008;**1**:273

[109] Lacambra M, Thai TA, Lam CC, Tse GM, et al. Granulomatous mastitis: The histological differentials. Journal of Clinical Pathology. 2011;**64**:405-411

[110] Bakaris S, Yuksel M, Ciragil P, Guven A, Ezberci F, Bulbuloglu E. Granulomatous mastitis including breast tuberculosis and idiopathic lobular granulomatous mastitis. Canadian Journal of Surgery. 2006;**49**(6):427-430

[111] Inoue Y, Suga M. Granulomatous disease and pathogenic microorganism. Kekkaku. 2008;**83**(2):115-130

[112] Altintoprak F, Karakece E, Kivilcim T, Dikicier E, Celebi F, Ciftci IH. Clinical study. Idiopathic granulomatous mastitis: An autoimmune disease? The Scientific World Journal. 2013:5. Article ID 148727. DOI: 10.1155/2013/148727

[113] Kessler E, Wolloc Y. Granulomatous mastitis: A lesion clinically simulating carcinoma. American Journal of Clinical Pathology. 1972;**58**(6):642

[114] Akcan A, Akyildiz H, Deneme MA, Akgun H, Aritas Y. Granulomatous lobular mastitis: A complex diagnostic and therapeutic problem. World Journal of Surgery. 2006;**30**:1403-1409

[115] Baslaim MM, Khayat HA, Al-Amoudi SA. Idiopathic granulomatous mastitis: A heterogeneous disease with variable clinical presentation. World Journal of Surgery. 2007;**31**:1677-1681

[116] Belaabidia B, Essadki O, el Mansouri A, Squalli S. Idiopathic granulomatous mastitis: Apropos of 8 cases and review of the literature. Gynécologie, Obstétrique & Fertilité. 2002;**30**(5):383-389

[117] De Sousa R, Patil R. Breast tuberculosis or granulomatous mastitis: A diagnostic dilemma. Annals of Tropical Medicine and Public Health. 2011;**4**:122-125

[118] Guarner J. Detection of microorganisms in granulomas that have been formalin-fixed: Review of the literature regarding use of molecular methods. Scientifica (Cairo). 2012:494571

[119] Falk V, Ludviksson K, Agren G. Genital tuberculosis in women. Analysis of 187 newly diagnosed cases from 47 Swedish hospitals during the ten-year period 1968 to 1977. American Journal of Obstetrics and Gynecology. 1980;**138**:974-977

[120] Carneiro PC, Graudenz MS, Zerbini MC, de Menezes Y, dos Santos LR, Ferraz AR. Granulomatous reaction associated with metastatic epidermoid cancer. The importance of using multiple methods in diagnostic pathology. Revista do Hospital das Clinicas; Faculdade de Medicina da Universidade de Sao Paulo. 1989;**44**:29-32

[121] Kervancioğlu S, Kervancioğlu R, Oźkur A, Sirikçi A. Primary tuberculosis of the breast. Diagnostic and Interventional Radiology. 2005;**11**(4):210-212

[122] Al-Marri MR, Aref E, Omar AJ. Mammographic features of isolated tuberculous mastitis. Saudi Medical Journal. 2005;**26**:646-650

[123] Romero C, Carreira C, Cereceda C, Pinto J, Lopez R, Bolaňos F. Mammary tuberculosis: Percutaneous treatment of a mammary tuberculous abscess. European Radiology. 2000; **10**(3):531-533

[124] Khandelwal R, Jam I. Breast tuberculosis mimicking a malignancy falsely over-stage the disease a rare case report with review of literature. Breast Disease. 2013;**34**(2):53-55

[125] Munjal K, Jain KV, Agrawal A, Bandi KP. Co-existing tubercular axillary lymphadenitis with breast carcinoma can falsely over-stage the disease. Case series. The Indian Journal of Tuberculosis. 2010;**57**:104-107

[126] Robinson A, Horne C, Weaver A. Coexistence of axillary tuberculous lymphadenitis with lymph node metastases from a breast carcinoma. Clinical Oncology. 2001;**1**(3):144-147

[127] Tulasi NR, Raju PC, Damodaran V, Randhika TS. A spectrum of coexistent tuberculosis and carcinoma in the breast and axillary lymph nodes: Report of five cases. Breast. 2006; **15**(3):437-439

[128] Balasubramanian SP, Rao MP, Jayaram S, Bose SM. Coexisting mammary tuberculosis and malignant disease. Canadian Journal of Surgery. 2001;**44**:224-225

[129] Fujii T, Kimura M, Yanagita Y, Koida T, Kuwano H. Tuberculosis of axillary lymph nodes with primary breast cancer. Breast Cancer. 2003;**10**:175-178

[130] Khurram M, Tariq M, Shahid P. Breast cancer with associated granulomatous axillary lymphadenitis: A diagnostic and clinical dilemma in regions with high prevalence of tuberculosis. Pathology, Research and Practice. 2007;**203**(10):699-704

[131] Naragam AP, Tati YS, Dara H, Kumar VA, Jada M, Shekhar Y, Dara H, Kawathekar P. Plasma cell mastitis mimicking as carcinoma of the breast: A case report and review of the literature IOSR. Journal of Dental and Medical Sciences. 2014;**13**(2):28-31. Ver. III

[132] Diallo R, Frevel T, Poremba C, Cirkel U, Metze D, Dockhom-Dworniczak B. Lupus vulgaris as the etiology of tuberculous mastitis. Pathologie. 1997;**18**(1):67-70

[133] Kao PT, Tu MY, Tang SH, Ma HK. Tuberculosis of the breast with erythema nodosum: A case report. Journal of Medical Case Reports. 2010;**4**:124

[134] Yoo H, Choi SH, Kim YJ, Cho YU, Choi SJ. Recurrent bilateral breast abscess due to nontuberculous mycobacterial infection. Journal of Breast Cancer. 2014;**17**(3):295-298

[135] Yukawa M, Watatani M, Isona S, Inoue M, et al. Management of granulomatous mastitis: A series of 13 patients who were evaluated for treatment without corticosteroids. International Surgery. 2015;**100**(5):774-782

[136] Challa VR, Srivastava A, Dhar A. Scrofulous swelling of the bosom masquerading as cancer. Indian Journal of Medical Microbiology. 2014;**32**(1):82-84

[137] Inaki J, Rodriguez V, Bodey GP. Causes of death in cancer patients. Cancer. 1974;**33**:568-573

[138] Chen YM, Chao JY, Tsai CM, Lee PY, Perng RP. Shortened survival of lung cancer patients initially presenting with pulmonary tuberculosis. Japanese Journal of Clinical Oncology. 1996;**26**:322-327

[139] Sheybani F, Sarvghad M, Naderi HR, Gharib M. Treatment for and clinical characteristics of granulomatous mastitis. Obstetrics and Gynecology. 2015;**125**(4):801-807

[140] O'Reilly M, Patel KR, Cummins R. Tuberculosis of the breast presenting as carcinoma. Military Medicine. 2000;**165**:800-802

[141] Daali M, Hssaida R, Hda A. Primary tuberculosis of the breast. Presse Médicale. 2001;**30**: 431-433

[142] Gupta V, Mohan H, Jain P, Singh S, Singla N. Tuberculous mastitis: A report of two cases in elderly females. Japanese Journal of Infectious Diseases. 2006:279-280

[143] Kumar P, Sharma N. Primary MDR -TB of the breast. The Indian Journal of Chest Diseases & Allied Sciences. 2003;**45**:63-65

[144] Imperiale A, Zandrino F, Calabrese M, Parodi G, Massa T. Abscesses of the breast. US-guided serial percutaneous aspiration and local antibiotic therapy after unsuccessful systemic antibiotic therapy. Acta Radiologica. 2001;**42**(2):161-165

[145] Mehendiratta V, Mccarty BC, Gomez L, Graviss AE, Musher MD. Computerized tomography (CT)-guided aspiration of abscesses. Outcome of therapy at a tertiary care hospital. Journal of Infection. 2007;**54**(2):122-128

[146] Gupta A, Gupta MM, Mankatala U, Khurana N. Primary tuberculosis of cervix mimicking carcinoma: A rare case. Journal of Mid-life Health. 2014;(2):96-97. DOI: 10.4103/0976-7800.133999

5

Insights into Recurrent Tuberculosis: Relapse Versus Reinfection and Related Risk Factors

Kogieleum Naidoo and Navisha Dookie

Abstract

Recurrent tuberculosis (TB) following successful treatment constitutes a significant challenge to TB control strategies. TB recurrence can be due to either reactivation of the same strain, i.e., relapse, or reinfection with a new strain. Recurrence due to reinfection has become an area of intense study due to its perceived significance in TB endemic settings with high rates of human immunodeficiency virus (HIV) coinfection. This review presents a descriptive analysis of recurrent TB disease and explores risk factors, immunopathogenesis, treatment, and preventative strategies. Currently available laboratory methods used to discriminate tuberculosis recurrence due to reinfection and relapse are discussed. We highlight risk factors for recurrence and strategies for early detection of TB recurrence. Enhanced treatment options such as intensified initial treatment, extension of treatment, and secondary preventative therapy for patients presenting with multiple risk factors are explored in this review. The potential value of identifying immunological correlates of risk and protection in recurrent TB is also briefly examined.

Keywords: recurrence, tuberculosis, relapse, reinfection, molecular typing

1. Introduction

Tuberculosis remains one of the most significant public health challenges globally, despite significant advances in tuberculosis (TB) control [1]. Approximately one-third of the world's population is estimated to harbor latent forms of the *Mycobacterium tuberculosis* (MTB) bacilli, creating a reservoir for future disease. The alarmingly high TB incidence and prevalence rates in countries that also have a high background prevalence of human immunodeficiency virus (HIV) have been persistent for more than a decade. The interplay between HIV infection and

TB has resulted in 10 times greater risk of TB reactivation from latent disease in coinfected individuals. In addition to the increased risk of TB reactivation disease, HIV coinfection has also been reported to substantially increase the rate of recurrent TB disease from reinfection due to the increased vulnerability of immune-compromised patients to TB infection [2, 3]. Recurrent TB disease occurs when patients who were previously treated for TB develop a new disease episode, due to either relapse (recurrence of the old infection) or reinfection (infection with a new strain) [4]. Recurrent TB disease is associated with poor treatment outcomes and higher mortality rates compared to primary TB infection [5]. Clinical, epidemiological, and/or microbiological data cannot be used to differentiate relapse and reinfection. Distinguishing between the two mechanisms requires evaluating the homology of the MTB strains isolated during the first and subsequent TB episode using molecular DNA fingerprinting technology [4].

In TB-endemic settings experiencing high rates of HIV coinfection, the rate of recurrent TB is significantly increased. Recurrence rates of up to 24.4% have been reported in HIV/TB-coinfected individuals, with most recurrences occurring within 2 years of successful treatment completion [5]. Prior to the development of DNA fingerprinting technology, primary TB disease was thought to impart some measure of immunity and subsequent TB infection was the result of reactivation of the strain from the original episode of infection [4]. However, with the advent of DNA fingerprinting techniques, numerous studies have explored the roles of relapse and reinfection in TB recurrence [6]. In countries with a high incidence of TB, reinfection has been reported as the main driver of recurrent TB, with molecular studies reporting up to 88% of TB recurrences due to reinfection in HIV-coinfected patients. In contrast, countries with a low TB incidence have reported TB relapse as the main cause of recurrent TB disease [7].

Current World Health Organization (WHO) guidelines use the term "relapse" to describe all TB recurrences during programmatic assessments. The term is largely generic and incorporates recurrence due to relapse or reinfection. The two mechanisms of TB recurrence exist as fundamentally independent forms of TB infection, have differing pathogenesis, and have different implications for patients and TB control programs [6, 7]. Relapse is associated with treatment failure and may be due to either clinical management complexities leading to subtherapeutic drug concentrations of key TB drugs due to drug–drug interactions or altered drug metabolism or from patient-related factors such as poor treatment adherence. Furthermore, relapse disease has been associated with an increased risk of acquiring drug-resistance in the infecting strain of MTB. Higher rates of TB relapse seen in HIV-infected patients may indicate the need for lengthier, more aggressive treatment to eliminate MTB infection compared to standard practice. High rates of reinfection are reflective of poor public health interventions that fail to reduce community transmission [3]. In the context of HIV coinfection, reinfection has been associated with failure to develop protective immunity after the first episode of TB resulting in this subset of patients bearing a higher susceptibility to reinfection with MTB [8]. The aim of the current review was to examine the disease burden due to recurrent TB disease and explore the risk factors, immunopathology, treatment, and prevention and the relative contribution of relapse versus reinfection to TB recurrence.

2. Epidemiology of recurrent TB

Population-based surveillance reports on the rates of recurrent TB following completion of anti-TB treatment are lacking. Recent estimates of recurrent TB across various regions indicate an average of 2290 cases/100000 person-years at 12 months following treatment completion. In high-incidence settings, this rate is as high as 7850 cases/100000 person-years [8]. An earlier report by Panjabi et al. analyzing 32 studies reported an overall recurrence rate of 3010 and 2290 per 100,000 person-years following 6 and 12 months of treatment, respectively, among controlled trials. They also reported that these rates were higher for observational studies compared to controlled trials. Rates were also reported to be higher in countries with high TB incidence [5]. Recurrence rates for specific regions have been emerging; many of which are demarcated as WHO high-burden countries. Glynn et al. reported a recurrence rate of 24.4 cases per 100 person-years in HIV-positive individuals and 4.7% per 100 person-years in their HIV-negative counterparts [9]. Charalambous et al. reported an overall recurrence rate of 7.89% per 100 person-years in the same setting among a mining population. The recurrence rate was higher in HIV-positive individuals at 8.86 cases per 100 person-years compared to 3.35 cases per 100 person-years in HIV-negative counterparts [10]. Narayanan et al. reported a recurrence rate of 14% among an HIV/TB-coinfected cohort of 306 patients from South India. Among the patients with recurrent TB, 88% of recurrent infections were due to reinfection [11]. Sun et al. reported a recurrence rate of 35 cases per 1000 person-years for patients with drug-sensitive TB and 65 cases per 1000 person-years among patients with drug-resistant TB [12]. Luzze et al. reported an overall recurrence rate of 8.4 cases per 100 person-years in a cohort from Uganda. The recurrence rate was also reported to be higher among HIV-positive individuals at 9.4 cases per 100 person-years compared to 6.7 cases per 100 person-years in HIV-negative counterparts [13]. Vree et al. reported a recurrence rate of 8.6% among a Vietnamese cohort of 244 patients [14]. Datiko et al. reported a recurrence rate of one case per 100 person-years (15 recurrent cases in 368 patients – 4.1%) among an Ethiopian cohort [15]. Moosazadeh et al. reported a recurrence incidence of 8.3% in Iran [16]. Crofts et al. reported the recurrence rate in England and Wales as 4.1 cases per 100 person-years; however, in HIV-positive individuals, this rate was reported as 7.6 cases per 100 person-years [17].

3. Definitions and terminology

Definitions of terms relating to recurrent TB disease that feature in this review are given below and some are illustrated in **Figure 1**.

3.1. Latent TB infection (LTBI)

LTBI is defined as a state of disease in which MTB persists within the host and is associated with damage that is evident at a cellular or tissue level but is not associated with the disease.

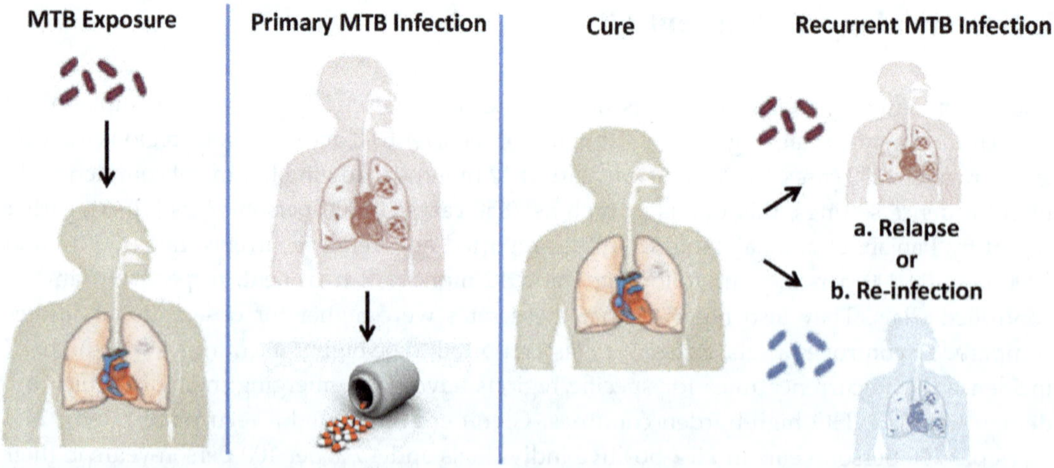

Figure 1. The continuum of *Mycobacterium tuberculosis* (MTB)–host interaction following MTB infection. Successful cure is achieved in ~95% of patients. In ~5% of patients, this cycle extends beyond successful treatment completion when the cycle of TB recurrence occurs either through (a) relapse of the original infection or (b) reinfection by new strain of MTB.

While this form of disease displays no clinical or radiological evidence of active disease, viable MTB bacilli are contained within tissues [18].

3.2. Primary TB disease

Primary TB is defined as disease occurring in a patient who has never been treated for TB or who has received less than 1 month of anti-TB treatment. In some instances, primary TB refers to the initial exposure of MTB; thereafter, the reactivation of TB disease following a period of clinical latency is referred to as postprimary or TB occurrence. In the current review, we refer to primary TB in accordance to the WHO definition [19].

3.3. Recurrent TB disease

Recurrent TB disease is defined as the diagnosis of a subsequent episode of TB following treatment completion or cure at the end of the most recent course of treatment. Recurrent TB disease occurs after the initial TB disease episode has been classified as clinically cured. According to WHO guidelines, cure is defined as smear and culture negative sputum samples from the last month of treatment and on at least one previous occasion [19].

3.4. TB relapse

Relapse disease is defined as a subsequent episode of TB disease due to the reactivation/reemergence of the original infecting strain of MTB, determined by genotypic homogeneity assessment of primary and recurrent MTB strains [4]. Given that MTB strains are highly homogenous by nature, combined with high rates of transmission, classification of relapse infection is challenging [20].

3.5. TB reinfection

Reinfection is defined as a subsequent episode of TB disease due to the exogenous infection with an MTB strain that is distinct from the organism that caused the original infection [4]. A challenge regarding detection of reinfection is that in high TB-endemic settings, patients maybe exposed to be reinfected with a very similar strain that caused the primary infection, making differentiation between relapse disease and reinfection difficult.

4. Clinical presentation of recurrent TB

The symptoms of recurrent TB have been reported to vary in clinical and radiologic symptoms and are clinically indistinguishable from primary TB disease [21]. In general, TB symptoms are usually gradual in onset and duration and may vary from a few weeks to months. However, in young children and patients with HIV coinfection, a more acute onset of disease has been recorded. Typical symptoms such as fever, night sweats, and weight-loss occur among approximately 75, 45, and 55% of patients, respectively. The presence of a persistent nonremitting cough has been cited as the most common symptom, recorded in approximately 95% of patients with TB. Patients with cavitary lung disease, synonymous with recurrent TB disease, typically present with chronic cough, mostly accompanied by fever and/or the presence of night sweats and weight loss. The associated cough may be productive or nonproductive in nature. The sputum produced by patients maybe mucoid, mucopurulent, and bloodstained or may have severe hemoptysis. Other symptoms include chest pain and dyspnoea. Chest X-ray plays a critical role in diagnosis of sputum smear-negative patients [22]. **Figure 1** depicts the radiological progression of initial drug-susceptible TB (**Figure 2a**), followed by a recurrent TB episode (**Figure 2b,** diagnosis, and **Figure 2c**, end of treatment for recurrent TB). Typical chest radiograph findings include old fibrotic lesions, often cooccurring with other nonspecific features of tuberculosis such as lobar opacities, consolidation, fibrosis, and interstitial infiltrates. Severely immune-suppressed

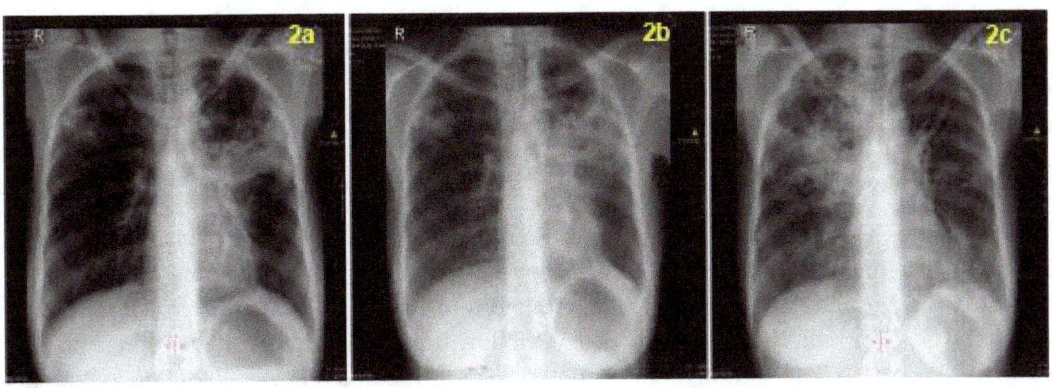

Figure 2. Chest X-rays of a patient with initial drug-sensitive TB, subsequently developed drug-resistant TB, depicting: (a) cavities and infiltrates in both lungs; (b) cavities and infiltrates on the right lung and fibrosis in the left lung; and (c) cavities, infiltrates, and patchy consolidation in right lung and consolidation in mid and lower zones of the left lung.

patients and young children are less likely to present with pathology on chest radiograph [22]. In the context of continuing disease due to poor adherence, recurrent TB is diagnosed by the clinical process, sputum smear microscopy, and chest radiograph [21]. Furthermore, the two mechanisms of recurrent TB are clinically indistinguishable and require specialized strain typing to differentiate between relapse and reinfection [4].

5. Methodology used to study recurrent TB

Discriminating TB reinfection from relapse through the study of the MTB genome using various laboratory methods is a key hallmark in the study of recurrent TB. DNA fingerprinting techniques are based on genomic variation, forming the basis of molecular epidemiological studies. The genome of the MTB complex is largely conserved with the presence of monomeric sequences repeated periodically, known as repetitive units. There are two types of repetitive units, namely, interspersed repeats (IR) and tandem repeats (TR). The former occur throughout the genome in the form of direct repeats and insertion sequences, while the latter are a series of head-to-tail direct uninterrupted repeats in the form of variable number tandem repeats (VNTR). The most common techniques used to distinguish between the two mechanisms of TB recurrence include *IS*6110-restriction fragment length polymorphism (*IS*6110-RFLP) analysis, mycobacterial interspersed repetitive-unit variable number of tandem repeats (MIRU-VNTR) typing, and spacer oligonucleotide genotyping (spoligotyping) [4, 23]. More recently, whole genome sequencing (WGS) has been used to compare strains representing different episodes of TB infection. One of the challenges associated with the former typing methods is the interpretation of similar isolates in the case of relapse disease. There is no standard for interpretation of changes in banding patterns when comparing specimens from different episodes of disease. It is suggested that identical bands or a difference of one band is good approximation for defining relapse. The use of WGS surmounts this issue by directly evaluating the number of single nucleotide polymorphism (SNP) differences between the disease episodes. There is still some uncertainty regarding the appropriate SNP cutoff value, which depends on the analysis platform and genome coverage. However, WGS is more robust as it excludes mixed infections and allows genomic associations with relapse and reinfection to be examined directly [8, 24, 25].

5.1. *IS*6110 RFLP typing

*IS*6110 RFLP is a well-validated method used extensively for MTB typing. This method relies upon the IS*6110* insertion element as a genetic marker was long recognized as the gold standard for studying the molecular epidemiology of MTB [26, 27]. The *IS*6110 insertion element has proven stable *in vitro* and *in vivo* with low transpositional frequency and is present in up to 25 copies in MTB. Strain identification using this method relies on variation in both the number and location of *IS*6110 elements in the MTB genome. The restriction endonuclease *Pvu*II cleaves the IS*6110* element once by recognizing a particular palindromic sequence. The result is thousands of DNA fragments of different lengths that are then separated according to size by gel electrophoresis. Notably, different molecular weight fragments arise because of the varying distances between insertion sequences, which create a specific banding pattern characteristic of that isolate. Dendograms are constructed to graphically represent the similarity coefficients between isolates, allowing them to be clustered into groups based on banding patterns. Visual inspection can then be used to decide which isolates among these groups are identical or differ by only one or two bands. The IS*6110* method has been standardized enabling comparison of fingerprints globally. Thus, IS*6110* RFLP genotyping can provide a comparison of the strains involved at the initial and recurrent TB episodes by comparing the fingerprint patterns. MTB isolates with identical *IS*6110 DNA fingerprints or slight variations in banding patterns identify relapse of a prior infection, while distinct fingerprints identify reinfection with a new strain of MTB [26–28]. Challenges of utilizing this typing technique includes lower discriminatory power in isolates with low copy numbers of the *IS*6110 element, usually less than six copies of the element, the high level of expertise required for the technique and analysis, and poor reproducibility of the technique. Furthermore, strains displaying identical *IS*6110 banding patterns have been reported to display unique genetic identities in the presence of a secondary technique [4].

5.2. MIRU-VNTR typing

MIRU-VNTR typing is a PCR-based technique followed by detection by capillary electrophoresis, which characterizes both the number and sizes of variable tandem repeats in 12 or more loci. The repeat number is highly variable in many loci and is therefore termed "variable number tandem repeat" loci. They consist of small repetitive sequences of 40- to 100-bp and are unique in nature. They are scattered in 41 locations in the genome of MTB and are present mainly in the intergenic regions. The principle of this method is PCR amplification of 12- to 24-VNTR loci using primers complementary to the flanking regions, followed by gel electrophoresis. The size of the PCR amplicon reflects the tandem repeat unit, which is then converted into a numerical code to get a digital format in which each digit represents the number of copies present at that locus. This method utilizes variations in repetitive sequences, which are not under selective pressure and evolve relatively rapidly making it an ideal tool for molecular epidemiological studies. The discriminatory power of MIRU-VNTR is proportional to the number of loci included. MIRU-VNTR typing using a standardized set of 24 loci is now the international standard and is currently employed in European countries and globally. This method is rapid, reproducible, and cheaper than RFLP typing. Historically, this method was widely used in its 12-loci format that had a lower discriminatory power compared to IS*6110* RFLP [4, 23].

5.3. Spoligotyping

Spoligotyping is a hybridization assay that detects variability in genomic direct repeat (DR) locus of the MTB complex. The DR region of MTB consists of multiple copies of a conserved 36 bp sequence region (the DRs), which are separated by multiple unique spacer sequences. This method involves PCR amplification of the entire DR locus using primers that are complementary to the flanking spacer sequences, followed by hybridization to a membrane with 43 spacer oligonucleotides. The resulting bands produce a dark band in the presence of a spacer or no band if a spacer is absent. The pattern is converted into a 43 digit binary code and subsequently converted into a 15 digit octal code. This code is unique and represents a specific banding pattern. This is a simple, high-throughput method that is cost-effective. It is, however, less discriminatory than RFLP typing. This method is ideal as a first-line screening tool, to be followed by other typing methods if needed [4, 23].

5.4. Whole genome sequencing

WGS analysis has been widely applied to the field of molecular epidemiology in the last decade. WGS plays a significant role in examining outbreaks and identifying transmission events where strains are genetically indistinguishable by conventional methods. WGS-based genotyping offers the optimal resolution of MTB complex isolates and holds the advantage of generating additional data, such as drug resistance [25]. Byrant et al. recently demonstrated the higher discriminatory power of WGS compared to MIRU-VNTR to differentiate relapse from reinfection. The decreasing cost of this platform, coupled with advances in genomics, makes WGS the most desirable single analysis tool for identification, prediction of drug resistance, and epidemiological typing. WGS also has a significant role in detecting MTB mixed strain infections. This method is set to become the gold standard for typing in the near future [24].

6. Relapse and reinfection

Published studies also vary in reported rates of TB disease due to reinfection from as low as <3–>60%. An earlier review by Lambert et al. failed to show a consistent trend when reporting whether TB recurrence is due to relapse versus reinfection [6]. Unsurprisingly, recurrence due to TB reinfection has been reported to be the main mechanism of recurrent TB disease in geographical regions with a high burden of TB disease; however, high rates of reinfection have also been reported from low- and moderate-incidence settings. Conversely, a poor association between reinfection and recurrent TB disease in high-burden settings has also been reported. This highlights that a consistent trend in recurrent TB disease is lacking [8, 10, 11, 24, 29–59]. Studies indicate that relapse generally occurs within a year following treatment, while reinfection predominates after the first year following treatment [8, 52]. In the context of HIV coinfection, there is a 2.4 times higher hazard ratio for recurrent TB disease, in comparison to HIV-uninfected individuals. HIV coinfection and antiretroviral treatment have been associated with an increased risk of recurrent TB due to reinfection [41, 47]. In a 13-year study conducted in Cape Town, South Africa, TB relapse rate peaked at 3.93% (95% confidence interval [CI], 2.35–5.96%) per annum 0.35 (95% CI, 0.15–0.45) years after treatment completion, whereas reinfection tuberculosis rate peaked at 1.58% (95% CI, 0.94–2.46%) per annum 1.20 (95% CI, 0.55–1.70) years after completion [52]. Reports of higher rates of TB reinfection may occur inadvertently likely due to laboratory contamination resulting in incorrect classification, mislabeling of isolates, mixed strain infections, varying clinical and radiological profile of patients, and length of follow-up. Varying lengths in the follow-up period make it difficult to make comparisons between studies. **Table 1** details published studies distinguishing reinfection from relapse in their reporting recurrent TB disease.

Author, publication year	Country	Study design	Number of patients analyzed	Recurrences (Total)	With fingerprinting results[a]	Reinfection (% of a)	Strain typing method	HIV status	Comment
Hawken et al. (1993)[c] [29]	Kenya	Prospective cohort	196	11	3	1 (33)	NA	HIV infected and uninfected	Increased recurrence rate (34-fold higher) in HIV-infected group compared to HIV-uninfected counterparts. Thiacetazone-containing regimen was used for treatment. Study not powered to determine the relative contribution of relapse or reinfection to TB recurrence.
Das et al. (1993)[c] [30]	Hong Kong	Retrospective analysis RCT	NA	Not reported	42	5 (12)	*IS*986-RFLP and phage typing	Not reported	Monthly sputum cultures were analyzed over a two-year period. Only 5 patients showed distinct differences in serial isolates. Detection of possible mixed infection, given the heterogeneity detected among serial samples. No HIV data or risk factors reported.
Godfrey-Faussett et al. (1994)[c] [31]	Kenya	Retrospective cohort	NA	Not reported	5	1 (20)	NA	HIV infected and uninfected	Study not powered to determine the relative contribution of relapse or reinfection to TB recurrence. No risk factors reported.
Das et al. (1995)[c] [32]	India	Retrospective analysis RCT	NA	30	13	3 (23)	*IS*6110-RFLP	Not reported	The main objective of the study was to determine the utility of *IS*6110-RFLP to distinguish between relapse and reinfection in recurrent TB.
Sahadevan et al. (1995)[c] [33]	India	Retrospective analysis RCT	52	44	29	9 (31)	*IS*6110-RFLP	Not reported	The main objective of the study was to modify the *IS*6110-RFLP assay using a direct repeat probe to increase its ability to distinguish between relapse and reinfection in recurrent TB.
El-Sadr et al. (1998)[c] [34]	USA	RCT	NA	2	1	1 (100)	NA	HIV infected	The main aim of the study was to determine the efficacy of levofloxacin

Author, publication year	Country	Study design	Number of patients analyzed	Recurrences (Total)	With fingerprinting results[a]	Reinfection (% of a)	Strain typing method	HIV status	Comment
								and uninfected	to the standard treatment regimen for drug-susceptible TB. The addition of levofloxacin resulted in low relapse rates, thus small sample size.
Vernon et al. (1999)[c] [35]	USA	RCT	71	8	7	0 (0)	*IS*6110-RFLP	HIV infected	This was an early study aimed at assessing the a once-weekly regimen of isoniazid and rifapentine with twice-weekly isoniazid and rifampin in the continuation phase of treatment for pulmonary TB in HIV-infected and -uninfected patients. The current report assessed only the HIV-infected cohort. Relapse TB was associated with an increase in rifamycin resistance.
Van Rie et al. (1999)[c] [36]	South Africa	Retrospective analysis-lab database	698	48	16	12 (75)	*IS*6110-RFLP	HIV uninfected	High-TB endemic setting. All patients in the cohort were reported to be HIV-uninfected. Reinfection was reported to occur within 7 to 8 months of previous cure. Reinfection in a high-endemic area in HIV-uninfected patients, probably due to the increased risk of developing recurrent TB after primary infection.
Johnson et al. (2000)[c] [37]	Uganda	Prospective cohort	291	17	4	0 (0)	*IS*6110-RFLP	HIV infected and uninfected	The main aim of the study was to assess the efficacy of an unsupervised, rifampicin-containing regiment for drug-susceptible TB in HIV-infected adults. No cases of reinfection. Relapse is probably an indication of the new regimen failing

Author, publication year	Country	Study design	Number of patients analyzed	Recurrences (Total)	With fingerprinting results[a]	Reinfection (% of a)	Strain typing method	HIV status	Comment
									or poor adherence in the current study.
Lourenco et al. (2000)[c] [38]	Brazil	Retrospective cohort	32	12	12	3 (25)	DRE-PCR and *IS*6110-RFLP	HIV infected	The study aimed to assess the relative contribution of relapse and reinfection in HIV-coinfected patients with recurrent TB. Study was not powered to assess the contribution of HIV. Among the three patients with reinfection, all were unique strains.
Caminero et al. (2001)[c] [39]	Gran Canaria Island	Retrospective population based-cohort	92	23	18	8 (44)	*IS*6110-RFLP	HIV infected and uninfected	The study setting has a moderate incidence of tuberculosis. Reinfection was attributed to TB recurrence in both HIV-infected and -uninfected patients. A dominant strain was reported for reinfection and relapse. Relapse was associated with increased drug resistance.
Bandera et al. (2001)[c] [40]	Italy	Prospective population based-cohort	2127	32	32	5 (16)	*IS*6110-RFLP	HIV infected and uninfected	Low TB incidence setting. Two of the five cases of reinfection were associated with drug resistance during recurrent TB episode, and three cases represented dominant strains circulating in the setting. Higher risk of relapse was described for HIV-infected and MDR-TB patients.
Sonnenberg et al. (2001)[c] [41]	South Africa	Prospective population based-cohort miners	65	65	39	14 (36)	*IS*6110-RFLP	HIV infected and uninfected	Thirteen of the fourteen recurrences occurred within 6 months of follow-up were attributed to relapse. HIV coinfection was cited as a strong risk factor for recurrence due to reinfection. Residual cavitation was also attributed to recurrent disease.

Author, publication year	Country	Study design	Number of patients analyzed	Recurrences (Total)	With fingerprinting results[a]	Reinfection (% of a)	Strain typing method	HIV status	Comment
Gracia de Viedma et al. (2002) [42]	Spain	Retrospective population based-cohort	2567	172	43	14 (33)	DRE-PCR; spoligotyping	HIV infected and uninfected	Low TB incidence and low exposure MTB, relapse was the main cause of recurrence. Patients displayed poor anti-TB treatment adherence. No association with HIV.
Fitzpatrick et al. (2002) [43]	Uganda	Retrospective population based-cohort	1100	40	40	9 (23)	Not reported	HIV infected and uninfected	Low HIV incidence setting, main cause of recurrence was relapse. Three of the four HIV-infected patients were reinfected with MTB. The remaining patient was sputum smear negative.
Lan et al. (2002) [44]	Vietnam	Retrospective population based-cohort	2901	168	39	0 (0)	*IS*6110-RFLP	Not reported	Primary MDR-TB was cited as a risk factor for relapse, associated with the Beijing strain. However, the study was not powered to detect risk factors related to relapse.
El Sahly et al. (2003) [45]	USA	Retrospective population based-cohort	Not reported	100	38	8 (21)	*IS*6110-RFLP and spoligotyping	HIV infected and uninfected	Low TB incidence setting. Relapse was the main driver of recurrence, with increased in drug resistance in the recurrent episode of TB. Only two of the eight patients with reinfection were HIV infected.
Jasmer et al. (2004) [46]	Canada, USA	RCT	1244	79	75	3 (4)	*IS*6110-RFLP	HIV infected and uninfected	High levels of reinfection despite Canada and USA having low TB incidence.
Verver et al. (2005) [47]	South Africa	RCT	447	61	31	24 (77)	*IS*6110-RFLP	HIV infected included	Recurrence following successful treatment as per definition of this review. Reinfection not stratified by HIV status.
Scaaf et al. (2005) [48]	South Africa	Prospective cohort	87	9	4	1 (25)	*IS*6110-RFLP	HIV infected	Pediatric population. Reinfection described in one patient; analysis of episode 1 and 3 of TB. Two further

Author, publication year	Country	Study design	Number of patients analyzed	Recurrences (Total)	With fingerprinting results[a]	Reinfection (% of a)	Strain typing method	HIV status	Comment
									cases of reinfection defined by epidemiologic data and DST.
Shen et al. (2006) [49]	China	Retrospective population based-cohort	202	54	52	32 (62)	*IS*6110-RFLP; MIRU-VNTR	Not reported	Data on HIV status not available; however, low HIV incidence setting (0.6 cases/100,000 person-years). No time interval defined between end of treatment and new episode of TB.
Cacho et al. (2007) [50]	Spain	Retrospective population based-cohort	645	20	8	1 (13)	*IS*6110-RFLP; MIRU-VNTR	HIV infected and uninfected	Patient with TB reinfection was HIV negative. Relapse was attributed to recurrent TB in this setting. No differences in risk factors reported for relapse and reinfection.
Charalambous et al. (2008) [10]	South Africa	Mining population	609	57	16	11 (69)	*IS*6110-RFLP	HIV infected and uninfected	Among the HIV-positive group, 10 of the 14 recurrences were due to reinfection. However, only two pairs available in the negative group. One case of reinfection and one case of relapse.
Narayanan et al. (2009) [11]	India	Prospective population based-cohort	Not reported	74	48	44 (92)	*IS*6110-RFLP; MIRU-VNTR; spoligotyping	HIV infected and uninfected	Reinfection was cited as the main cause of recurrence in HIV-infected patients (88%), while relapse was the main cause of recurrence in HIV-uninfected counterparts (91%).
Bang et al. (2009) [51]	Denmark	Retrospective population based-cohort	4154	73	73	19 (26)	*IS*6110-RFLP	Not reported	The risk of TB recurrence by reinfection increased with time. No data available for risk factors contributing to recurrence.
Marx et al. (2010) [52]	South Africa	Retrospective population based-cohort	309	203	130	66 (51)	*IS*6110-RFLP	HIV infected and uninfected	Relapse and reinfection not stratified by HIV status. Relapse occurred early after treatment completion, while reinfection occurred ≥1 year of treatment completion.

Author, publication year	Country	Study design	Number of patients analyzed	Recurrences (Total)	With fingerprinting results[a]	Reinfection (% of a)	Strain typing method	HIV status	Comment
Crampin et al. (2010) [53]	Malawi	Long-term cohort	584	53	39	13 (33)	*IS*6110-RFLP	HIV infected and uninfected	Reinfection was cited as the main cause of recurrence in HIV-infected patients (52%), while relapse was the main cause of recurrence in HIV-uninfected counterparts (93.7%).
Vargese et al. (2012) [54]	Saudi Arabia	Retrospective population-based cohort	Not reported	223	223	39 (17)	MIRU-VNTR	Not reported	14% of reinfection cases were associated with resistance to ≥1 first-line drug.
Bryant et al. (2013) [24]	Malaysia, South Africa, and Thailand	Sub-study of RCT	Not reported	50	36	3 (9)	MIRU-VNTR and WGS	HIV infected and uninfected	Main objective of the substudy was to determine the role of WGS to distinguish relapse from reinfection.
Guerra-Assuno et al. (2014) [8]	Malawi	Prospective population-based cohort	1471	139	75	20 (26)	*IS*6110-RFLP and WGS	HIV infected and uninfected	Reinfection was most common in HIV-infected patients. Relapse was associated with an increased prevalence of isoniazid resistance.
Interrante et al. (2015) [55]	USA	Population-based cohort	3039	136	136	20 (15)	*IS*6110-RFLP; MIRU-VNTR	HIV infected and uninfected	18 of the 136 cases of recurrence TB were HIV infected. Of these, four cases were attributed to reinfection.
Schiroli et al. (2015) [56]	Italy	Prospective cohort study	4682	83	83	19 (23)	*IS*6110-RFLP; MIRU-VNTR	HIV infected and uninfected	No causal association with HIV status. Increased drug resistance in patients with recurrent TB.
Korhonen et al. (2016) [57]	Finland	Population-based cohort	8299	48	21	3 (14)	WGS based spoligotyping	HIV infected and uninfected	Low rate of HIV coinfection in cohort (1/21). The difference in the number of SNPs in relapse isolates was reported to be 0–6. In the presence of dominant strain types, reinfection cannot be ruled out. In one case of relapse, the difference in the number of SNPs was reported to be 38 over a 2-year period.

Author, publication year	Country	Study design	Number of patients analyzed	Recurrences (Total)	With fingerprinting results[a]	Reinfection (% of a)	Strain typing method	HIV status	Comment
Shen et al. (2017) [58]	China	Retrospective population-based cohort	13,417	710	141	59 (42)	*IS*6110-RFLP; MIRU-VNTR	Not reported	Low HIV prevalence in the study setting. Patients with cavitation, diabetes, and initial drug resistance were at high risk for recurrent TB. Reinfection contributed to a significant number of cases.
Whitney et al. (2017) [59]	Southern Africa	Substudy of RCT	Not reported	51	35	3 (9)	MIRU-VNTR and WGS	Not reported	Main objective of the substudy was to determine the role of WGS to distinguish relapse from reinfection. The difference in the number of SNPs in relapse isolates was reported to be 0–5.

[a]Total number of recurrent TB episodes within the cohort.

[b]Percentage of recurrent TB episodes caused by reinfection (calculated from a).

[c]Adapted from the systematic review by Lambert et al. [6]
Abbreviations: DRE-PCR, double repetitive element-polymerase chain reaction; DST, drug susceptibility profile; MDR-TB, multidrug resistant-tuberculosis; MIRU-VNTR, mycobacterial interspersed repetitive unit-variable number tandem repeats; MTB, *Mycobacterium tuberculosis*; RCT, randomized controlled trial; RFLP, restriction fragment length polymorphism; SNP, single nucleotide polymorphism.

Table 1. Studies conducted on recurrent tuberculosis infections, distinguishing the contribution reinfection versus relapse.

7. Risk factors for recurrent TB

Trinh et al. outlined risk factors for TB recurrence in three categories: (i) treatment response associated with relapse, (ii) individual vulnerability associated with both relapse and reinfection, and (iii) repeat exposure associated with reinfection. Risk factors contributing to each of these categories are detailed below and outlined in **Table 2** (adapted from Trinh et al. [3]).

7.1. Treatment response: relapse

7.1.1. Treatment regimen, adherence, and drug resistance

Incomplete bacteriologic cure, which is usually caused by irregular medication intake, is the most common cause of relapse. Inadequate treatment regimens, poor treatment adherence, and unrecognized drug resistance have been cited as risk factors for relapse TB infection. Regimens with low bactericidal potency, inadequate treatment duration, inappropriate drug choice, and undetected drug resistance all contribute to treatment failure and relapse disease. The use of standardized regimens in the absence of full drug susceptibility testing contributes to inadequate regimen choice and further impacts on the development of drug resistance and relapse [3, 6, 60]. Earlier studies reporting on the association between inadequate treatment regimen and risk for recurrent TB cited the use of thiacetazone-containing regimens. Thiacetazone is an antitubercular drug that was used widely in combination with isoniazid for the treatment of TB. This agent has since been replaced by the widespread use of standardized

TB recurrence risk		
Treatment response: relapse	**Individual vulnerability: relapse or reinfection**	**Repeat exposure: reinfection**
1. Treatment regimen • Inadequate treatment • Undetected drug resistance 2. Treatment adherence • Poor compliance • Drug shortage 3. Drug PK/PD* and pharmacogenomic determinants • Poor drug penetration • Variable PK values • Genetic mutations that alter drug metabolizing enzymes	1. Individual Vulnerability • HIV infection (CD4 count) • Previous TB disease and residual lung damage • Greater area of lung tissue involved • Positive sputum culture at 2 months of treatment • Diabetes Mellitus • Extremes of Age • Vulnerable groups and social risk factors • Infection with strains that have an increased propensity for drug resistance 2. Reduced local defenses • Cigarette smoking • Air pollution • Silicoses • Chronic lung disease	1. Epidemic control • High TB prevalence 2. Infection control • Clinics/hospitals/prisons • Public transport • Places of socialization 3. TB contacts • Household contacts • Social or work contacts • Overcrowding or poor living conditions

*PK = pharmacokinetics; PD = pharmacodynamics.

Table 2. Risk factors for TB recurrence, adapted from Trinh et al. [3].

regimens containing rifampicin [21, 61]. Poor treatment adherence has also been reported to drive the development of drug resistance and thus relapse. Poor adherence to anti-TB treatment is associated with increased treatment duration, complex multidrug regimens, as well as social risk factors. Other issues linked to regimen choice and adherence include substandard drug quality and drug stock outs, and these are associated with poorly resourced, high TB-endemic countries [3]. Recurrent TB is also associated with an increased risk of developing drug resistance. Studies have reported an increase in acquired rifamycin-resistant TB in patients that received rifamycin-based directly observed therapy. In both studies, the key risk factor for rifamycin-resistance acquisition was HIV coinfection with advanced immunosuppression. In a cohort of 93 relapse patients with no prior evidence of MDR-TB, Chiang et al. reported that the prevalence of overall drug resistance was 33.3% and the prevalence of MDR-TB in the relapse patients was 12.9% [62]. Similarly, Sun et al. reported higher rate of TB recurrence in MDR-TB patients. In a cohort of 100 MDR and 150 non-MDR TB patients, recurrence rates of 65/1000 and 35/1000 person-years, respectively, were reported. The increased prevalence of drug resistance in relapse patients is exacerbated by the inefficacy of standardized retreatment regimens and underscores the need for increased MDR-TB case detection for retreatment patients [12].

7.1.2. Drug pharmacodynamics (PD) and pharmacokinetics (PK)

Host-specific factors such as PD, PK, and pharmacogenomics impact on the response to anti-TB treatment. Current anti-TB treatment dosing is based on the patient's body weight [63]. Drug concentrations and pharmacokinetics vary among patients, resulting in adverse reactions due to toxicity as well as suboptimal drug concentrations that impact on the development of drug resistance and relapse. Plasma concentrations of HIV and anti-TB drugs have been reported to display wide interindividual variability associated with genetic mutations in the respective drug-metabolizing enzymes or transporter proteins [64–66].

7.2. Individual vulnerability: relapse and reinfection

7.2.1. Individual vulnerability

7.2.1.1. HIV infection

HIV coinfection has been reported to increase the rate of recurrent TB disease, especially in high TB-endemic settings where TB recurrence rates of up to 24.4% have been reported. A cohort study in Malawi showed that the rates of tuberculosis relapse were similar between HIV-positive and -negative individuals [53]. Similar results were found in a study of South African mineworkers [41]. In contrast, several studies have reported a nearly three-fold higher incidence of recurrent TB among HIV-positive individuals as compared to their negative counterparts. In a review of 32 studies, Panjabi et al. reported excessive rates of recurrent TB following the completion of treatment using standardized regimens. Among the controlled trials included in the review, the overall recurrence rates (per 100,000 person-years) were 3010 (95% confidence interval 2230–3970) and 2290 (95% confidence interval 1730–2940), respectively, at 6 and 12 months following treatment completion. Recurrence rates were reported to be higher for observational studies compared to controlled trials in countries with higher TB incidence rates. In the studies reviewed, recurrence rates were found to be higher among HIV-infected (6.7, 95% confidence interval 5.9–7.6) compared to HIV-uninfected (3.3 95% confidence interval 2.8–3.9) individuals. In the HIV-infected group, recurrent TB was associated with low initial CD4 T-cell count and anti-TB treatment less than 37 weeks of duration. While the association of low initial CD4+ T-cell count and TB recurrence was unclear in this review, the authors reported that small sample sizes lacked sufficient power to detect differences in recurrence rates between patients with high and low CD4+ T-cell counts [5]. An earlier study by Pulido et al. was the only study in the analysis that reported a statistically significant relationship in a multivariate analysis. A complimentary explanation is that patients with severe immunosuppression secondary to HIV die from other causes before TB recurs. Studies also reported that anti-TB treatment for less than 37 weeks was the most influential predictor of TB recurrence. The risk of TB recurrence in patients with low CD4+ T-cell counts was four times higher than that in patients with higher CD4+ T-cell counts. This also highlights that the six-month standard treatment regimen may be suboptimal at preventing recurrent TB in patients with low initial CD4+ T-cell counts [67]. Chaisson et al. reported similar findings in their review of two studies, which compared the rates of recurrent TB among HIV-infected and HIV-uninfected individuals [7]. In an Indian cohort, Narayanan et al. reported higher rates of recurrent TB in HIV-infected individuals compared with the HIV-uninfected group (14% versus 9%). In addition, recurrence due to reinfection was reported in 88% of the HIV-infected group and 9% of the HIV-uninfected group ($p < 0.05$). Among the recurrent isolates, patients from the HIV-infected group were associated with more clustering of strains and increased drug resistance [11].

7.2.1.2. Previous TB disease and residual lung damage

The severity of lung disease indicated by the presence of cavities and, in particular, residual cavities is a significant risk factor for recurrent TB disease. Lung cavities persisting at the end of treatment has been reported as a dominant correlate of recurrent disease in many studies [5]. Sonnenberg et al., in a study of South African mineworkers, found that residual cavitation was a risk factor for tuberculosis relapse [41]. The association between residual cavitation and recurrent disease has been attributed to poor penetration of anti-TB drugs into the cavity walls surrounding fibrotic tissue. It has also been postulated that MTB strains, like other nontuberculous mycobacteria, may have increased propensity for the infection of previously damaged tissue. The relationship between residual lung cavitation with recurrent TB disease warrants further investigation. Future studies should be aimed to assess the number and size of cavities present before and at the end of recurrent TB disease [5].

7.2.1.3. Greater area of lung tissue involved in infection

Several studies have reported that the extent of lung tissue involved in disease was a predictor of recurrent TB disease. However, no standard measure was applied to establish the amount of lung tissue involved in disease, and thus measures of lung area varied between studies [5]. Mallory et al. divided lung tissue into three areas, recording the number of zones with lesions. The authors report a dose–response association between the number of lung zones with fibrosis and the likelihood of recurrence to strongly suggestive of a relationship [68]. Tam et al. scored lung involvement by combining the total area of lung tissue with lesions [69].

7.2.1.4. Positive sputum culture at 2 months of treatment

Numerous studies reflect evidence in support of a positive sputum bacteriologic status during anti-TB treatment and recurrent TB disease. These findings suggest that a positive sputum culture at 2 months of treatment is predictive of recurrence. This association has been attributed to an inadequate response to the intensive phase of anti-TB treatment [5]. Horne et al. conducted a systematic review and meta-analysis to assess the accuracy of positive sputum smear or culture for predicting treatment failure or relapse in pulmonary TB. The authors demonstrated that both sputum smear and culture during tuberculosis treatment have low sensitivity and modest specificity for predicting failure and relapse. Although the study represented a diverse group of patients, the individual studies had similar performance characteristics [70]. Gillepsie et al. reiterated the poor predictability of culture conversion for long-term outcomes. While two-month culture conversion is associated with relapse-free cure, this correlation is not strong enough to reliably predict outcomes for individual patients or definitively guide the selection of regimen in drug development [71].

7.2.1.5. Diabetes mellitus

Diabetes mellitus (DM) is recognized as a risk factor for the reactivation of TB infection and relapse infection following the completion of treatment. Diabetics have been reported to have three times higher risk of developing pulmonary TB compared to nondiabetics [72, 73]. Numerous studies have reported that DM coinfection adversely affects TB treatment outcomes, which included treatment failure, death, and relapse. In addition to the interaction between DM and TB, the high reported prevalence of DM in MDR-TB is alarming, with approximately 10–23% of MDR-TB patients having DM. A proposed hypothesis for this association is that altered immunity accompanied with DM has an effect on MDR-TB transmission, as with other immunodeficiency disease. A recent systematic review aimed to quantitatively evaluate the propensity for patients with DM and TB to cluster according to the genotype of the infected MTB strain. While the meta-analysis failed to show an association between TB transmission patterns in DM patients, among the 4076 patients analyzed, 13% had DM with 27% of these patient isolates displaying clustering. Further work is needed to address this phenomenon. These factors highlight the need for continual monitoring of DM patients who complete treatment for incident TB and possible use of secondary isoniazid prophylaxis treatment. In addition, comanagement for DM-TB patients will be significant in reducing relapse in these patients [74].

7.2.1.6. Extremes of age

Young adults (15–44 years) have been reported to have the highest risk for recurrent disease [75]. Children under 15 years and adults over 65 years have a lower risk compared to young adults. Age is linked to default on treatment; however, no particular age has been singled out in association with recurrence [21]. It is postulated that children have lower bacterial load as well as increased supervision and attention to care, indicated by higher rates of treatment completion. There are limited data available on recurrence in children. Scaaf et al. reported 11 recurrences of TB disease in a cohort of 87 children. Of the eighty-seven children described in the study, nine had a second episode of TB, and two of which had a third episode of confirmed TB. Full epidemiological profiling could not be conducted, as clinical isolates representing the first episode of TB were not available for five of the cases [48].

7.2.1.7. Vulnerable groups and social risk factors

Vulnerable groups with increased susceptibility to TB infection and recurrent TB include HIV-coinfected patients, children, health care workers (HCWs), prisoners, homeless persons, drug users, and close contacts of TB patients. HIV coinfection, discussed above, is associated with high rates of recurrent TB. Children contribute a significant proportion of the TB disease burden and suffer severe tuberculosis-related morbidity and mortality, particularly in endemic areas. HCWs are placed at a higher risk for the acquisition of nosocomially acquired TB. Risk factors include poor or malfunctioning infection control measures and poor utilization of personal protective equipment. There is also a significant risk of secondary hospital outbreaks related to undetected and untreated TB. Prisoners, homeless persons, and drug users are at higher risk for TB and recurrent infections as they represent underserved populations. These populations are also more likely to be coinfected with HIV and are more difficult to manage and treat adherently. Imprisonment has been recognized as a significant risk factor for TB transmission. Household contacts of TB patients have been reported to be at high risk for developing TB, including drug-resistant TB. Preventative therapy remains the most significant tool to reduce the risk of TB infection among high-risk individuals [3, 79].

7.2.1.8. Infection with certain strain types

Infection with strains of the Beijing genotype has been associated with unfavorable TB outcomes. The Beijing genotype has gained particular attention due to reports on its association with drug-resistant TB in outbreaks and population-based studies [3]. Huyen et al. demonstrated that the Beijing genotype was associated with an increased rate of relapse in Vietnam. Among a cohort of 1068 patients that were followed up for 18 months, 23 cases of relapse occurred, linked to this genotype [83]. Nguyen et al. reported similar findings for the same settings. However, this strain type has been reported to account for 40% of TB cases in Vietnam, and this may represent high transmission rates rather than the success of the strain [84].

7.2.2. Reduced local defenses

7.2.2.1. Tobacco smoking

A systematic review by Lin et al. demonstrated that tobacco smoke is consistently associated with increased risk of TB infection. In comparison to nonsmokers, smoking increases the risk of developing active TB and mortality. Smoking has been reported to affect baseline severity, bacteriologic response, treatment outcome, and relapse in TB. Smoking has also been reported to alter the lung immune responses to MTB, contributing to a higher susceptibility to individual TB infection. Chronic exposure to tobacco and air pollutants impairs the normal clearance of secretions on the bronchial mucosal surface and may allow MTB to evade the early host immune defenses. Smoke also inhibits the activity of alveolar macrophages by reducing the phagocytic ability of the cells. Lower levels of pro-inflammatory cytokines have also been reported for smokers [76]. Leung et al. evaluated the impact of smoking on TB outcomes by monitoring 16,435 patients receiving anti-TB treatment at chest clinics in Hong Kong. Overall, 16.7% of negative treatment outcomes were attributed to smokers, with the key contributor being default and death in smokers. Among 13,349 patients who were successfully treated for TB, 426 cases of relapse were detected. They reported a clear gradient (hazard ratios of 1.00, 1.33, and 1.63) of relapse risk from nonsmokers to previous smokers and current smokers, with an overall population attributable risk of 19.4% (current smokers: 12.2%; previous smokers: 7.2%) [77].

7.2.2.2. Air pollution

In addition to tobacco smoke, environmental exposures have been associated with an increased risk for developing TB. Air quality, which is impacted by atmospheric pollution and carbon monoxide, has been reported to induce bacillary reactivation and to increase the incidence of TB [76]. De Castro Fernandes et al. reported that air pollution was directly related to TB incidence in Brazil. Other studies conducted in the US and Russia also reported a link between the concentration of smoke, suspended particulate matter, and TB in relation to carbon dioxide and nitric oxide levels. Air pollution generated by traffic in Taiwan, linked to sulfur dioxide, ozone, and carbon monoxide, was linked to culture-confirmed TB. Similarly, a study conducted in South Korea revealed that exposure to sulfur dioxide increased the risk of TB by 7%. Indoor air pollution, resulting from the use of solid fuels for cooking, has been recognized as a risk factor for TB disease. The role of these factors in recurrent TB requires further study [78].

7.2.2.3. Chronic lung disease

Chronic lung diseases, including chronic obstructive pulmonary disease (COPD), asthma, and interstitial lung diseases such as silicosis, have been recognized as risk factors for the development of tuberculosis. Studies have demonstrated that 25–30% of silicosis patients develop TB with a relative risk for TB of 2.8 in silicosis patients when compared to the general population. However, there are limited data on the role of chronic lung disease in recurrent TB [79]. Pettit et al. reported an increased risk of TB recurrence with chronic lung disease (OR 5.28, 95% CI 1.16–2404, $P = 0.03$). However, a major limitation of the study was the low recurrence rate in the cohort, as the study was conducted in a low TB-incidence setting. Conversely, reports now suggest that a history of TB may lead to chronic lung disease, particularly COPD and bronchiectasis [80]. A recent systematic review by Byrne et al. reported a strong and consistent positive association between a history of TB and the presence of chronic respiratory diseases, including COPD and bronchiectasis. This suggests that the development of chronic lung disease following TB increases the risk of recurrent TB infection. In addition, tobacco smoking is an attributable risk factor for the development of COPD and thus may be a link in the development of TB and recurrent TB [80].

7.3. Repeat exposure: reinfection

7.3.1. Epidemic control, infection control, and close TB contacts

On a public health level, recurrent tuberculosis accounts for a considerable proportion of TB cases in weak TB control programs and contributes to ongoing transmission of infection to close contacts in the home environment, community, and health care facilities. In high-incidence settings, recurrence has been attributed mainly to reinfection, with up to 75% of cases being attributed to reinfection. Reinfection represents a constant risk over time in patients with a history of TB. High reinfection rates have important implications for TB control strategies and underscore the need to reduce transmission in the community and the urgent need for rapid diagnosis and treatment of TB [3, 7, 8]. Coupled with comorbidities such HIV and diabetes that result in reduced immunity, such populations become more susceptible to infection and reinfection [5, 74]. Recent studies have indicated that transmission events are most likely to occur with the community and not within the household. A recent report on an XDR-TB cohort in South Africa demonstrated that 19% of patients that were discharged were linked to secondary case of TB [81]. Shah et al. reported that XDR-TB in the KwaZulu-Natal province of South Africa was linked to transmission of disease as opposed to inadequate drug treatment for MDR-TB. The authors demonstrated person-to-person and hospital-based epidemiological links [82]. Taken together, these studies highlight that epidemic control requires an increased focus on interrupting transmission and the need to establish community-based containment strategies, including voluntary long-term community stay facilities and palliative care in tuberculosis-endemic settings [81, 82].

8. Immunopathogenesis of recurrent TB

MTB has evolved with the human host over decades and has successfully evaded natural immune defenses, progressing to a stage of relative dormancy. Successful control of the TB epidemic would be best achieved with an effective preventative vaccine; however, the incomplete understanding of natural correlates of protection that an effective vaccine should emulate has hampered vaccine development. The continuum of the host-pathogen interaction following MTB infection to TB disease extends across the innate immune, adaptive immune, and quiescent and active replicating phases of infection. In approximately 5% of patients, this cycle extends beyond successful treatment completion when the cycle of TB recurrence may occur. In this subset of patients, persistence of MTB results in relapse, whereas in others, reinfection with MTB results in subsequent disease. Biomarkers indicative of the spectrum of TB disease have been described; however, there are limited reports on biomarkers of recurrent TB [85]. The matter of whether or not the first episode of TB imparts some measure of immunity has not been explicitly established but is assumed to have an impact [86].

Thobakgale et al. conducted a study in a cohort of HIV-coinfected patients with a history of previous successful TB treatment, which aimed to identify innate immune correlates associated with TB recurrence. Production of interleukin-1 (IL-1) beta by innate immune cells following ex-vivo stimulation with Toll-like receptor (TLR) and Bacillus Calmette-Guérin (BCG) stimulants correlated with differential TB recurrence outcomes. Elevated IL-1 beta production by monocytes following TLR stimulation was protective against TB recurrence. In contrast, production of IL-1 beta by monocytes and myeloid dendritic cells following stimulation with BCG was associated with an increased risk for recurrent TB. These findings highlight significant differences in the host immune response to TB and require validation in larger cohort of patients [87]. Sivro et al. studied the role of plasma cytokine correlates of TB recurrence in a cohort of HIV-coinfected patients with a history of previous successful TB treatment. The study reported higher levels of plasma levels of interleukin-6 (IL-6), IL-1 beta, and soluble IL-1 receptor antagonist were associated with increased risk of TB recurrence, while plasma interferon beta levels decreased the risk of TB recurrence. These findings highlight that the markers of systemic inflammation, which are also involved in the rapid progression of HIV, predict TB recurrence in HIV-coinfected patients [88].

Gene expression profiling of ex-vivo whole blood specimens has demonstrated transcriptomic changes in patients with recurrent TB as compared to healthy counterparts, including significant changes in gene expression during successful treatment. Mistry et al. identified a gene signature that identified a set of genes in patients with recurrent TB that clearly distinguished this group from patients who remained cured [89]. Cliff et al. reported on the expression of 668 genes in patients who experience recurrent TB in comparison to those who remained cured, with the differences lasting up to 4 weeks following TB diagnosis. The upregulated genes were involved in cytotoxic cell-mediated killing. These findings suggest that patients who subsequently relapse exhibit altered immune responses, including robust cytolytic responses to MTB *in vitro* at diagnosis, compared to patients who achieved cure [90]. Thompson et al. reported on several clinically significant host-blood RNA signatures that predicted TB treatment outcomes, stratifying patients according to their risk of treatment failure. The signature correlated with pulmonary inflammatory states measured by PET-CT scanning and can complement current sputum-based testing methods for a rapid and accurate alternate testing method [91].

De Steenwinkel et al. reported on the differences between primary and recurrent TB in relation to changes in mycobacterial load in infected organs, immunopathology, and plasma cytokine levels using a murine model. In comparison to primary TB, recurrent TB was associated with lower mycobacterial load in the lung, spleen, and liver. Significantly lower levels of tumor necrosis factor-alpha, interferon-alpha, IL-6, MIG/CXCL9, IP-10/CXCL10, and IL-17 were observed for recurrent TB. In addition, memory Th-1 cells were locally and systemically expanded and congregated in the lung during recurrent TB, promoting efficient control of MTB growth [92].

9. Treatment of recurrent TB

Current WHO guidelines advocate the use of the standard six-month TB treatment regimen for all new and retreatment drug-susceptible TB cases. This regimen comprises a two-month intensive treatment of isoniazid, rifampicin, pyrazinamide, and ethambutol, followed by a four-month continuation phase of isoniazid and rifampicin. They further recommend the use of rapid molecular-based drug susceptibility testing (DST) to guide regimen choice for all retreatment TB patients. However, in settings where rapid DSTs are not available, empiric treatment is advised based on the following recommendations. Patients with a high likelihood of MDR-TB should be initiated on an empiric MDR-TB regimen using clinical discretion or if the patients have relapsed or defaulted on treatment after a second or subsequent course of treatment. The second recommendation is a retreatment regimen of 2 months of isoniazid, rifampicin, pyrazinamide, ethambutol, and streptomycin, followed by 1 month of isoniazid, rifampicin, pyrazinamide, and ethambutol and finally 5 months of isoniazid, rifampicin, and ethambutol [93].

It is well recognized by many that a stratified medicine approach would be a desirable approach for the retreatment of TB. However, the challenge associated with a stratified medicine approach is in identifying groups that are eligible for a longer treatment regimen [94, 95]. There are many identifiable risk factors associated with recurrence, such as a baseline cavitation and month-two smear status that may indicate the need for increasing treatment duration. However, the recent REMoxTB and RIFQUIN studies, which evaluated new regimens aimed at shortening treatment duration for drug-susceptible TB, reported a relapse risk of 2.8 and 3.2%, respectively, with an 18-month follow-up period [96]. Among the factors attributed to poor success of the new regimens in the REMoxTB study, it was suggested that baseline cavitation modified the differences between the results. In contrast, 91% (n = 386) of the patients on the standard 6-month regimen with baseline cavitation had a favorable outcome at the end of the follow-up period [71]. A systematic review by Menzies et al. related to treatment outcomes of rifampicin-containing regimens of various durations showed only a modest benefit in regimens given for nine or more months in comparison to the standard six-month treatment. Thus, the benefit of a stratified treatment approach remains debatable [97].

In the context of recurrence due to relapse or reinfection disease, a different treatment approach is required. In the case of reinfection, this can be considered as a new primary infection, and thus, standard regimens may be effective. In contrast, relapse is associated with an increased risk of drug resistance due to the persistence of the original infecting strain under suboptimal treatment. Collectively, all the factors mentioned here underscore the significance an individualized treatment approach guided by DST [92, 93].

10. Preventative therapy for recurrent TB

Active TB disease has been shown to be preventable by the use of primary preventative therapy (pPT), which aims to prevent the first episode of TB in individuals in whom active TB has been excluded. The average preventative effect of pPT in HIV-uninfected individuals is a 60% reduction in the incidence of recurrent TB, while in HIV-infected individuals, the average effect is a 30% reduction in recurrent TB [98, 99]. A potential approach to prevent recurrent TB is secondary preventative therapy (sPT), by continuing the use of anti-TB therapy following completion of treatment for TB. sPT aims to reduce the incidence of recurrent TB in TB patients who have completed treatment for their most recent episode of TB [100]. The World Health Organization (WHO) recommends the use of isoniazid preventative therapy (IPT) in patients with HIV infection.

The TEMPRANO (trial of early antiretrovirals and isoniazid preventative therapy in Africa) study demonstrated that the use of 6 months of IPT combined with early antiretroviral therapy reduced the risk of severe HIV-related comorbidities by 44% and all-cause mortality by 33% [101]. Kabali et al. reported reduced mortality in tuberculin skin test (TST)-positive patients with CD4+ T-cell counts >200 cells/mm^3 in a Tanzanian cohort [102]. Charalambous et al. demonstrated a 49% reduction in mortality that remained significant even in patients who had a past history of TB. However, in high-burden countries and in TST-positive patients, a 36-month course of IPT has been recommended. The 36-month IPT course demonstrated a 74%

reduced risk of active TB and 68% reduction in mortality compared to the 6-month course [103]. The REMEMBER (reducing early mortality and early morbidity by empirical tuberculosis treatment regimens) study aimed to assess whether empirical TB treatment will reduce early mortality compared with IPT in patients with advanced HIV disease initiating antiretroviral therapy. Overall, empirical TB therapy did not reduce early mortality compared to IPT. However, the low mortality rate in the study underscores the need for TB screening and IPT in patients with HIV [104].

In their review of four studies, Bruin et al. reported the effect of sPT for the prevention of recurrent TB in HIV-infected individuals and the context in which the preventative approach may be applied. All four studies reported that sPT decreased incidence of recurrent TB in comparison to nontreatment groups. Relative reductions varied from 55.0 to 82.1%. However, only one of the four studies reported a significant effect on overall survival [100]. Perriens et al. described the use of isoniazid (INH) and rifampicin (RIF) twice weekly for an additional 6 months in comparison to a placebo. Patients receiving sPT were reported to be significantly less likely to develop recurrent TB compared to the placebo group (relative risk 0.21, $p < 0.01$) [105]. Haller et al. assessed the effectiveness of INH and sulphadoxine-pyrimethamine as sPT. The relative rate for the incidence of recurrent TB in patients receiving additional treatment ($n = 134$) and those not ($n = 129$) was 0.30 (95% confidence interval: 0.09–0.94) [106]. Fitzgerald et al. assessed the use of INH for an additional year following the completion of initial treatment compared to a placebo group. The intervention significantly reduced the incidence of recurrent TB from 7.8 per 100 person-years to 1.4 per 100 person-years (relative risk 0.18, confidence interval: 0.04–0.83) [107]. Churchyard et al. assessed the effect of INH in combination with cotrimoxazole versus cotrimoxazole only or no intervention in HIV-infected gold miners in South Africa. The rate ration for the development of recurrent TB in comparing the groups with INH and the group without INH was 0.45 (95% confidence interval: 0.26–0.78) [108]. As with pPT, the ideal duration and drug choice remain unclear. In all four studies, the duration of treatment varied from 6 to 24 months. The duration of effectiveness of sPT could not be assessed due to the short follow-up periods of the studies. None of the studies included made a distinction between relapse and reinfection as the mechanism of recurrent TB. Furthermore, Haller et al. and Fitzgerald et al. diagnosed recurrent TB by clinical assessment only, which could indicate overestimation of recurrent TB [106, 107].

11. Conclusion and future perspectives

Recurrent TB poses a major threat to TB control programs, especially given the persistent vulnerability of HIV-infected patients to tuberculosis, and the higher propensity of recurrent disease being due to resistant MTB strains. In the absence of large-scale population-based surveillance reports, the overall rate of recurrent TB following completion of treatment is significantly underestimated. Current estimates are based on a combination of randomized controlled trials and observational studies, with reliability estimates of the former limited by study follow-up time, and the latter prominently demonstrating higher rates of recurrence. Under clinical trial conditions, adherence rates are better; treatment facilities are more accessible and incorporate adequate follow-up after treatment, leading to improved treatment outcomes and lower rates of recurrence. In contrast, observational studies reflect the operating environment of most high-burden TB facilities.

Distinguishing between relapse and reinfection is of paramount importance in addressing the burden of recurrent TB disease. High rates of relapse demand renewed interventions to improve individual patient care while high rates of reinfection demand improved infection and epidemic control measures. Urgent attention is required to address challenges of adherence, such as social and health care worker support systems and step-down management facilities. With the heightened risk or recurrent TB in HIV, TB screening should be conducted at all ART follow-up visits, and TB preventative therapy should be implemented in all HIV-positive patients completing TB treatment. Enhanced infection control strategies should be implemented in clinical and community settings to reduce ongoing transmission of TB. There has been considerable disparity in the studies reporting on the role of relapse versus reinfection. Further large-scale studies are required to address the role of relapse and reinfection as well as the role of mixed infections in recurrent TB.

This review highlights well-established principles in TB control. TB recurrence rates are grossly underestimated and are highest in those with extensive pulmonary disease and cavitary disease and in those with comorbidities such as HIV infection and diabetes. Active case findings among these patients within 12 months of completing treatment would enable early detection of TB recurrence. Enhanced treatment options, such as intensified initial treatment, extension of treatment, and secondary preventative therapy for patients presenting with multiple risk factors will prevent recurrent TB infection. Understanding the immunological correlates that offer protection against recurrent TB will also play a role in host-directed therapy and reducing recurrent TB.

Author details

Kogieleum Naidoo[1,2]* and Navisha Dookie[1]

*Address all correspondence to: kogie.naidoo@caprisa.org

1 Centre for the AIDS Programme of Research in South Africa (CAPRISA), University of KwaZulu-Natal, Durban, South Africa

2 South African Medical Research Council (SAMRC) – CAPRISA HIV-TB Pathogenesis and Treatment Research Unit, Durban, South Africa

References

[1] World Health Organization. Global Tuberculosis Report. 2017 [cited Nov 30, 2017]. Available from: http://www.who.int/tb/publications/global_report/en/

[2] Kwan CK, Ernst JD. HIV and tuberculosis: A deadly human syndemic. Clinical Microbiology Reviews. 2011;**24**(2):351-376. DOI: 10.1128/CMR.00042-10

[3] Trinh QM, Nguyen HL, Nguyen VN, et al. Tuberculosis and HIV co-infection-focus on the Asia-Pacific region. International Journal of Infectious Diseases. 2015;**32**:170-178. DOI: 10.1016/j.ijid.2014.11.023

[4] Mathema B, Kurepina NE, Bifani PJ, et al. Molecular epidemiology of tuberculosis: Current insights. Clinical Microbiology Reviews. 2006;**19**(4):658-685. DOI: 10.1128/CMR.00061-05

[5] Panjabi R, Comstock GW, Recurrent GJE. Tuberculosis and its risk factors: Adequately treated patients are still at high risk. The International Journal of Tuberculosis and Lung Disease. 2007;**11**(8):828-837

[6] Lambert ML, Hasker E, Van Deun A, et al. Recurrence in tuberculosis: Relapse or reinfection? The Lancet Infectious Diseases. 2003;**3**:282-287

[7] Chaisson RE, Churchyard GJ. Recurrent tuberculosis: Relapse, reinfection, and HIV. The Journal of Infectious Diseases. 2010;**201**(5):653-655

[8] Guerra-Assunção JA, Houben RMGJ, Crampin AC, et al. Recurrence due to relapse or reinfection with *Mycobacterium tuberculosis*: A whole-genome sequencing approach in a large, population-based cohort with a high HIV infection prevalence and active follow-up. The Journal of Infectious Diseases. 2015;**211**(7):1154-1163

[9] Glynn JR, Murray J, Bester A, et al. High rates of recurrence in HIV-infected and HIV-uninfected patients with tuberculosis. The Journal of Infectious Diseases. 2010;**201**(5):704-711

[10] Charalambous S, Grant AD, Moloi V, et al. Contribution of reinfection to recurrent tuberculosis in South African gold miners. The International Journal of Tuberculosis and Lung Disease. 2008;**12**:942-948

[11] Narayanan S, Swaminathan S, Supply P, et al. Impact of HIV infection on the recurrence of tuberculosis in South India. The Journal of Infectious Diseases. 2010;**201**:691-703

[12] Sun Y, Harley D, Vally H, et al. Impact of multidrug resistance on tuberculosis recurrence and long-term outcome in China. PLoS. 2017;**12**(1):e0168865

[13] Luzze H, Johnson DF, Dickman K, et al. Relapse more common than reinfection in recurrent tuberculosis 1–2 years post treatment in urban Uganda. The International Journal of Tuberculosis and Lung Disease. 2013;**17**(3):361-367

[14] Vree M, Huong NT, Duong BD, et al. Survival and relapse rate of tuberculosis patients who successfully completed treatment in Vietnam. The International Journal of Tuberculosis and Lung Disease. 2007;**11**(4):392-397

[15] Datiko DG, Lindtjørn B, et al. Tuberculosis recurrence in smear-positive patients cured under DOTS in Southern Ethiopia: Retrospective cohort study. BMC Public Health. 2009;**9**(348)

[16] Moosazadeh M, Bahrampour A, Nasehi M, et al. The incidence of recurrence of tuberculosis and its related factors in smear-positive pulmonary tuberculosis patients in Iran: A retrospective cohort study. Lung India. 2015;**32**(6):557-560

[17] Crofts JP, Andrews NJ, Barker RD, et al. Risk factors for recurrent tuberculosis in England and Wales, 1998–2005. Thorax. 2010;**65**:310-314

[18] Achkar JM, Jenny-Avital ER. Incipient and subclinical tuberculosis: Defining early disease states in the context of host immune response. The Journal of Infectious Diseases. 2011;**204**(4):S1179-S1186

[19] World Health Organization. Definitions and reporting framework for tuberculosis – 2013 revision. 2013 [cited Sep 4, 2017]. Available from: http://apps.who.int/iris/bitstream/10665/79199/1/9789241505345_eng.pdf

[20] Gan M, Liu Q, Yang C, et al. Deep whole-genome sequencing to detect mixed infection of *Mycobacterium tuberculosis*. PLoS One. 2016;**11**:e0159029

[21] Akpabio US. A description of patients with recurrence of pulmonary tuberculosis in TB hospital, Ermelo [dissertation]. University of Stellenbosch; 2009

[22] Heemskerk D, Caws M, Marais B, et al. Tuberculosis in Adults and Children. London: Springer; 2015. Available from: https://www.ncbi.nlm.nih.gov/books/NBK344402/ DOI: 10.1007/978-3-319-19132-4

[23] Ei PW, Aung WW, Lee JS, et al. Molecular strain typing of mycobacterium tuberculosis: A review of frequently used methods. Journal of Korean Medical Science. 2016;**31**:1673-1683

[24] Bryant JM, Harris SR, Parkhill J, et al. Whole-genome sequencing to establish relapse or re-infection with *Mycobacterium tuberculosis*: A retrospective observational study. The Lancet Respiratory Medicine. 2013;**1**:786-792

[25] Roetzer A, Diel R, Kohl TA, et al. Whole genome sequencing versus traditional genotyping for investigation of mycobacterium tuberculosis outbreak: A longitudinal molecular epidemiological study. PLoS Medicine. 2013;**10**:e1001387

[26] Cave M, Eisenach KD, Templeton G, et al. Stability of DNA fingerprint pattern produced with IS6110 in strains of *Mycobacterium tuberculosis*. Journal of Clinical Microbiology. 1994;**32**:262-266

[27] Warren RM, Victor TC, Streicher EM, et al. Patients with active tuberculosis often have different strains in the same sputum specimen. American Journal of Respiratory and Critical Care Medicine. 2004;**169**:610-614

[28] Van Embden JD, Cave MD, Crawford JT, et al. Strain identification of mycobacterium tuberculosis by DNA fingerprinting: Recommendations for a standardized methodology. Journal of Clinical Microbiology. 1993;**31**:406-409

[29] Hawken M, Nunn P, Gathua S, et al. Increased recurrence of tuberculosis in HIV-1-infected patients in Kenya. Lancet. 1993;**342**:332-337

[30] Das S, Chan SL, Allen BW, et al. Application of DNA fingerprinting with IS986 to sequential mycobacterial isolates obtained from pulmonary tuberculosis patients in Hong Kong before, during and after short-course chemotherapy. Tubercle and Lung Disease. 1993;**74**:47-51

[31] Godfrey-Faussett P, Githui W, Batchelor B, et al. Recurrence of HIV-related tuberculosis in an endemic area may be due to relapse or reinfection. Tubercle and Lung Disease. 1994;**75**:199-202

[32] Das S, Paramasivan CN, Lowrie DB, et al. IS6100 restriction fragment length polymorphism typing of clinical isolates of *Mycobacterium tuberculosis* from patients with pulmonary tuberculosis in Madras, South India. Tubercle and Lung Disease. 1995;**76**:550-554

[33] Sahadevan R, Narayanan S, Paramasivan CN, et al. Restriction fragment length polymorphism typing of clinical isolates of *Mycobacterium tuberculosis* from patients with pulmonary tuberculosis in Madras, India, by use of direct-repeat probe. Journal of Clinical Microbiology. 1995;**33**:3037-3039

[34] El Sadr WM, Perlman DC, Matts JP, et al. Evaluation of an intensive intermittent-induction regimen and duration of short-course treatment for human immunodeficiency virus-related pulmonary tuberculosis. Terry Beirn Community Programs for Clinical Research on AIDS (CPCRA) and the AIDS Clinical Trials Group (ACTG). Clinical Infectious Diseases. 1998;**26**:1148-1158

[35] Vernon A, Burman W, Benator D, et al. Acquired rifamycin mono-resistance in patients with HIV-related tuberculosis treated with once-weekly rifapentine and isoniazid. Tuberculosis Trials Consortium. Lancet. 1999;**353**:1843-1847

[36] Van Rie A, Warren R, Richardson M, et al. Exogenous reinfection as a cause of recurrent tuberculosis after curative treatment. The New England Journal of Medicine. 1999;**341**: 1174-1179

[37] Johnson JL, Okwera A, Nsubuga P, et al. Efficacy of an unsupervised 8-month rifampicin-containing regimen for the treatment of pulmonary tuberculosis in HIV-infected adults. Uganda-Case Western Reserve University Research Collaboration. The International Journal of Tuberculosis and Lung Disease. 2000;**4**:1032-1040

[38] Lourenco MC, Grinsztejn B, Fandinho-montes FC, et al. Genotypic patterns of multiple isolates of *M. tuberculosis* from tuberculous HIV patients. Tropical Medicine & International Health. 2000;**5**:488-494

[39] Caminero JA, Pena MJ, Campos-Herrero MI, et al. Exogenous reinfection with tuberculosis on a European island with a moderate incidence of disease. American Journal of Respiratory and Critical Care Medicine. 2001;**163**:717-720

[40] Bandera A, Gori A, Catozzi L, et al. Molecular epidemiology study of exogenous reinfection in an area with a low incidence of tuberculosis. Journal of Clinical Microbiology. 2001;**39**:2213-2218

[41] Sonnenberg P, Murray J, Glynn JR, et al. HIV-1 and recurrence, relapse, and reinfection of tuberculosis after cure: A cohort study in South African mineworkers. Lancet. 2001; **358**(9294):1687-1693

[42] Garcia de Viedma D, Marin M, Hernangomez S, et al. Tuberculosis recurrences: Reinfection plays a role in a population whose clinical/epidemiological characteristics do not favor reinfection. Archives of Internal Medicine. 2002;**162**:1873-1879

[43] Fitzpatrick LK, Okwera A, Mugerwa R, et al. An investigation of suspected exogenous reinfection in tuberculosis patients in Kampala, Uganda. The International Journal of Tuberculosis and Lung Disease. 2002;**6**:550-552

[44] Lan NT, Lien HT, Tung Le B, et al. *Mycobacterium tuberculosis* Beijing genotype and risk for treatment failure and relapse, Vietnam. Emerging Infectious Diseases. 2003;**9**: 1633-1635

[45] El Sahly HM, Wright JA, Soini H, et al. Recurrent tuberculosis in Houston, Texas: A population-based study. The International Journal of Tuberculosis and Lung Disease. 2004;**8**:333-340

[46] Jasmer RM, Bozeman L, Schwartzman K, et al. Recurrent tuberculosis in the United States and Canada: Relapse or reinfection? American Journal of Respiratory and Critical Care Medicine. 2004;**170**:1360-1366

[47] Verver S, Warren RM, Beyers N, et al. Rate of reinfection tuberculosis after successful treatment is higher than rate of new tuberculosis. American Journal of Respiratory and Critical Care Medicine. 2005;**171**:1430-1435

[48] Schaaf HS, Krook S, Hollemans DW, et al. Recurrent culture-confirmed tuberculosis in human immunodeficiency virus-infected children. Pediatric Infectious Disease. 2005; **24**(8):685-691

[49] Shen G, Xue Z, Shen X, et al. Recurrent tuberculosis and exogenous reinfection, Shangai, China. Emerging Infectious Diseases. 2006;**12**(11):1776-1778

[50] Cacho J, Pérez Meixeira A, Cano I, et al. Recurrent tuberculosis from 1992 to 2004 in a metropolitan area. The European Respiratory Journal. 2007;**30**(2):333-337

[51] Bang D, Andersen AB, Thomsen VO, et al. Recurrent tuberculosis in Denmark: Relapse vs. re-infection. The International Journal of Tuberculosis and Lung Disease. 2010;**14**(4): 447-453

[52] Marx FM, Dunbar R, Enarson DA, et al. The temporal dynamics of relapse and reinfection tuberculosis after successful treatment: A retrospective cohort study. Clinical Infectious Diseases. 2014;**58**(12):1676-1683

[53] Crampin AC, Mwaungulu JN, Mwaungulu FD, et al. Recurrent TB: Relapse or reinfection? The effect of HIV in a general population cohort in Malawi. Acquired Immune Deficiency Syndrome. 2010;**24**(3):417-426

[54] Varghese B, al-Omari R, Grimshaw C, et al. Endogenous reactivation followed by exogenous re-infection with drug resistant strains, a new challenge for tuberculosis control in Saudi Arabia. Tuberculosis. 2013;**93**(2):246-249

[55] Interrante JD, Haddad MB, Kim L, et al. Exogenous reinfection as a cause of late recurrent tuberculosis in the United States. Annals of the American Thoracic Society. 2015;**12**(11): 1619-1626

[56] Schiroli C, Carugati M, Zanini F, et al. Exogenous reinfection of tuberculosis in a low-burden area. Infection. 2015;**43**(6):647-653

[57] Korhonen V, Smit PW, Haanperä M, et al. Whole genome analysis of *Mycobacterium tuberculosis* isolates from recurrent episodes of tuberculosis, Finland, 1995–2013. Clinical Microbiology and Infection. 2016;**22**(6):549-554

[58] Shen X, Yang C, Wu J, et al. Recurrent tuberculosis in an urban area in China: Relapse or exogenous reinfection? Tuberculosis. 2017;**103**:97-104

[59] Witney AA, Bateson AL, Jindani A, et al. Use of whole-genome sequencing to distinguish relapse from reinfection in a completed tuberculosis clinical trial. BMC Medicine. 2017;**15**(1):71

[60] Picon PD, Basanesi SL, Caramori MLA, et al. Risk factors for recurrence in tuberculosis. Jornal Brasileiro de Pneumologia. 2007;**33**(5):572-578

[61] Johnson JL, Okwera A, Vjecha MJ, et al. Risk factors for relapse in human immunodeficiency virus type 1 infected adults with pulmonary tuberculosis. The International Journal of Tuberculosis and Lung Disease. 1997;**1**(5):446-453

[62] Chiang CY, Hsu CJ, Huang RM, et al. Anti-tuberculosis drug resistance among retreatment tuberculosis patients in a referral center in Taipei. Journal of the Formosan Medical Association. 2004;**103**(6):411-415

[63] Blumberg HM, Burman WJ, Chaisson RE, et al. American Thoracic Society/Centers for Disease Control and Prevention/Infectious Diseases Society of America: Treatment of tuberculosis. American Journal of Respiratory and Critical Care Medicine. 2003;**167**: 603-662

[64] Satyaraddi A, Velpandian T, Sharma SK, et al. Correlation of plasma anti-tuberculosis drug levels with subsequent development of hepatotoxicity. The International Journal of Tuberculosis and Lung Disease. 2014;**18**:188-195

[65] Pasipanodya JG, Srivastava S, Gumbo T, et al. Meta-analysis of clinical studies supports the pharmacokinetic variability hypothesis for acquired drug resistance and failure of antituberculosis therapy. Clinical Infectious Diseases. 2012;**55**:169-177

[66] Srivastava S, Pasipanodya JG, Meek C, et al. Multidrug-resistant tuberculosis not due to noncompliance but to between-patient pharmacokinetic variability. The Journal of Infectious Diseases. 2011;**204**:1951-1959

[67] Pulido F, Pena J-M, Rubio R, et al. Relapse of tuberculosis after treatment in human immunodeficiency virus-infected patients. Archives of Internal Medicine. 1997;**157**: 227-232

[68] Mallory KF, Churchyard GJ, Kleinschmidt I, et al. The impact of HIV infection on recurrence of tuberculosis in South African gold miners. International Journal of Tuberculosis and Lung Disease. 2000;**4**:455-462

[69] Tam CM, Chan SL, Kam KM, et al. Rifapentine and isoniazid in the continuation phase of a 6-month regimen. Final report at 5 years: Prognostic value of various measures. The International Journal of Tuberculosis and Lung Disease. 2002;**6**:3-10

[70] Horne DJ, Royce SE, Gooze L, et al. Sputum monitoring during tuberculosis treatment for predicting outcome: Systematic review and meta-analysis. The Lancet Infectious Diseases. 2010;**10**(6):387-394

[71] Gillespie SH, Crook AM, McHugh TD, et al. Four-month moxifloxacin-based regimens for drug-sensitive tuberculosis. The New England Journal of Medicine. 2014;**371**:1577-1587

[72] Sola E, Rivera C, Mangual M, et al. Diabetes mellitus: An important risk factor for reactivation of tuberculosis. Endocrinology, Diabetes & Metabolism. 2016;**2016**. pii: 16-0035

[73] Lee PH, Lin HC, Huang ASE, et al. Diabetes and risk of tuberculosis relapse: Nation-wide nested case-control study. PLoS One. 2014;**9**(3):e92623

[74] Blanco-Guillot F, Delgado-Sánchez G, Mongua-Rodríguez N, et al. Molecular clustering of patients with diabetes and pulmonary tuberculosis: A systematic review and meta-analysis. PLoS One. 2017;**12**(9):e0184675

[75] Kim L, Moonan PK, Heilig CM, et al. Factors associated with recurrent tuberculosis more than 12 months after treatment completion. The International Journal of Tuberculosis and Lung Disease. 2016;**20**(1):49-56

[76] Lin HH, Ezzati M, Murray M. Tobacco smoke, indoor air pollution and tuberculosis: A systematic review and meta-analysis. PLoS Medicine. 2007;**4**(1):e20

[77] Leung CC, Yew WW, Chan CK, et al. Smoking adversely affects treatment response, outcome and relapse in tuberculosis. The European Respiratory Journal. 2015;**45**(3):738-745

[78] De Castro Fernandes FM, De Souza Martins E, Arnaud Sampaio Pedrosa DM, et al. Relationship between climatic factors and air quality with tuberculosis in the Federal District, Brazil, 2003–2012. Brazilian Journal of Infectious Diseases. 2017;**21**(4):369-375

[79] Ai JW, Ruan QL, Liu QH, et al. Updates on the risk factors for latent tuberculosis reactivation and their managements. Emerging Microbes & Infections. 2016;**5**:e10

[80] Byrne AL, Marais BJ, Mitnick CD et al. Tuberculosis and chronic respiratory disease: A systematic review. International Journal of Infectious Diseases. 2015;**32**:138-146

[81] Pietersen E, Ignatius E, Streicher EM, et al. Long-term outcomes of patients with extensively drugresistant tuberculosis in South Africa: A cohort study. Lancet. 2014;**383**(9924): 1230-1239

[82] Shah NS, Auld SC, Brust JCM, et al. Transmission of extensively drug-resistant tuberculosis in South Africa. The New England Journal of Medicine. 2017;**376**:243-253

[83] Huyen MN, Buu TN, Tiemersma E, et al. Tuberculosis relapse in Vietnam is significantly associated with *Mycobacterium tuberculosis* Beijing genotype infections. The Journal of Infectious Diseases. 2013;**207**(10):1516-1524

[84] Nguyen TLH, Maeda S, Keicho N, et al. Sub-lineages of *Mycobacterium tuberculosis* Beijing genotype strains and unfavorable outcomes of anti-tuberculosis treatment. Tuberculosis. 2015;**95**(3):336-342

[85] Dheeda K, Schwander SK, Zhu B, et al. The immunology of tuberculosis: From bench to bedside. Respirology. 2010;**15**(3):1440-1843

[86] Cardona PJ. Reactivation or reinfection in adult tuberculosis: Is that the question? International Journal of Mycobacteriology. 2016;**5**(4):400-407

[87] Thobakgale C, Naidoo K, McKinnon LR, et al. Interleukin 1-beta (IL-1β) production by innate cells following TLR stimulation correlates with TB recurrence in ART-treated HIV-infected patients. Journal of Acquired Immune Deficiency Syndromes. 2017;**74**(2):213-220

[88] Sivro A, McKinnon LR, Yende-Zuma N, et al. Plasma cytokine predictors of tuberculosis recurrence in antiretroviral-treated HIV-infected individuals from Durban, South Africa. Clinical Infectious Diseases. 2017;**65**(5):819-826

[89] Mistry R, Cliff JM, Clayton CL, et al. Gene-expression patterns in whole blood identify subjects at risk for recurrent tuberculosis. The Journal of Infectious Diseases. 2007;**195**: 357-365

[90] Cliff JM, Cho J, Lee J, et al. Excessive cytolytic responses predict tuberculosis relapse after apparently successful treatment. The Journal of Infectious Diseases. 2016;**213**:485-495

[91] Thompson EG, Du Y, Malherbe ST, et al. Host blood RNA signatures predict the outcome of tuberculosis. Tuberculosis. 2017;**107**:48-58

[92] De Steenwinkel JEM, Knegt GJ, Ten Kate MT, et al. Relapse of tuberculosis versus primary tuberculosis; course, pathogenesis and therapy in mice. Tuberculosis. 2013;**93**: 213-221

[93] World Health Organization. Treatment of Tuberculosis Guidelines. 4th ed. [cited Nov 30, 2017]. Available from: http://www.who.int/tb/publications/tb_treatmentguidelines/en/

[94] Johnston JC, Khan FA, Dowdy DW. Reducing relapse in tuberculosis treatment: Is it time to reassess WHO treatment guidelines? The International Journal of Tuberculosis and Lung Disease. 2015;**19**(6):624

[95] Nunn AJ, Phillips PPJ, Ibrahim A. Reducing relapse in tuberculosis treatment. The International Journal of Tuberculosis and Lung Disease. 2015;**19**(10):1263-1264

[96] Jindani A, Harrison TS, Nunn AJ, et al. High-dose rifapentine with moxifloxacin for pulmonary tuberculosis. The New England Journal of Medicine. 2014;**371**:1599-1608

[97] Menzies D, Benedetti A, Paydar A, et al. Effect of duration and intermittency of rifampin on tuberculosis treatment outcomes: A systematic review and meta-analysis. PLoS Medicine. 2009;**6**:e1000146

[98] Smieja MJ, Marchetti CA, Cook DJ, et al. Isoniazid for preventing tuberculosis in non-HIV infected persons. Cochrane Database of Systematic Reviews. 2000;(2):CD001363

[99] Akolo C, Adetifa I, Shepperd S, et al. Treatment of latent tuberculosis infection in HIV infected persons. Cochrane Database of Systematic Reviews. 2010;CD000171

[100] Bruins WS, van Leth F. Effect of secondary preventive therapy on recurrence of tuberculosis in HIV-infected individuals: A systematic review. Infectious Diseases. 2017;**49**(3): 161-169

[101] The Trial of Early Antiretrovirals and Isoniazid Preventive Therapy in Africa. Agence National de Recherche sur le Sida et les h'epatites virales 12136 Study Group. A trial of early antiretrovirals and isoniazid preventive therapy in Africa. The New England Journal of Medicine. 2015;**373**:808-822

[102] Kabali C, von Reyn CF, Brooks DR, et al. Completion of isoniazid preventive therapy and survival in HIV-infected, TST positive adults in Tanzania. The International Journal of Tuberculosis and Lung Disease. 2011;**15**:1515-1521

[103] Charalambous S, Grant AD, Innes C, et al. Association of isoniazid preventive therapy with lower early mortality in individuals on antiretroviral therapy in a workplace programme. Acquired Immune Deficiency Syndrome. 2010;**24**(5):S5-S13

[104] Hosseinipour MC, Bisson GP, Miyahara S, et al. Empirical tuberculosis therapy versus isoniazid in adult outpatients with advanced HIV initiating antiretroviral therapy (REMEMBER): A multicountry open-label randomised controlled trial. Lancet. 2016; **387**(10024):1198-1209

[105] Perriens JH, St Louis ME, Mukadi YB, et al. Pulmonary tuberculosis in HIV-infected patients in Zaire. A controlled trial of treatment for either 6 or 12 months. The New England Journal of Medicine. 1995;**332**:779-784

[106] Haller L, Sossouhounto R, Coulibaly IM, et al. Isoniazid plus sulphadoxine-pyrimethamine can reduce morbidity of HIV-positive patients treated for tuberculosis in Africa: A controlled clinical trial. Chemotherapy. 1999;**45**:452-465

[107] Fitzgerald DW, Desvarieux M, Severe P, et al. Effect of post-treatment isoniazid on prevention of recurrent tuberculosis in HIV-1-infected individuals: A randomized trial. Lancet. 2000;**356**:1470-1474

[108] Churchyard GJ, Fielding K, Charalambous S, et al. Efficacy of secondary isoniazid preventive therapy among HIV-infected Southern Africans: Time to change policy? Acquired Immune Deficiency Syndrome. 2003;**17**:2063-2070

6

Determinants of Survival of Patients with Tuberculosis in Developing Countries

Abiola Olaleye and Andy Beke

Abstract

Tuberculosis (TB), a major disease of public health importance, continues to cause significant morbidity and mortality to populations around the world. In 2016, it accounted for 1.7 million deaths worldwide. While the mortality rate among patients undergoing TB treatment has been declining over the years, TB death rates remains high in developing countries. This chapter discusses the epidemiology of TB mortality, the pathogenesis of TB highlighting susceptibility to mortality, and the interaction of factors which determine an individual's risk to death on account of TB. Furthermore, the chapter proposes the need for a strategic research agenda on reduction of TB burden, focusing on the factors that enable or impede political will towards translating knowledge into effective action.

Keywords: tuberculosis, survival, determinants, patients, developing, countries

1. Introduction

Tuberculosis (TB) remains a disease of public health importance affecting vulnerable populations. TB is the leading cause of death from a single infectious agent worldwide. The burden of the disease is enormous with an estimated 10.4 million new cases and 1.7 million TB deaths reported in 2016. Furthermore, more than one-fifths of reported deaths occurred among those who were HIV-infected [1]. While TB-mortality rate among HIV-negative people was 17 per 100,000 population, it was 5 per 100,000 among people living with HIV. In addition, 12% of incident cases of TB occurred among HIV-positive people while one in ten of new TB cases occurred among children in the same year [1]. According to WHO, the 30 countries most affected by TB include Angola, Bangladesh, Brazil, Cambodia, China, Congo, Central African Republic, DPR Korea, DR Congo, Ethiopia, India, Indonesia, Kenya, Lesotho, Liberia,

Mozambique, Myanmar, Namibia, Nigeria, Pakistan, Papua New Guinea, Philippines, Russian Federation, Sierra Leone, South Africa, Thailand, UR Tanzania, Viet Nam, Zambia, and Zimbabwe [1].

TB mortality burden is continues to pose challenges to socioeconomic development in developing countries as South East Asia, Western Pacific, and African regions accounted for more than 90% of TB-deaths in 2016 [1].

Analysis of cohorts of patients on tuberculosis treatment enables public health programmes to describe the survival of patients and factors associated with mortality experience among patients. While treatment outcomes vary among different cohorts of TB patients, patients with drug resistance TB and those with coexisting debilitating conditions experience worst outcomes. Furthermore, survival of TB patients depends on several medical, demographic and socio-economic factors. This chapter focuses on the epidemiology of TB mortality, and the determinants of survival of TB patients – the factors which represent the most important opportunities for prevention of TB-related deaths in developing countries.

2. Epidemiology of TB mortality

Mycobacterium tuberculosis—the causative organism of TB, is the leading cause of death from a single infectious agent after Human Immunodeficiency Virus (HIV). About 45,000 TB-related deaths occurred in Europe in 2011 and its estimated mortality rate was 5.0 per 100,000 population [2]. While 330 TB-related deaths and an estimated TB-mortality rate of 0.5 per 100,000 population were reported in the United Kingdom, TB-death rates were 0.4, 1.0, 8.9, 15.0, and 16.0 per 100,000 population in Germany, France, Belarus, Russia, and Ukraine respectively [3]. In the United States, more than 50,000 TB-related deaths were reported from 1990 to 2006, accounting for 0.13% of the total number of deaths in the country [4]. While TB was reported as the underlying cause of death in about 40% of the 39,694,210 total deaths that occurred, it was reported as one of the contributing causes of death in more than 60% of the total deaths [1]. The overall mean annual mortality rate was 1.16 per 100,000 person-years during this period [1]. Similarly, 7% of the 301 persons with TB reported to Connecticut TB Control Program from 2007 to 2009 died on account of the disease [5]. Furthermore, 11% of the 40, 125 patients with culture-confirmed TB died on account the disease in California from 1994 to 2008 [3]. In 2014, more than 5% of the 9406 patients with TB in the US died due to the disease [6].

Although TB is a major public health problem worldwide, its mortality in developing countries is alarming. An estimated 2.5 million TB deaths were reported in China from 1990 to 2015 and 2% of these deaths occurred in 2015 [7]. Furthermore, TB-mortality rates were 32 and 44 per 100,000 population in 2016 in India and Pakistan, respectively [1]. While 16% of those who had TB died of the disease in Zimbabwe was in 2013 [8], TB-related mortality rates were estimated at 29, 56, 83, 104, and 222 per 100,000 population in Ethiopia, Ghana, Swaziland, Nigeria, and South Africa respectively in 2016 [1]. In addition, the estimated TB-related mortality rate in in Africa was 72 per 100,000 population while it was 3.4 per 100,000 population in European region and 2.3 per 100,000 population in the WHO Region of the Americas in 2016 [1].

2.1. Global trends in TB mortality

Tuberculosis, often referred to as "consumption," "phthisis," or the "white plague," accounted for the highest number of deaths in Europe and America during the eighteenth and nineteenth centuries. While 70–90% of urban populations of Europe and North America were infected with TB in the late nineteenth century, four-fifths of people infected with TB died of it [9]. Through the knowledge made available by the work of Villemin, Koch, von Pirquet, TB mortality began to decline in the early and mid-nineteenth century [10–12]. TB Decline in TB mortality in these parts of the world was associated with improvement in socio-economic conditions of the populations.

In the United Kingdom, the rapid decline in TB mortality was cited as one of the most important health gains of the twentieth century [13]. Using all certified causes of death (both underlying cause and elsewhere on certificates), TB-mortality in the Oxford region declined from 39.7 deaths per million population in 1979 to 9.0 in 2008. In England, TB-mortality rates fell from 18.5 per million population in 1995 to 12.2 in 2008 [13].

TB mortality has been dropping rapidly since 1900 in developed countries, especially after the development of new anti-tuberculosis drugs. In the United States, 74,842 TB-related deaths were reported in 1933 [14]. This had declined by 22.9% by 1942 and a further decline was reported in the following decade such that only 25,080 TB-related deaths were reported in 1952 [12]. Furthermore, TB-mortality rates were 59.6, 43.1, and 16.1 per 100, 000 population in 1933, 1942, and 1952 respectively in the United States [12]. While 644 TB-deaths were reported in 2006, the estimated number of TB-related deaths was 610 in 2016 [1]. In essence, TB-mortality declined in the US from 59.6 per 100, 000 in 1933 to 0.19 per 100, 000 in 2016 [1, 12].

Due to poor vital registration systems, records on TB-mortality trends in developing countries are limited. A significant increase in TB mortality was recorded from 1990 and 2000 worldwide. However, the increase was more obvious in developing countries (**Figure 1**). In 2004, TB-mortality rate in Bangladesh was 51 per 100,000 population, while it was 81 per 100,000 in 2014 [8, 15]. Similarly, TB-death rates in Nigeria and South Africa in 2004 were 82 and 135

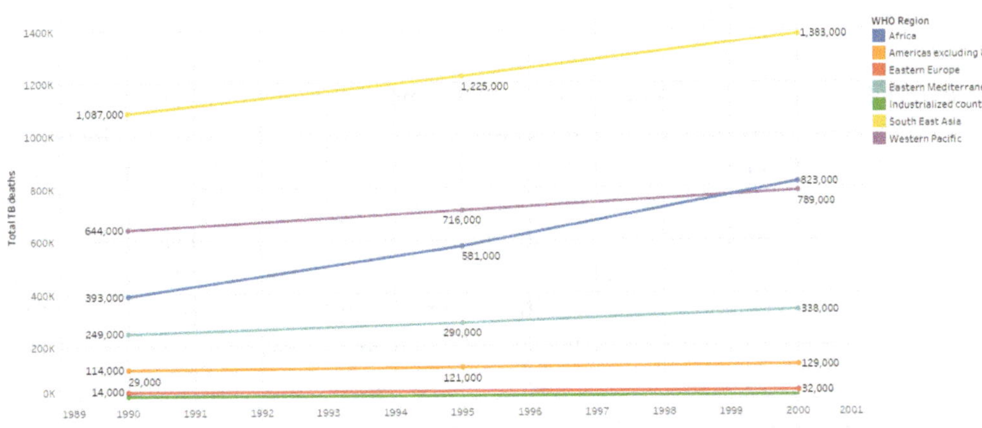

Figure 1. Global trends in TB mortality from 1990 to 2000. Data source: Global tuberculosis report 2013. WHO/HTM/TB/2013.11. Geneva: WHO; 2013.

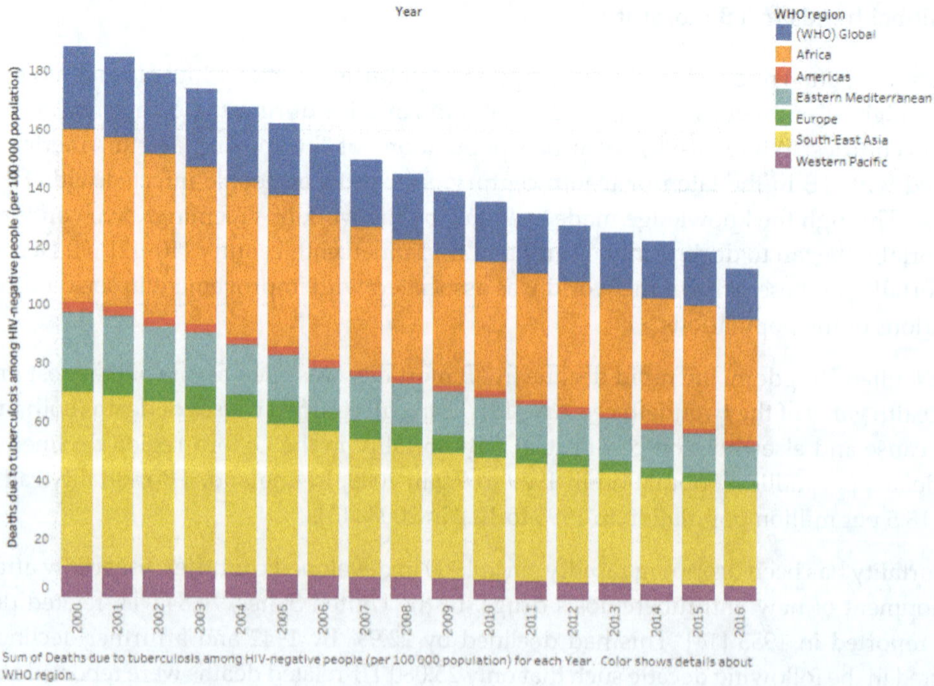

Figure 2. Global trends in TB mortality from 2000 to 2016. Data source: WHO. Global Health Observatory data repository. Tuberculosis [Internet]. Geneva: WHO; 2017 Dec 1 [cited 2018 Feb 12]. Available from: http://apps.who.int/gho/data/node.main.1315?lang=en.

per 100,000 population respectively. By 2014, the mortality rates had increased to 170 per 100,000 in Nigeria while it decreased to 24 per 100,000 in South Africa [7, 14]. Furthermore, TB mortality rates declined significantly between 2000 and 2016 (**Figure 2**).

3. Pathogenesis of TB infection

Tuberculosis (TB) is an old disease of mankind from time immemorial. An evidence of TB spine was found in Egyptian mummies of several thousand years BC, while Babylonian and Chinese writings also referred to the disease [16]. TB is an infection caused by the rod-shaped, non-spore-forming bacterium called *Mycobacterium tuberculosis*, a member of a group called M. tuberculosis complex (MTBC). Other members of this complex include *M. bovis, M. microti, M. africanum, M. caprae, M. canetti* and *M. pinnipedii*. MTBC members are closely related genetically. The genome of *M. bovis* differs from that of M. tuberculosis by less than 0.05% [17]. While *M. bovis* primarily affects cattle, it can also TB disease in other mammals include man [18].

TB infection leads to a complex interaction with the immune system of the human host. This interaction is often moderated by a number of factors with influence survival of TB patients.

3.1. Transmission

TB is transmitted from a person with active TB disease to an uninfected person through the air by droplet nuclei—particles measuring 1–5 μm in diameter containing MTBC [19]. These droplet nuclei are produced when persons with pulmonary or laryngeal TB cough, sneeze, speak, or sing. Iatrogenic transmission of TB may also occur during aerosol treatments, sputum induction, bronchoscopy, or during tissue or secretion processing in hospitals or laboratories. Droplet nuclei can remain airborne for long periods of time after expectoration. The transmission of TB depends on a number of factors including the number of tubercle bacilli present in droplets, its virulence and exposure to ultraviolet light, the extent of ventilation, and the immune status of exposed persons. After inhalation of an infectious droplet nucleus, it settles in the respiratory tract and reaches a respiratory bronchiole or alveolus where the tubercle bacilli may establish an infection depending on the bacterial virulence and the inherent mycobactericidal capacity of the alveolar macrophage. With the activation of the host defenses, phagocytosis by alveolar macrophages often initiates a cascade of events resulting in either a successful control of the infection, which is usually followed by latent tuberculosis. The invading mycobacterium may overwhelm host defense mechanisms followed by progression to active disease, known as primary progressive tuberculosis [19]. Within the alveolar macrophage, the tubercle bacillus continues growing slowly and dividing almost every 25–32 h for 2–12 weeks such that they reach 10^3–10^4 thereby eliciting a cellular immune response which is often detected by a positive reaction to a tuberculin test. For an immunocompetent person, the formation of granulomas around the invading mycobacterium occurs at this time.

Prior to the development of cellular immunity, tubercle bacilli may be disseminated via the lymphatics to the hilar lymph nodes and the bloodstream. When these bacilli reach more distant sites, they may give rise to extra pulmonary TB infection of the brain meninges, larynx, lymph nodes, spine, and kidney.

3.2. Pathophysiology

Granulomas formed by accumulation of T lymphocytes and microphages limit mycobacterial replication and spread [20]. Although the environment provided by granuloma formation destroys macrophages and produces early solid necrosis at the center of the lesion, tubercle bacilli often adapt to enhance their survival [20]. The formation of caseous necrosis, a soft-cheese structure with low oxygen levels, low pH, and limited nutrients in the following 2–3 weeks creates a condition that limits further mycobacterial growth. Latent tuberculosis is established at this stage. While tuberculous lesions undergo fibrosis and calcification thereby controlling the infection, the tubercle bacilli within the lesions may begin to multiply rapidly if the immune system of the individual deteriorates [21].

For an immunocompromised person, granuloma formation also occurs following infection with MTBC. However, the granulomas formed are unable to contain the infection. Hence, this progresses to primary progressive tuberculosis [21]. The necrotic tissue of the granuloma liquefies and the fibrous wall breaks down. Furthermore, the semiliquid necrotic matter may drain into surrounding structures including the bronchi, and nearby blood vessels leaving an empty, air-filled cavity at the middle of the initial lesion. In addition, discharge of the necrotic material into a vessel may lead to extra pulmonary TB and mortality from TB may be related to this.

4. Factors associated with survival among TB patients in developing countries

The management of patients suspected of TB disease involves clinical assessment and treatment (**Figure 3**). Of the treatment outcomes, Cured and Completed treatment are considered as successful outcomes while the remaining ones are often referred to as poor treatment outcomes [1, 22].

Although deaths on account of TB disease occur worldwide, developing countries account for more than 90% of TB mortality in recent times. Hence, the focus of this section will be on developing countries. Several factors influence susceptibility of TB infection, its severity as well as mortality.

Factors associated with survival among TB patients in developing countries can be discussed using a framework proposed by the Commission on Social Determinants of Health (CSDH) established by WHO (**Figure 4**) [23].

Factors associated with survival among patients with TB disease can be classified into patient and community/social factors. In the context of the CSDH framework, most of the patient factors can be described in terms of the health system while community/social factors are related to the structural determinants of health and health inequities. Patient characteristics include age, sex, alcohol use, cigarette smoking, previous history of TB treatment, HIV co-infection, and comorbid conditions, TB diagnostic methods, and treatment regimens. On the other hand, structural determinants of health associated with TB survival include the presence of education, employment, access to health care and protection from catastrophic expenditure associated with TB morbidity.

4.1. Age

Aging affects the immune system at multiple levels including reduced production of B and T cells and diminished function of mature lymphocytes in secondary lymphoid tissues. Furthermore, aging causes a profound alteration in the composition and quality of the mature lymphocyte pool and alters the patterns of gene expression in mature B and T cells. Compared to young people, elderly individuals respond to immune challenge in a less efficient manner [24].

Old age increases the likelihood of death from TB. Evidence for this has been reported in previous studies. While several age cut-points have been used in studies to show vulnerability, TB infection in people over the age of 60 years is associated with increased mortality. A retrospective study among adult patients with clinically and/or bacteriologically diagnosed TB in Argentina reported increased mortality among people who were older than 50 years [22]. A similar study conducted in South Africa reported that patients who were 60 years or

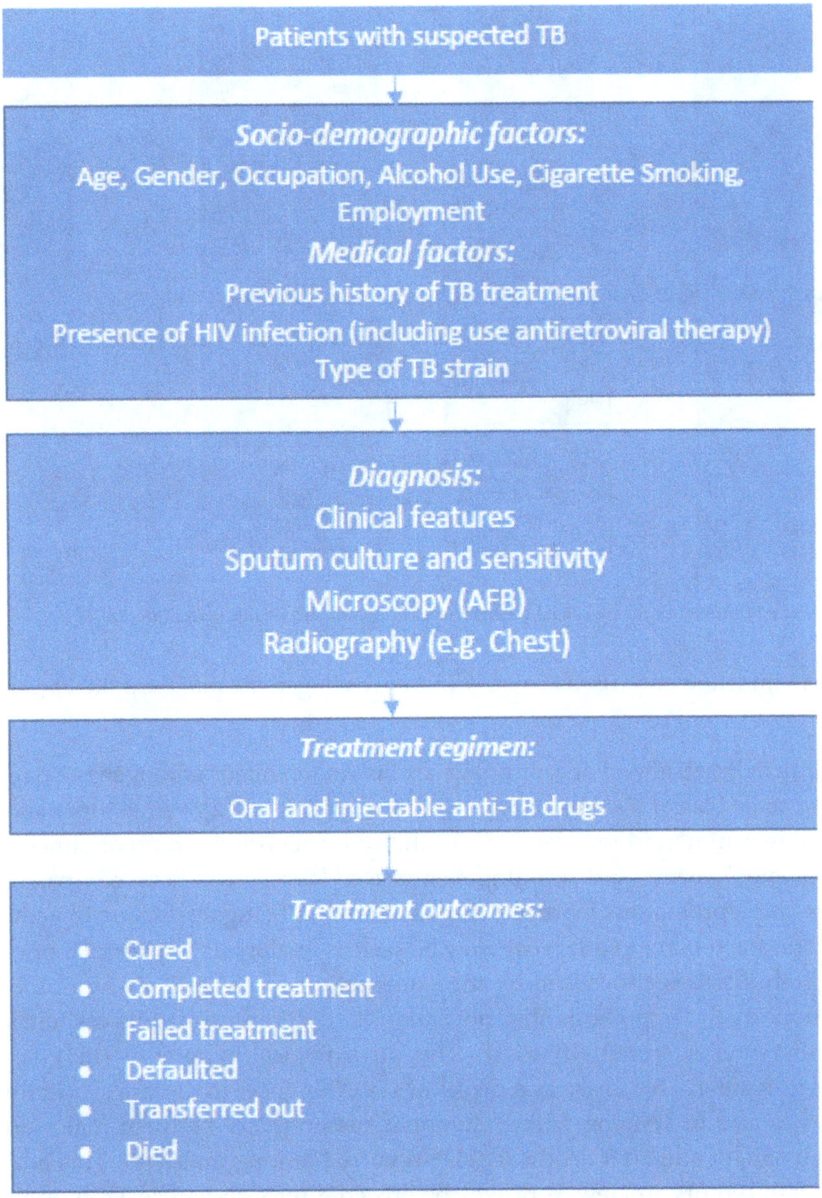

Figure 3. Clinical assessment and treatment of TB patients.

older were twice more likely to die from TB than the younger ones [25]. In addition, patients aged 65 years and above were two times more likely to die from TB than other patients in a study in Zimbabwe [26].

4.2. Sex

Infectious diseases including TB generally affect males more than females. Studies have shown that interactions between sex hormones and the immune system render males more

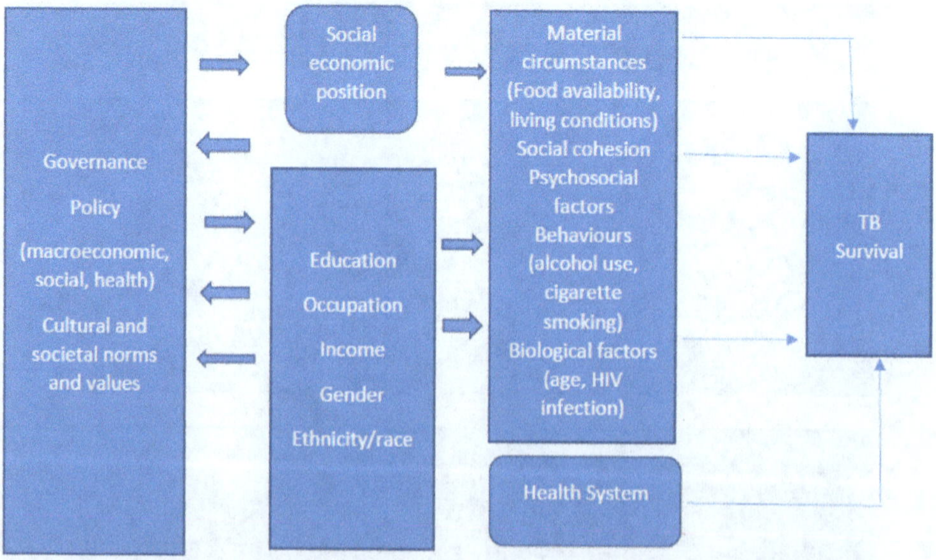

Figure 4. Conceptual framework for the social determinants of health and health inequities [23].

susceptible to infection and disease, with differences in genetic make-up likely playing a role [27, 28].

A recent study in Brazil aimed at examining sex bias in ten major pathogens also reported the characteristic male bias of a male-to-female ratio of almost 2:1 [2]. While tuberculoid leprosy is slightly more common in females (0.85:1), the study reported a ratio of almost 3:1 for the severe lepromatous form. Host immune response to leprosy has been compared to that in tuberculosis and lepromatous leprosy was considered as being analogous to active tuberculosis. Furthermore, tuberculoid leprosy may be seen as analogous to latent TB or cured or TB [29]. Since both diseases are caused by the same pathogen—Mycobacterium, the male bias observed supports the hypothesis that physiological differences may be responsible for the observed differential susceptibility to TB. This physiological hypothesis (PH) has also been found to be relevant in TB disease as a driver of sex differences in disease susceptibility [1, 2]. TB mortality is also in keeping with differential susceptibility between males and females as more than 65% of adult TB deaths in 2016 occurred among males [1]. This is also similar to the twentieth century in New York which showed a male-to-female TB mortality ratio of approximately 2:1 [30].

A consistent finding in literature shows that males are more likely to die from tuberculosis than females. A study in Ethiopia, showed that males are twice more likely to have poor treatment outcome (including death) following TB treatment [31]. In addition, a systematic review and meta-analysis consisting of multidrug resistant-TB (MDR-TB) data from 31 treatment programmes from 21 countries showed that males are less likely to have a successful outcome after treatment [32]. Although there was no association between sex and survival among patients in a study in South Africa, male patients were more likely to have unfavorable TB treatment outcomes [33].

4.3. Education

Educational status is an important factor which moderates health care seeking behavior and adherence to prescribed medications. The level of educational achievement may protect against acquiring TB infection through promotion of healthy habits. In addition, education been recognized as a marker of economic status. Hence, low level education may be associated with lack of access to resources, overcrowding and poor hygienic conditions which may also contribute to increased mortality. In a study in Peru, MDR-TB patients who attended formal school for 6 or less years had about threefold increase in TB mortality risk [34]. Similarly, attendance or completion of primary school level was associated with TB treatment failure [35]. While educational status may be a significant factor influencing survival in most health conditions, only a few studies reported it as a determinant of survival among patients with TB in developing countries [32, 34].

4.4. Occupation

Occupations which compromise structural and/or functional integrity of the lungs predispose individuals to the transmission of TB as well as to higher risk of mortality on account of the disease. While exposures to dust inside the mines damage the structure and function of the lungs (e.g., silicosis), associated social conditions outside the mines (e.g., crowding) drive HIV and TB epidemics. This makes mining a strong predictor of TB mortality. Studies in Southern Africa have reported the strong association between mining and TB mortality [36, 37].

4.5. Smoking

Smoking is one of the most important risk factors associated with incidence, morbidity, recurrence and mortality from TB. Smoking has been associated with a fourfold increase in TB mortality risk [38].

4.6. Previous history of TB treatment

Previous TB treatment has been associated with TB mortality. A prospective study among smear positive TB patients with Iranian nationality who had successful TB treatment showed that those who had previous history of TB treatment were almost three times more likely to die [39]. Similarly, patients with a previous history of TB treatment were almost seven times more likely to die than treatment-naive patients in another study in Iran [40]. This may be related to development of resistance following treatment default, failure, or loss to follow up.

4.7. Type of TB strain

Multidrug-resistant tuberculosis (MDR-TB), a form of TB disease resistant to both isoniazid and rifampicin is a global problem. Increasing incidence of this type of TB is a reflection of the health care system of a country. It arises as a result of weak TB treatment programmes coupled with poor adherence to anti-TB therapy. While the extent and burden of the disease varies among countries, it often overwhelms the capacity of the health system in many high burden resource-poor countries.

Studies have consistently shown that MDR-TB is a strong predictor of TB mortality. In 2016, it was responsible for a large percentage of TB mortality worldwide [1]. MDR-TB was associated with almost eightfold increase in mortality risk in a retrospective study in Peru [32]. Other studies have also shown similar findings. Furthermore, MDR-TB associated hazard ratio (HR) estimates in TB mortality increase in previous studies were in the range of 7.8–8.5 [41, 42].

Extensively drug-resistant tuberculosis (XDR-TB), a variant of MDR-TB resistant to any fluoroquinolone and at least one of three injectable second-line drugs (i.e., amikacin, kanamycin, or capreomycin) in addition to isoniazid and rifampin. XDR-TB has also been associated with high death rates while on treatment.

There are multiple causes for the increased risk of multidrug-resistant TB strains. MDR-TB infection often occur with other co-morbid conditions including HIV infection, diabetes, renal disease, and Substance Use Disorders [43]. In addition, MDR-TB has been associated with high rates of treatment failure and relapse which increases TB mortality. With high toxicity of anti-tuberculosis drugs used in the treatment of MDR-TB and the extended duration of use, an increase in toxicity profile of patients and consequent adverse effects may be related to increased mortality experienced among MDR-TB patients.

4.8. HIV co-infection

Studies have shown that HIV/TB co-infection is associated with increased TB mortality risk before, during, or after TB treatment. In most cases, deaths are usually caused by complications of HIV infection rather than TB disease itself. However, a synergistic interaction occurs between TB and HIV infection which speeds up the progression of illness and increasing mortality risk. HIV infection enhances the reactivation and progression of latent *Mycobacterium tuberculosis* to active TB disease, and the active TB disease accelerates HIV disease progression in infected patients. Furthermore, HIV infection alters the clinical presentation of TB and complicates TB treatment follow-up [44].

In Malawi, HIV positive patients were 2.5 times more likely to die from TB infection in a prospective cohort study among TB patients [45]. Another study in Malawi also reported almost fourfold increase in TB mortality among HIV/TB co-infected patients compared to HIV seronegative TB patients [46]. Furthermore, HIV co-infection was associated with almost sixfold increase in TB mortality in a study in Ethiopia [35].

Among patients who were HIV/TB co-infected, being on antiretroviral therapy (ART), initiation of cotrimoxazole prophylactic therapy (CPT), being ambulatory, and having high CD4 counts were factors associated with survival in several studies. Patients who were on ART were 0.35 times less likely to die from TB compared to those who were not on ART [47].

While MDR-TB infection is associated with increased mortality risk for both HIV-seropositive and seronegative patients, HIV/MDR-TB co-infection increases the risk of death. A study in Thailand reported that patients who were HIV positive patients infected with MDR-TB were twice more likely to die compared to HIV seropositive patients who had non-MDR-TB co-infection [48]. Similarly, HIV/TB co-infected patients who delayed initiation of ART 6 or months or more after TB diagnosis were 2.6 times more likely to die compared with those who initiated ART in less than 6 months following TB diagnosis [47].

4.9. Extra pulmonary TB

Although extra pulmonary TB is not as common as pulmonary disease, its occurrence has consistently been shown in literature as a predictor of TB mortality. Patients with extra pulmonary TB including TB meningitis, TB pericarditis, TB peritonitis, bilateral or extensive pleural effusion due to TB, Potts disease, TB of the genitourinary tract, and TB of the intestine were twice more likely to die on account of the disease than patients with pulmonary disease in a study in Brazil [49]. Furthermore, patients who had extra pulmonary TB were three times more likely to die than those who had pulmonary TB [50]. Similarly, miliary TB has also been associated with poor outcomes [51].

4.10. Co-morbid conditions

Co-morbid conditions including malnutrition, chronic renal disease, chronic liver disease, drug induced immunosuppression, and diabetes mellitus are predictors of mortality among TB patients.

4.10.1. Diabetes

The synergistic interactions between diabetes mellitus and TB are well documented in literature [52]. Diabetes alters host immunity to TB which leads to higher baseline mycobacterial burdens and longer times to achieve culture conversion with treatment. While treatment failure or death was reported in 41% of patients with TB and diabetes in case-control study, these outcomes were only reported in 13% of those with TB alone. Furthermore, seven of the eight patients in the TB and diabetes group died of respiratory failure related to TB [53].

4.10.2. Malnutrition

Malnutrition has been cited as a predictor of mortality among TB patients. Malnourished patients were 27 times more likely to have unfavorable TB outcome and death in a study in South Africa [54].

4.10.3. Chronic renal disease

The presence of end stage renal disease requiring dialysis was associated with sevenfold increase in TB mortality risk in a previous study [55].

4.10.4. Drug-induced immunosuppression

The presence of drug induced immunosuppression was associated with increased TB mortality risk with adjusted odds ratio of 3.2 [51].

4.11. Poor adherence to anti-Koch therapy

Studies have shown that TB patients with poor adherence to medications are more likely to die compared to other patients. A retrospective study involving patients in 48 clinics in Rwanda among patients treated in 48 clinics in Rwanda showed that poor treatment adherence was associated with more than threefold increase in TB mortality [56].

4.12. Neighbourhood and social factors

Neighbourhood factors refer to issues within the society that contribute to TB mortality which are not directly related to a patient's individual condition but a constellation of factors which affect a patient's access to care, treatment enablers, emergency services, and attitudes of the general population to health. These include societal norms and values, policy, and governance issues within and outside the health system (**Figure 4**).

Neighbourhoods play a role in TB morbidity and mortality as good housing may influence air quality and disease transmission. Access to nutritious foods may also be important for immune responses and recovery from TB infection. In addition, Service characteristics of neighbourhoods can create and support employment opportunities which may reinforce socioeconomic disparities in health.

The level of the commitment of health authorities at the local, regional, and national levels towards TB treatment, care and support influences the survival of patients [1]. For instance, the failure of a TB treatment programme to follow up on patients on treatment may contribute to increased mortality. In addition, failure of the health system to screen and test HIV positive patients for TB may also affect their survival.

Social protection is one of the functions of the health system. However, unemployment, low status occupation, low annual income, high cost of travel to the health care facility for TB treatment, poor living conditions, low literacy level, and high out-of-pocket expenditure on TB treatment have been described as factors associated with poor treatment adherence, unfavorable TB treatment outcomes, and death. Furthermore, a strong correlation was reported between TB treatment outcomes and overall health system performance in a study in South Africa where TB treatment centers with higher health system performance rating also had higher percentage of successful treatment outcomes [57].

4.13. Climatic factors and TB seasonality

Studies have shown that seasonal variation in the incidence of TB disease occurs in many developing countries. In India and Hong Kong, TB seasonality was highest among young children. However, seasonality of notified TB cases was more pronounced among males in Mongolia and South Western Cameroon [58]. In Southern Africa, most significant declines in the diagnoses of pulmonary TB occurred in December, followed by April–May. While these may not be unrelated to climatic factors, changes in health-seeking behavior and fluctuations in clinical activities were cited as responsible factors [59]. In China, increased incidence of TB was associated with increased temperature, precipitation, and wind speed [60].

Seasonality of TB disease may be related to differences in TB risk factors at certain seasons. A study in Peru showed the complex interaction of social determinants of TB infection, exposure to infection and increased transmission. Overcrowding, increased indoor time, and poorer ventilation, poorer nutrition, lower immunity, health-seeking behavior, and education interact in a complex way to an increase in TB disease at certain seasons than others. Vitamin D deficiency, more likely to occur in winter, was also associated with TB seasonality [61].

5. Conclusion

The burden of TB and the mortality on account of the disease has been discussed. While differences in mortality between population groups due to society's characteristics have been noted, factors associated with reduced survival among TB patients have been highlighted. Furthermore, it is important to note that changes in social and cultural environments of people are associated with changes in their risks of acquiring TB infection, and the risk of dying from the disease. Although associations between social factors and TB morbidity and mortality are well known, there is paucity of studies regarding the underlying processes linking social determinants and TB treatment outcomes and effective ways to intervene. While TB morbidity and mortality have reduced significantly in many parts of the third world in recent times, limited progress achievement are been recorded in other countries. A crucial obstacle in this regard is often the lack of political will. A strategic research agenda on reduction of TB burden should focus on the factors that enhance or impede political will to translate knowledge into effective action.

Author details

Abiola Olaleye* and Andy Beke

*Address all correspondence to: kayodeolaleye2012@gmail.com

School of Health Systems and Public Health, University of Pretoria, Pretoria, South Africa

References

[1] World Health Organization (WHO). Global Tuberculosis Report 2017. WHO/HTM/TB/2017.23. Geneva: WHO; 2017

[2] European Centre for Disease Prevention and Control/WHO Regional Office for Europe. Tuberculosis surveillance and monitoring in Europe 2017. WHO; 2017

[3] Pascopella L, Barry PM, Flood J, De Riemer K. Death with tuberculosis in California, 1994-2008. Open Forum Infectious Diseases. 2014;**1**(3):ofu090. DOI: 10.1093/ofid/ofu090 eCollection 2014 Dec

[4] Jung RS, Bennion JR, Sorvillo F, Bellomy A. Trends in tuberculosis mortality in the United States, 1990-2006: A population-based case-control study. Public Health Reports. 2010;**125**(3):389-397

[5] Kattan JA, Sosa LE, Lobato MN. Tuberculosis mortality: Death from a curable disease, Connecticut, 2007-2009. The International Journal of Tuberculosis and Lung Disease. 2012;**16**(12):1657-1662. DOI: 10.5588/ijtld.12.0169

[6] Centers for Disease Control and Prevention (CDC). Reported Tuberculosis in the United States, 2015. Atlanta: US Department of Health and Human Services, CDC; 2016

[7] Zhu S, Xia L, Yu S, Chen S, Zhang J. The burden and challenges of tuberculosis in China: Findings from the Global Burden of Disease Study 2015. Scientific Reports. 2017;**7**(1):14601. DOI: 10.1038/s41598-017-15024-1

[8] Global tuberculosis report 2014. WHO: Geneva; 2014. WHO/HTM/TB/2014.08

[9] Daniel TM. The history of tuberculosis. Respiratory Medicine. 2006;**100**(11):1862-1870 Epub 2006 Sep 1

[10] Grigg ERN. The arcana of tuberculosis with a brief epidemiologic history of the disease in the USA. American Review of Tuberculosis and Pulmonary Diseases. 1958;**78**:151-172

[11] Grigg ERN. The arcana of tuberculosis with a brief epidemiologic history of the disease in the USA. Part III. American Review of Tuberculosis and Pulmonary Diseases. 1958;**78**:426-453

[12] Dubos R, Dubos J. Tuberculosis, Man, and Society. The White Plague. Boston: Little, Brown, and Company; 1952

[13] Duncan ME, Goldacre MJ. Mortality trends for tuberculosis and sarcoidosis in English populations, 1979-2008. The International Journal of Tuberculosis and Lung Disease. 2012;**16**(1):38-42. DOI: 10.5588/ijtld.11.0077

[14] Iskrant AP, Rogot E. Trends in tuberculosis mortality in continental United States. Public Health Reports. 1953;**68**(9):911-920

[15] Global tuberculosis control: surveillance, planning, financing. WHO report 2006. Geneva: World Health Organization 2006. WHO/HTM/TB/2006.362

[16] Gutierrez MC, Brisse S, Brosch R, Fabre M, Omaïs B, Marmiesse M, et al. Ancient origin and gene mosaicism of the progenitor of Mycobacterium tuberculosis. PLoS Pathogens. 2005;**1**(1):e5 Epub 2005 Aug 19

[17] Iwamoto T, Sonobe T, Hayashi K. Loop-mediated isothermal amplification for direct detection of Mycobacterium tuberculosis complex, M. Avium, and M. Intracellulare in sputum samples. Journal of Clinical Microbiology. 2003;**41**(6):2616-2622. DOI: 10.1128/JCM.41.6.2616-2622.2003

[18] Lombardi G, Botti I, Pacciarini ML, Boniotti MB, Roncarati G, Dal Monte P. Five-year surveillance of human tuberculosis caused by Mycobacterium bovis in Bologna, Italy:

An underestimated problem. Epidemiology and Infection. 2017;**145**(14):3035-3039. DOI: 10.1017/S0950268817001996 Epub 2017 Sep 7

[19] Edwards D, Kirkpatrick CH. The immunology of mycobacterial diseases. The American Review of Respiratory Disease. 1986;**134**(5):1062-1071. DOI: 10.1164/arrd.1986.134.5.1062

[20] Frieden TR, Sterling TR, Munsiff SS, Watt CJ, Dye C. Tuberculosis. Lancet. 2003;**362**:887-899

[21] Knechel NA. Tuberculosis: Pathophysiology, clinical features, and diagnosis. Critical Care Nurse. 2009;**29**(2):34-43; quiz 44. DOI: 10.4037/ccn2009968

[22] Zerbini E, Greco A, Estrada S, Cisneros M, Colombo C, Beltrame S, et al. Risk factors associated with tuberculosis mortality in adults in six provinces of Argentina. Medicina (B Aires). 2017;**77**(4):267-273

[23] Solar O, Irwin A. A conceptual framework for action on the social determinants of health. Social Determinants of Health Discussion Paper 2 (Policy and Practice). Geneva: WHO; 2010

[24] Linton PJ, Dorshkind K. Age-related changes in lymphocyte development and function. Nature Immunology. 2004;**5**(2):133-139

[25] Olaleye AO, Beke AK. Survival of smear-positive multidrug resistant tuberculosis patients in Witbank, South Africa: A retrospective cohort study. Infectious Diseases (London). 2016;**48**(6):422-427. DOI: 10.3109/23744235.2016.1153806 Epub 2016 Mar 8

[26] Takarinda KC, Sandy C, Masuka N, Hazangwe P, Choto RC, Mutasa-Apollo T, et al. Factors associated with mortality among patients on TB treatment in the Southern Region of Zimbabwe, 2013. Tuberculosis Research and Treatment. 2017;**2017**:6232071. DOI: 10.1155/2017/6232071 Epub 2017 Mar 2

[27] Nhamoyebonde S, Leslie A. Biological differences between the sexes and susceptibility to tuberculosis. The Journal of Infectious Diseases. 2014;**209**(Suppl 3):S100-S106. DOI: 10.1093/infdis/jiu147

[28] Guerra-Silveira F, Abad-Franch F. Sex bias in infectious disease epidemiology: Patterns and processes. In: Nishiura H, editor. PLoS One. 2013;**8**(4):e62390. DOI: 10.1371/journal.pone.0062390

[29] Teles RMB, Graeber TG, Krutzik SR, Montoya D, Schenk M, Lee DJ, et al. Type I interferon suppresses type II interferon–triggered human anti-mycobacterial responses. Science. 2013;**339**(6126):1448-1453. DOI: 10.1126/science.1233665

[30] Frieden TR, Lerner BH, Rutherford BR. Lessons from the 1800s: Tuberculosis control in the new millennium. Lancet. 2000;**355**(9209):1088-1092. DOI: 10.1016/S0140-6736(00)02048-1

[31] Melese A, Zeleke B. Factors associated with poor treatment outcome of tuberculosis in Debre Tabor, Northwest Ethiopia. BMC Research Notes. 2018;**11**:25. DOI: 10.1186/s13104-018-3129-8

[32] Johnston JC, Shahidi NC, Sadatsafavi M, Fitzgerald JM. Treatment outcomes of multidrug-resistant tuberculosis: A systematic review and meta-analysis. PLoS One. 2009;**4**(9):e6914. DOI: 10.1371/journal.pone.0006914

[33] Olaleye AO, Beke AK. Predictors of drug sensitive tuberculosis treatment outcomes among hospitalized patients in South Africa: A multinomial logit model. Infectious diseases (London). 2017;**49**(6):478-481. DOI: 10.1080/23744235.2017.1280618 Epub 2017 Jan 27

[34] Chung-Delgado K, Guillen-Bravo S, Revilla-Montag A, Bernabe-Ortiz A. Mortality among MDR-TB cases: Comparison with drug-susceptible tuberculosis and associated factors. PLoS One. 2015;**10**(3):e0119332. DOI: 10.1371/journal.pone.0119332

[35] Abdelbary BE, Garcia-Viveros M, Ramirez-Oropesa H, Rahbar MH, Restrepo BI. Predicting treatment failure, death and drug resistance using a computed risk score among newly diagnosed TB patients in Tamaulipas, Mexico. Epidemiology and Infection. 2017;**145**(14):3020-3034. DOI: 10.1017/S0950268817001911 Epub 2017 Sep 14

[36] Stuckler D, Steele S, Lurie M, Basu S. "Dying for gold": The effects of mineral mining on HIV, tuberculosis, silicosis and occupational diseases in southern Africa. International Journal of Health Services. 2013;**43**(4):639-649. DOI: 10.2190/HS.43.4.c

[37] Dharmadhikari A, Smith J, Nardell E, Churchyard G, Keshavjee S. Aspiring to zero tuberculosis deaths among southern Africa's miners: Is there a way forward? International Journal of Health Services. 2013;**43**(4):651-664

[38] Getachew T, Bayray A, Weldearegay B. Survival and predictors of mortality among patients under multi-drug resistant tuberculosis treatment in Ethiopia: St. Peter's specialized tuberculosis hospital, Ethiopia. International Journal of Pharmaceutical Sciences and Research (IJPSR). 2013;**4**(2):776-787

[39] Moosazadeh M, Bahrampour A, Nasehi M, Khanjani N. Survival and predictors of death after successful treatment among smear positive tuberculosis: A cohort study. International Journal of Preventive Medicine. 2014;**5**(8):1005-1012

[40] Alavi-Naini R, Moghtaderi A, Metanat M, Mohammadi M, Zabetian M. Factors associated with mortality in tuberculosis patients. Journal of Research in Medical Sciences. 2013;**18**(1):52-55

[41] Kliiman K, Altraja A. Predictors and mortality associated with treatment default in pulmonary tuberculosis. The International Journal of Tuberculosis and Lung Disease. 2010;**14**(4):454-463

[42] Lockman S, Kruuner A, Binkin N, Levina K, Wang Y, Danilovitsh M, et al. Clinical outcomes of Estonian patients with primary multidrug-resistant versus drug-susceptible tuberculosis. Clinical Infectious Diseases. 2001;**32**(3):373-380

[43] Shah NS, Richardson JR, Moodley P, Moodley S, Babaria P, Ramtahal M, et al. Second-line drug resistance among extensively drug-resistant tuberculosis patients in rural South Africa. Emerging Infectious Diseases. 2011;**17**:510-513

[44] Mayer KH, Dukes HC. Synergistic pandemics: Confronting the global HIV and tuberculosis epidemics. Clinical Infectious Diseases. 2010;**50**(Suppl 3):S67-S70. DOI: 10.1086/651475

[45] Harries AD, Nyangulu DS, Kang'ombe C, Ndalama D, Glynn JR, Banda H, et al. Treatment outcome of an unselected cohort of tuberculosis patients in relation to human immunodeficiency virus serostatus in Zomba Hospital, Malawi. Transactions of the Royal Society of Tropical Medicine and Hygiene. 1998;**92**(3):343-347

[46] Hargreaves NJ, Kadzakumanja O, Whitty CJ, Salaniponi FM, Harries AD, Squire SB. 'Smear-negative' pulmonary tuberculosis in a DOTS programme: Poor outcomes in an area of high HIV seroprevalence. The International Journal of Tuberculosis and Lung Disease. 2001;**5**(9):847-854

[47] Sileshi B, Deyessa N, Girma B, Melese M, Suarez P. Predictors of mortality among TB-HIV co-infected patients being treated for tuberculosis in Northwest Ethiopia: A retrospective cohort study. BMC Infectious Diseases. 2013;**13**:297. DOI: 10.1186/1471-2334-13-297

[48] Manosuthi W, Chottanapand S, Thongyen S, Chaovavanich A, Sungkanuparph S. Survival rate and risk factors of mortality among HIV/tuberculosis-coinfected patients with and without antiretroviral therapy. Journal of Acquired Immune Deficiency Syndromes. 2006;**43**(1):42-46

[49] de Faria Gomes NM, da Mota Bastos MC, Marins RM, Barbosa AA, Soares LC, de Oliveira W de Abreu AM, Souto Filho JT. Pulmonary Medicine. 2015;**2015**:546106. 10.1155/2015/546106. Epub 2015 Oct 27

[50] Djouma FN, Noubom M, Ngomba AV, Donfack H, Kouomboua PSM, Saah MAF. Determinants of death among tuberculosis patients in a semi urban diagnostic and treatment centre of Bafoussam, West Cameroon: A retrospective case-control study. The Pan African Medical Journal. 2015;**22**:253. DOI: 10.11604/pamj.2015.22.253.6576

[51] Ranzani OT, Rodrigues LC, Waldman EA, Carvalho CRR. Estimating the impact of tuberculosis anatomical classification on treatment outcomes: A patient and surveillance perspective analysis. PLoS One. 2017;**12**(11):e0187585. DOI: 10.1371/journal.pone.0187585

[52] Dooley KE, Chaisson RE. Tuberculosis and diabetes mellitus: Convergence of two epidemics. The Lancet Infectious Diseases. 2009;**9**(12):737-746. DOI: 10.1016/S1473-3099(09)70282-8

[53] Bermejo M, Gil S, Velasco M, Prado A, Garcia C, Guijarro M. Tuberculin test in diabetic patients in a health center. Atencion Primaria. 1995;**16**:154-157

[54] Hicks RM, Padayatchi N, Shah NS, Wolf A, Werner L, Sunkari VB, et al. Malnutrition associated with unfavorable outcome and death among South African MDR-TB and HIV co infected children. The International Journal of Tuberculosis and Lung Disease. 2014;**18**(9):1074-1083. DOI: 10.5588/ijtld.14.0231

[55] Rao VK, Iademarco EP, Fraser VJ, Kollef MH. The impact of comorbidity on mortality following in-hospital diagnosis of tuberculosis. Chest. 1998;**114**(5):1244-1252

[56] Kayigamba FR, Bakker MI, Mugisha V, De Naeyer L, Gasana M, Cobelens F, van der Loeff MS. Adherence to tuberculosis treatment, sputum smear conversion and mortality: A retrospective cohort study in 48 Rwandan clinics. PLoS One 2013;**8**(9):e73501. 10.1371/journal.pone.0073501. eCollection 2013

[57] Loveday M, Padayatchi N, Wallengren K, Roberts J, Brust JCM, Ngozo J, et al. Association between health systems performance and treatment outcomes in patients co-infected with MDR-TB and HIV in KwaZulu-Natal, South Africa: Implications for TB programmes. PLoS One. 2014;**9**(4):e94016. DOI: 10.1371/journal.pone.0094016

[58] Fares A. Seasonality of tuberculosis. Journal of Global Infectious Diseases. 2011;**3**(1):46-55. DOI: 10.4103/0974-777X.77296

[59] Ballif M, Zürcher K, Reid SE, Boulle A, Fox MP, Prozesky HW, et al. Seasonal variations in tuberculosis diagnosis among HIV-positive individuals in southern Africa: Analysis of cohort studies at antiretroviral treatment programmes. BMJ Open. 2018;**8**(1):e017405

[60] Rao H-X, Zhang X, Zhao L, Yu J, Ren W, Zhang X, et al. Spatial transmission and meteorological determinants of tuberculosis incidence in Qinghai Province, China: A spatial clustering panel analysis. Infectious Diseases of Poverty. 2016;**5**:45. DOI: 10.1186/s40249-016-0139-4

[61] Wingfield T, Schumacher SG, Sandhu G, Tovar MA, Zevallos K, Baldwin MR, et al. The seasonality of tuberculosis, sunlight, vitamin D, and household crowding. The Journal of Infectious Diseases. 2014;**210**(5):774-783. DOI: 10.1093/infdis/jiu121

7

Urinary Tract Tuberculosis

Gerardo Amaya-Tapia and
Guadalupe Aguirre-Avalos

Abstract

Urinary tract tuberculosis (UTTB) is an insidious disease with non-specific constitutional symptoms that are often unrecognized and lead to delayed diagnosis. Advanced UTTB may cause loss of kidney function. In the majority of literature, UTTB is reviewed together with genital tuberculosis because often both sites are involved simultaneously; "Genitourinary tuberculosis" (GUTB) is the most common term used in the literature. However, the term may cause confusion because the clinical presentation and diagnosis approach is very different, and does not always occur simultaneously. UTTB is the term used here as we encountered tuberculosis involvement of urinary tract only. This book chapter is a comprehensive review of the epidemiology, pathophysiology, clinical presentation, diagnosis approach, and current treatment of this disease.

Keywords: tuberculosis, urinary tract infection, renal tuberculosis, extra-pulmonary tuberculosis, genitourinary tuberculosis

1. Introduction

Throughout history, tuberculosis (TB) has been identified as a respiratory disease, with prominent symptoms as cough, fever, and wasting. Current clinical experience reveals that the lungs are involved in 80–90% of all TB patients not infected by human immunodeficiency virus (HIV). Extra-pulmonary forms are more common in people co-infected with HIV where genitourinary tuberculosis (GUTB) represents 27% [1].

GUTB is a term coined by Wildbolz in 1937 [2]; it is a worldwide disease, but shows a more destructive behavior in developing countries. The kidney is the most common site of GUTB [3], and it usually affects adults between the second and fourth decades of life and is reported as being rare in children [4, 5]. Clinical renal TB is a chronic process that can start many years after the initial lung infection [6].

Renal involvement in TB can be part of a disseminated infection or a localized GUTB disease. With renal disease progression, extensive areas of papillary necrosis can cause formation of cavities that destroy the renal parenchyma and can migrate into the collecting system. Advanced disease may cause obstructive uropathy, bladder defects, and loss of kidney function [7].

UTTB is underdiagnosed in most health care centers; the clinicians must have a high degree of suspicion for UTTB in patients presenting with non-specific symptoms, culture-negative, pyuria, and for whom imaging studies show some typical findings of UTTB. Acid fast bacilli (AFB) microscopy and Lowenstein Jensen (LJ) culture are the tests most used in health institutions. AFB stain has a poor sensitivity and false positive can result from mycobacteria external genital colonization or by the presence of precipitates that resemble AFB. Although, LJ cultures have a better sensitivity, it may require around 8 weeks to obtain growth and identification [8]. In addition to other forms of extra-pulmonary tuberculosis, the amplification tests of deoxyribonucleic acid (DNA) have been used with good results, increasing the sensitivity, specificity and shortening the time to obtain the results. However, UTTB diagnostic requires a comprehensive approach and not just the use of a single test.

The initial treatment for TB in adults consists of the association of three or four different drugs, an intensive phase of 2 months of isoniazid (INH), rifampin (RIF), pyrazinamide (PZA), and ethambutol (EMB) followed by a continuation phase of 4 months of INH and RIF [9].

2. Epidemiology

The 2017 edition of the World Health Organization global TB report includes data available from 201 countries and territories that account for over 99% of the world's population. In 2016, a total of 6.3 million new cases of TB were reported and extra-pulmonary TB represented 15% of the cases notified, ranging from 8% in the Western Pacific Region to 24% in the Eastern Mediterranean Region [10]. According to other registers, of the total TB cases reported, the most frequent types of extra-pulmonary TB were lymphatic (14.8–40.4%), pleural (7.8–19.8%), bones and/or joints (3.5–11%), and GUTB (1.7–6.5%) [11, 12]. Involvement of the kidneys is the most common form of tuberculosis of the genitourinary tract [13].

In UTTB, a history of pulmonary TB is present in 17.7–25.8% [14–16]. The time interval between the onset of primary pulmonary TB and development of GUTB has a mean interval of 3–10 years in more than 50% of patients [14, 15]. In frequency, renal involvement is the most common finding following by ureteric and bladder involvement [16]. Simultaneous involvement of kidney, ureter, and bladder has been reported until a 25.8% [15, 16]. The incidence of active pulmonary TB concurrent with UTTB varied from 10 to 25.8%.

The proportion of immune-compromising conditions, such as malignancy, diabetes mellitus, chronic renal failure, and immunosuppressive drug use, are found as 46.7% [14]. The incidence of TB has been estimated to be as much as 10-fold higher among renal failure patients than among the general population [17].

3. Pathogenesis

Pulmonary infection is the primary focus in most cases of TB. After exposition, the bacilli remain stored in macrophages, where they slowly multiply, UTTB is the result of hematogenous spread from the lungs. Once the bacilli reach the circulation system, it can be distributed to all parts of the body, especially those sites with adequate conditions for its multiplication and with local immune deficiencies [18, 19]. The lymphatic nodes, encephalus, and urinary tract are some of the most frequent sites involved [20, 21].

The kidneys, and possibly the prostate and seminal vesicles, are often the primary sites of GUTB. All other genital organs, including the epididymis and bladder, become involved by ascent or descent of *Mtb* from a source elsewhere in the genitourinary tract [22]. *Mtb* bacilli are shed into the urine; they spread into the urinary tract, involving the renal pelvis, ureters and bladder; the urinary tract mucosa may be ulcerated, thin and without contractility [4]. In most patients, acquired cellular immunity develops and there is inhibition of bacilli multiplication and containment of the disease by the formation of microscopic granulomas, leading caseous necrosis with local tissue destruction [18].

The infection occurs initially in the medullary region, where granulomatous lesions can occur. If, in the course of primary infection, cell-mediated immunity develops and the proliferation of organisms is limited by competitive macrophages, this results in the formation of granulomas in which dormant bacilli can be maintained for long periods, leading caseous necrosis with local tissue destruction. When the bacilli are spilling down into the nephrons, they are trapped in the loop of Henle, establishing new foci of infection [18]. The multiple focus of microscopic necrosis lead macroscopic lesions that rapidly involve the renal papilla, causing fibrosis that can cause ureteral damage, with dilations intercalated with strictures, which constitutes an important TB sign on the pyelogram [23].

Sites of the urinary tract where there are natural narrow strictures, such as the calyceal neck, the pelvi-ureteric junction, and the uretero-vesical junction are the sites that suffer strictures more frequently. Steroid therapy may be useful in the early stages of scarring and could reduce the risk of stenosis that can lead to urinary obstruction and irreversible kidney damage [24]. A mass lesion may result from massive destruction and coalescence of granulomas, if they do not rupture into the adjoining calyx [25].

Hypercalcemia may occur, usually secondary to abnormal cortisol production by granulomatous tissue [26]. Although calcification is unusual in the early stages of the disease, nearly every end-stage tuberculosis kidney contains calcification. Hydronephrosis or hydrocalicosis may be the final stage, and may lead to a non-functioning, calcified kidney of any size; this process is called autonephrectomy [24].

4. Clinical presentation

UTTB has an insidious onset, no specific symptoms with atypical presentations [27], which lead to difficulty and delay the diagnosis in most health care centers [19, 20, 22, 28]. The majority

Ref	Author, country	Year*	Patients no.	Fever	Flank pain	Dysuria	Hematuria	Pyuria	Renal failure
[13]	Krishnamoorthy, India	2017	110	NR	27.3	25.5	11	NR	1.8
[14]	Altiparmak, Turkey	2015	79	43	38	51	79.1	67.1	19
[15]	Wagaskar, India	2016	31	29	45.1	32	19.4	NR	35.4
[16]	Zhang, China	2016	120	22.5	49.1	60.8	25	NR	NR
[35]	García-Rodríguez, Spain	1994	81	34.6	56.8	67.9	4.9	19.8	1.2
[36]	Gokce, Turkey	2002	174	19.5	43.5	43.1	39.6	NR	NR
[37]	Ye, China	2016	193	NR	49.2	61.1	63.2	19.2	NR

*Year of publication; NR, not reported.

Table 1. Clinical and laboratory features in UTTB (percent).

of patients present local symptoms such as frequent voiding, dysuria, pyuria, pain (back, flank or abdominal), and microscopic or macroscopic hematuria [4, 28–31]. Systemic symptoms of fever, night sweats, weight loss, and anorexia are less common [4, 29–31].

In a series of 115 cases with GUTB, the most common symptoms were reported to be flank pain, nicturia, frequent voiding and dysuria [32]. Figueiredo and Lucon [33] reported that storage symptoms (urinary frequency, urgency, urgency incontinence, nocturia), dysuria, and hematuria were the most common symptoms on admission, affecting 50.5, 37.9 and 35.6% of cases, respectively. Loin pain and fever were reported less frequent (34.4 and 21.9%, respectively).

Lower urinary symptoms occur whenever the disease spreads down to the ureters and bladder. Urinary symptoms suggestive of urinary tract infection, accompanied by pyuria and hematuria with no bacterial growth, suggest UTTB [7, 21, 34]. Pyuria and/or microscopic hematuria are present in more than 90% of cases. Heavy proteinuria and cellular casts are not generally seen and the plasma creatinine concentration is usually normal [21]. Advanced disease may cause obstructive uropathy, bladder defects, and loss of kidney function [7]. **Table 1** summarized the most frequent findings in large recent series of UTTB.

5. Case report

A 43-year-old woman was admitted to the hospital for fever, dysuria, and gross hematuria. She has a history of 2 years with progressive malaise, weight loss, and recurrent episodes of fever and dysuria that were treated with different antibiotics. Renal TB was diagnosed 1.5 years prior, receiving treatment during 6 months, improving her clinical conditions. However, despite anti-TB therapy, she continued having recurrent episodes of fever and dysuria. She also reports having intermittent diarrhea for 1 year and fever with flank pain for 3 months. Her physical examination revealed a chronically ill woman with fever and oral candidosis. Cardiothoracic examination was normal with the exception of tachycardia. Abdominal examination revealed diffuse abdominal tenderness with flank pain, and lower limb edema was noted. Laboratory studies revealed urinalysis with pyuria and hematuria. Two serologies for antibodies to HIV were positive. The smear of urine staining with Ziehl-Neelsen (ZN) demonstrated AFB, and mycobacteria cultures were performed. Her chest x-ray showed diffuse bilateral infiltrates consistent with pulmonary tuberculosis (**Figures 1** and **2**). Renal ultrasonography (USG) showed both kidneys enlargement with marked dilation of renal pelvis and calyces. The findings on conventional urography were stricture sites of the ureters and renal pelvis with severe hydronephrosis and ureter distortion (**Figures 3** and **4**). An abdominal computed tomography (CT) showed a large abscess in psoas muscle (**Figures 5** and **6**). Initial empiric antimicrobial therapy with ceftriaxone, ciprofloxacin, and anti-TB therapy were started. The abscess was aspirated by external incision with complete drainage. Cultures for pyogenic bacteria of the psoas abscess and urine were both negatives. A polymerase chain reaction (PCR) test for *Mtb* in urine was positive (**Figure 7**). The patient was discharged home after 8 days of hospital stay.

The patient was re-admitted to the hospital 6 days after home stay. She continues with fever and abdominal discomfort. On the hospital day seven, her condition started to deteriorate

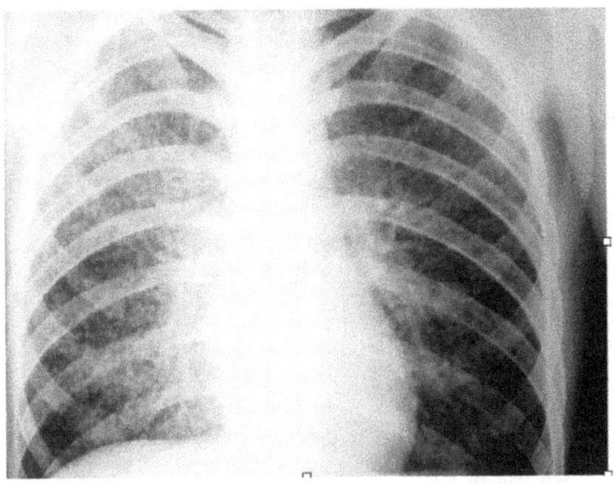

Figure 1. Chest radiograph showing diffuse micro-nodular infiltrates in both lung fields.

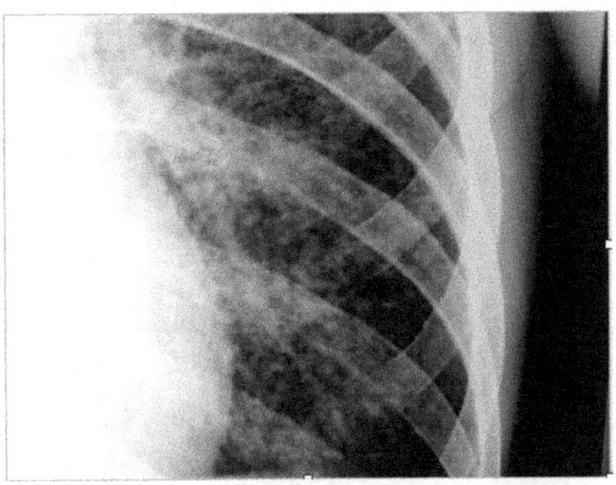

Figure 2. Magnified view of the left down lobe shows multiple micro-nodular infiltrates.

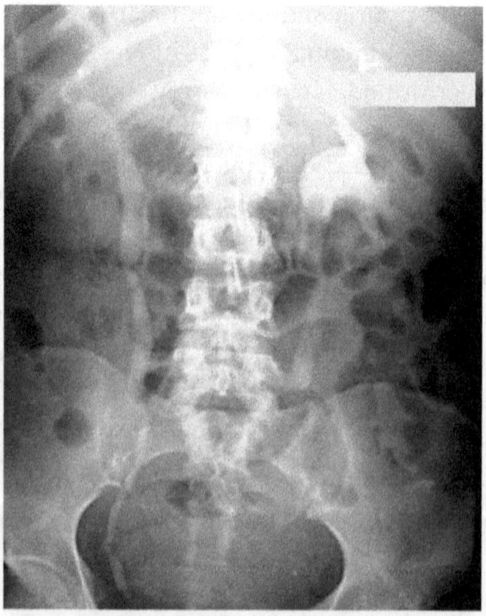

Figure 3. Intravenous urography revealing a non-functioning left kidney. Important deformity and dilatation of the collecting system, with ureteral tortuosity.

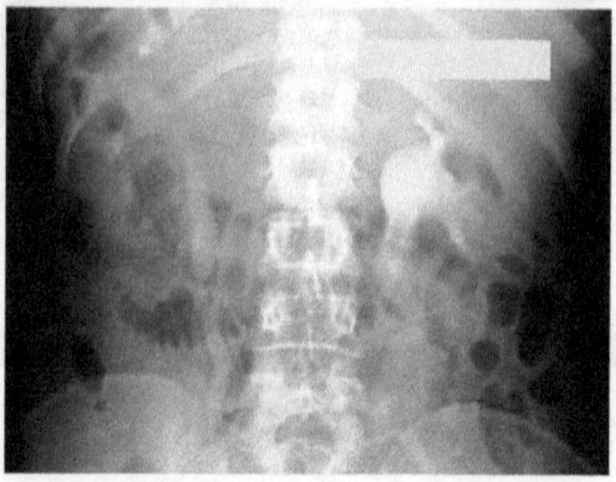

Figure 4. Left renal pelvis with severe hydronephrosis and ureteral distortion.

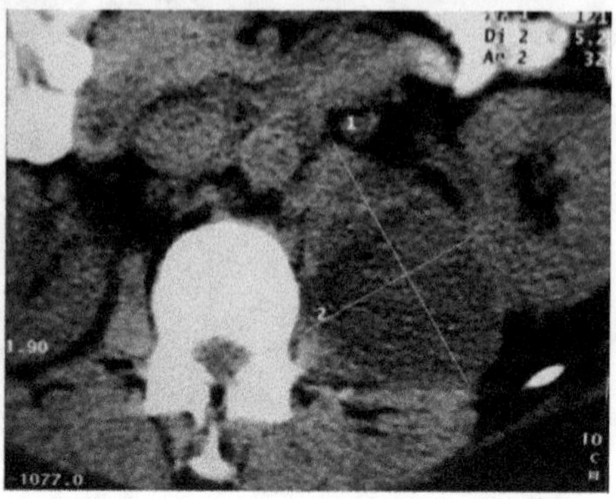

Figure 5. Axial CT revealing involvement of left psoas muscle and para-aortic space with displacement of the left kidney.

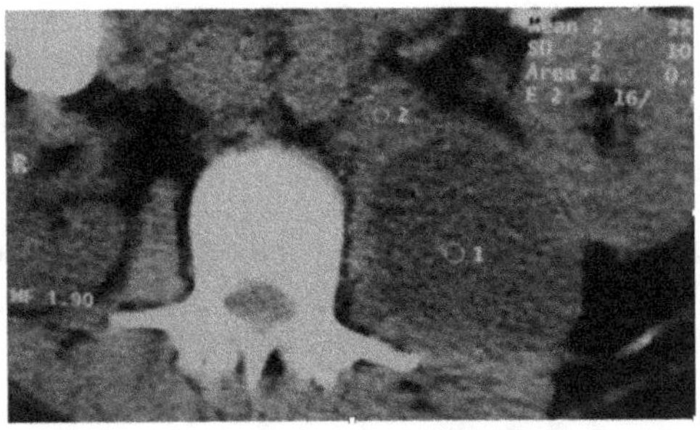

Figure 6. Axial CT revealing left psoas muscle abscess of 7 × 5 cm (1) and para-aortic lymph nodes (2).

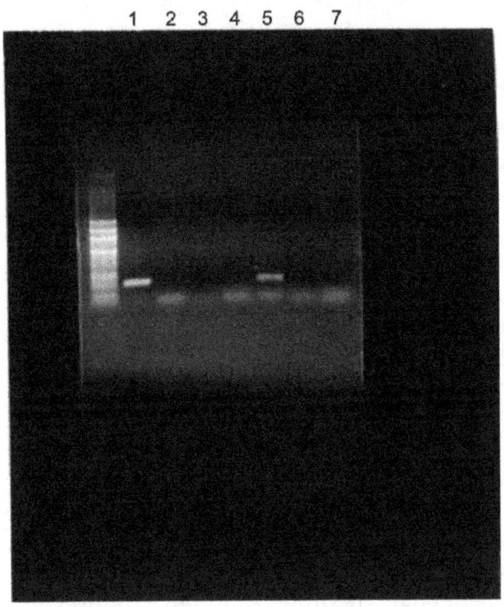

Figure 7. A representative image of PCR showing a DNA product of 200 base pairs for the first amplification. A positive control on the first line with a positive test on line 5.

and she died despite aggressive support Mycobacterial culture media subsequently yielded *Mtb* susceptible to all primary anti-TB drugs.

6. Diagnostic approach

The diagnosis of UTTB is a challenge owing to the insidious onset of UTTB with few and non-specific symptoms, technical difficulties to isolate *Mtb* and the long time required to confirm the diagnosis by classical conventional methods of cultivation, lack of awareness of physicians, and poor care-seeking behavior [33, 38].

The diagnosis of UTTB is usually performed in patients with clinical manifestations or abnormal urinalysis with findings that suggest UTTB. Urinalysis may vary from mild changes, such as proteinuria and leukocyturia, to extreme pyuria, sometimes accompanied by hematuria. There are some characteristics in urine examination that suggest a diagnosis of renal TB, such as acid pH, leukocyturia and/or hematuria, associated with negative urine culture for the usual bacteria that causes urinary tract infection [23].

There are several diagnostic methods for this entity. Here, we review the most common procedures used: (1) ZN staining and cultures isolation for *Mtb* in urine, (2) PCR for *Mtb*, (3) imaging studies, and (4) histopathological evidence for TB [14].

6.1. ZN stain and cultures for *Mtb* in urine

AFB can be seen in centrifuged urine by ZN staining, but it has low sensitivity when only few bacilli are seen. Also, it can be the result of urine contamination by non-pathogenic *Mycobacterium* spp., which can lead to false positive results [21].

Culture and identification provide a specific diagnosis, but might not be available for 2–3 weeks or longer. Multiple samplings should be obtained to increase test sensitivity; at least three different samples on LJ solid culture medium are recommended to maximize the likelihood of a positive result. Urine cultures are regularly negative, unless there is severe bladder dysfunction. Among patients with active renal TB, 30–40% of single urine specimens will be positive by *Mycobacterium* culture [39, 40]. BACTEC showed to be a better culture method compared to LJ, with a sensitivity of 37.5% and a specificity of 100% and the mean detection time for *Mtb* was 24.0 days by L-J medium culture versus only 12.8 days by BACTEC [41, 42].

6.2. Polymerase chain reaction for *Mtb*

The PCR assay has been extensively used as diagnosis in many forms of extra-pulmonary TB [43, 44], including some UTTB case reports [45, 46].

As a rapid and sensitive diagnostic method, PCR for *Mtb* identification in the urine has become the ideal diagnostic tool in recent years. It allows to make a diagnosis even when there are few bacilli and AFB detection is not possible. The sensitivity of AFB detection by ZN technique is between 42.1 and 52.1%. The sensitivities of culture methods vary from 10 to 90% while PCR in detecting *Mtb* in urine have a sensitivity that varies from 25 to 93% and a high specificity of 95–100% [38, 47–50]. In a prospective study in 42 patients where PCR was used, it showed a better sensitivity than the urine culture (80.9% against 30.9%); the author concludes that the PCR is far superior diagnosis technique for UTTB with high sensitivity and specificity, avoiding the retard of the start of therapy [51].

In the recent years, there has been important effort to increase the PCR for *Mtb* detection capacity, to avoid false positives by contamination and to determine his utility in different clinical samples [52–54]. In comparison with the traditional PCR of a single amplification, nested PCR consists of performing a second DNA step in order to increase sensitivity. According to the amount of DNA that is obtained, the nested PCR can enhance the sensitivity in approximately 1000 times than the PCR of a single amplification [55–57].

In a study with 417 clinical samples (including 28 of urine), the nested PCR for *Mtb* had a sensitivity of 97% and a specificity of 92% including positive results in some patients with negative culture. The authors concluded that the nested PCR is superior in sensitivity and rapidity than the traditional methods [57]. Nested PCR display a better sensitivity than the first DNA amplification, increasing the detection limit from 10 pg to 10 fg that is equivalent to two cells in the second amplification. The great amount of DNA in the second step of the nested PCR make easy the detection; it has been reported that during the first amplification, many positive samples gave a relatively weak or doubtful band. In contrast, in the second amplification a a strong positive band was observed [57].

6.3. Imaging studies

Although it is usually stated that imaging studies are only suggestive of the disease and should not be used for the confirmation or exclusion of UTTB [58], the intravenous urography (IVU) has been the image study more used for this entity; anatomical alterations of the collecting system can be seen with some facility. USG, CT, and magnetic resonance imaging (MRI) are less invasive methods that are better for detecting lesions in organs and tissues, including tumors, abscesses and calcifications; these can be done in addition to the IVU [59].

6.3.1. Plain radiograph

UTTB commonly results from hematogenous spread from a pulmonary focus; nevertheless, only 36.5% of patients with UTTB have a previous diagnosis of TB or abnormal imaging studies [5]. Chest radiograph will be normal in half the patients [60]. But, only 10% of chest radiograph will show signs of active TB [60, 61].

The greatest use of simple radiography is to demonstrate calcifications that can represent infections in extra-pulmonary sites, such as lymph nodes, liver, and spleen. Also, simple radiography can identify psoas abscesses and abnormalities of the spine [4, 62]. In UTTB, calcified lesions are mainly located in renal and upper collector system in 24–44% of cases [61], and this finding may be the first sign that TB is present [60]. Fine calcifications that were previously unidentifiable are now much better seen with CT [59].

Calcifications can be small calcifications, multiple, or large single calcifications [63]. These are usually amorphous calcifications located in the renal parenchyma or can take the form of the collecting system where they lodge and tend to be granular or curvilinear [22, 64]. The calcified caseous tissue in the kidneys may look like ground glass, known as "putty kidney". Premkumar et al. [65] termed "putty kidney" if the uniform calcification was greater than 1 cm in diameter.

Apperson et al. [66] emphasized the difficulty of differentiating calcifications from calculi in renal TB. In their cases of renal TB, 9.3% had discrete calculi and 8.7% had parenchymal calcification.

6.3.2. Intravenous urography

IVU has been considered the radiographic procedure of choice due to its ability to show the collector system like no other, and less frequently modern techniques such as computerized axial tomography and magnetic resonance are also used [67]. Early findings are best demonstrated on contrast-enhanced tomography which is replacing IVU as the investigation of choice in that situation. In a retrospective study conducted in Spain, IVU guided the diagnosis in 28/32 cases (87.5%), with calculus lesions, bladder alterations, hydronephrosis, calcifications and ureteral stenosis as the most common alterations [68]. However, 10–15% of patients with active UTTB may have normal urographic findings [69].

Early alterations of UTTB are located mainly in calyces, UVI can show minimal calyceal dilation and loss of calyceal sharpness [61]. Although the calyceal damage is an early sign of UTTB, papillary necrosis could be the first sign observed [59]. As the disease progresses, the irregularity of the calices increases and may have a moth-eaten appearance [4, 25]. Other advanced manifestations include extensive cavitation, fibrotic strictures, cortical scars, mass lesions, calcification, autonephrectomy, perinephric abscess, and fistula formation [60].

6.3.3. *Ultrasonography*

USG is a readily available technique for demonstrating the various morphologic abnormalities found in renal TB [18, 70] and is a convenient method for guiding needles for fine-needle aspiration cytology (FNAC) [71, 72]. USG has convenient, low-priced, and non-invasive advantages; a disadvantage is that a mass may be missed if its echogenicity is similar to the renal parenchyma.

Traditionally, USG has been considered of less value than IVU or CT in UTTB cases [6, 73]. USG has limitations in detecting subtle urothelial lesions, as well as isoechoic parenchymal masses and is not useful for evaluating renal function [65, 69]. However, a well-detailed study can provide valuable information. In a large retrospective study, the coincidence rate of USG in the diagnosis of renal TB was 58.9% [74]. As the disease progresses, both an infiltrative pattern affecting the tissues and a pattern that affects the collecting system can be observed. In the first case, papillary destruction, calcifications, infected debris, hypoechoic masses or abscesses can be observed, in the second case dilated calyces, small renal pelvis, hydronephrosis, distortion of renal morphology, deformity of the ureters, and bladder atrophy can be found [75, 76].

On the USG, renal abscess is presented as a semi-solid echogenicity and a thick ill-defined wall that can extend and drain, causing perinephric abscess that later may cause a cutaneous fistula [21, 68].

6.3.4. *Computed tomography*

CT is useful both in the diagnosis of renal TB and in assessing its severity in terms of loss of renal function and involvement of other organs in the abdomen [77]. It directly visualizes the renal parenchyma, irrespective of renal function and, in addition, assesses extrarenal spread of the disease. The CT nephrogram is not as dependent on renal function as is an IVU. CT is also useful in identifying renal scars, mass lesions, and urothelial thickening, all of which are common findings in renal TB [78].

In general, CT shows more details of pathologic anatomy due to the availability of axial images for review and is superior to retrograde pyelography, IVU, and USG in detecting multiple small urothelial lesions [79]. It can detect calcification with greater accuracy, precision, and sensitivity [61] and is the most sensitive modality for identifying renal calcifications, which occur in over 50% of cases of GUTB [80]. CT is also the best modality for demonstrating the extent, nature, and distribution of calcification within the abnormal kidney [65]. The implementation of CT urography with multidetector technology improves the assessment of renal and urinary tract lesions using reformatted images [17].

The disadvantages of CT include its inability to identify very early changes of TB such as small parenchymal and subtle papillary necrosis. UTTB is characterized by a vast presentation that is of great diagnostic value [19, 62, 81]. In early disease, CT can detect obstruction of a single major or a group of minor calyces as well as abnormalities in the collector system (dilatation or contraction of the renal pelvis). In advance disease, the kidneys are small with replacement of parenchyma by one or more low density areas. Parenchyma or calyces calcifications are seen at 37% [81]. Newer scanners, if used meticulously, may be able to identify small granulomas. The needs to use contrast and radiation issues, especially in young patients, are other limitations of CT studies that are not encountered on USG [78].

6.3.5. Magnetic resonance imaging

MRI provides morphological details of the kidneys as well as excellent delineation of the ureters [67]. It allows characterization of various renal masses and can provide valuable information contributing to their clinical management [82, 83]. It is particularly useful in pediatric or pregnant patients or when ionizing radiation and iodinated contrast cannot be administered. Non-contrast MRI is especially useful in patients with renal failure [67].

Magnetic resonance urography (MRU) comprises an evolving group of techniques with the potential for optimal non-invasive evaluation of urinary tract abnormalities. Both static-fluid (non-contrast, heavily T2W sequences) and excretory MRU (performed during the excretory phase of enhancement after intravenous gadolinium) can be combined with conventional MRI for comprehensive evaluation of the urinary tract. MRU demonstrates the ureters in their entirety and is useful for confirming the presence of stenosis [84]. It is most successful in patients with moderately to severely dilated or obstructed collecting systems and in impaired renal function situations [84, 85]. MRU performed with a distended urinary bladder allows better visualization of the upper urinary tract [86]. Time-resolved dynamic contrast-enhanced MRU has been used in the evaluation of ureteral peristalsis in GUTB [87]. In view of the possibility of nephrogenic systemic, fibrosis/nephrogenic, fibrosing dermopathy, caution should be exercised while administering gadolinium in patients with compromised renal function [88]. There are very few articles available in the literature on MRU in renal TB and hence the appearance of the same is still not widely known.

6.3.6. Fine-needle aspiration cytology

Sonographically guided FNAC is useful as a means of diagnosing of renal and genital (epididymitis and epididymo-orchitis) abscess or masses, and is of value in defining the granulomatous nature of sonographically visible lesions [72]. Histologic findings of renal or genital TB are similar to those of TB elsewhere in the body (granuloma formation, non-specific inflammatory infiltrate). The granulomas appear with central Langerhans cells surrounded by lymphocytes, fibrocytes, and epithelioid cells, which later progress to central caseous formation and varying degrees of fibrosis and calcification. AFB may be detected on FNAC smears in up to 60% of these patients [72, 89].

The advantages of USG-guided FNAC are that it is rapid, inexpensive, versatile, does not require the injection of any contrast medium, and can be easily repeated when necessary [90]. USG-guided FNAC is now widely accepted as a safe diagnostic procedure in various neoplastic and non-neoplastic disorders [91, 92].

7. Treatment

A multidisciplinary approach with infectious disease and urology teams is crucial to provide optimal patient care; tuberculosis medications remain the cornerstone of treatment and surgical management is reserved for specific indications. There is lack of standardized treatment regimen for UTTB, it is accepted that pulmonary and extra-pulmonary TB should be treated with the same regimens.

The objectives of TB therapy are (1) to rapidly reduce the number of actively growing bacilli in the patient, thereby decreasing severity of the disease and preventing death (2) to eradicate populations of persisting bacilli in order to achieve durable cure (prevent relapse) after completion of therapy; and (3) to prevent acquisition of drug resistance during therapy.

7.1. Medical treatment

Clinical judgment and the index of suspicion for TB are critical in making a decision to initiate treatment [9, 14]. Therapy should be initiated promptly even before the results of AFB smear microscopy, molecular tests, and mycobacterial culture are known. It is particularly important in cases admitted with episodes of cystitis concomitant with sterile pyuria and progressive renal parenchymal damage not related to other clinical diseases [14]. If the diagnosis has been made while renal function still remains, it may be possible to arrest the fall in glomerular filtration rate or even produce improvement, using a combination of anti-TB treatment and corticosteroids [21].

Fibrotic alterations can be decreased by use of corticosteroids in association with anti-TB drugs. However, despite these strategies, patients with advanced disease or those with a delayed diagnosis might require surgery [93]. The use of corticosteroids in addition to stenting for ureteral obstruction is discussed in the literature, and its efficacy in this setting remains unclear [94].

Regarding the duration of the UTTB treatment, the expert recommendation is that a standard daily 6-month regimen is adequate [12, 29, 31, 95, 96]. In countries where new cases of tuberculosis are resistant to organisms (resistant to isoniazid ≥4%), it is recommended to use four drugs in the intensive phase: INH, RIF, PZA, and EMB [97–101].

Two regimens can be used. The first-line regimen, which is used for 6 months, is with INH, RIF, PZA, and EMB administered daily or 5 days per week for 2 or 3 months, followed by INH and RIF daily or 5 days per week for 3 or 4 months [93]. The second-line regimen, which is recommended for TB caused by drug-susceptible organisms when directly observed therapy (DOT) is difficult to achieve, it consist of INH, RIF, PZA, and EMB daily or 5 days per week for 2 or 3 months, followed by INH and RIF 3 times a week, for 3 or 4 months (**Tables 2** and **3**) [9].

Intensive phase		Continuation phase		
Drugs	**Interval and dose (minimum duration)**	**Drugs**	**Interval and dose (minimum duration)**	**Range of total doses**
INH	7 d/wk for 56 doses	INH	7 d/wk for 126	182–130
RIF	(8 wk), or	RIF	doses (18 wk), or	
PZA	5 d/wk for 40 doses		5 d/wk for 90	
EMB	(8 wk)		doses (18 wk)	

DOT, directly observed therapy; EMB, ethambutol; INH, isoniazid; PZA, pyrazinamide; RIF, rifampin.

Table 2. Recommended drug regimen for tuberculosis caused by drug-susceptible organisms.

Intensive phase		Continuation phase		
Drugs	**Interval and dose (minimum duration)**	**Drugs**	**Interval and dose (minimum duration)**	**Range of total doses**
INH	7 d/wk for 56 doses	INH	3 times weekly for 54 doses (18 wk)	110–94
RIF	(8 wk), or	RIF		
PZA	5 d/wk for 40 doses			
EMB	(8 wk)			

DOT, directly observed therapy; EMB, ethambutol; INH, isoniazid; PZA, pyrazinamide; RIF, rifampin.

Table 3. Recommended drug regimen for tuberculosis caused by drug-susceptible organisms when DOT is difficult to achieve.

Pyridoxine (vitamin B6) is given with INH to all persons at risk of neuropathy (e.g., pregnant women; breastfeeding infants; persons infected with HIV; patients with diabetes, alcoholism, malnutrition, or chronic renal failure; or those who are of advanced age) [102, 103]. Although there is no studies that compare 5 with 7 daily doses, experts believe that the treatment of intensive phase with 5-days-a-week is as effective as 7-days-a-week [9].

Some authors propose that prolonged anti-TB treatment effectively sterilizes caseous and calcified masses of the involved kidney, whereas others believe that the sequestered caseous material should be removed to shorten the duration of medical therapy and to prevent late TB reactivation [28, 104].

Adequately controlled, randomized studies specific to UTTB comparing different treatment regimens have not been performed. Such studies would establish if short-course therapies are adequate to ensure eradication of UTTB, including patients with prostatic infection. There is little information about the vigilance and follow-up of patients with UTTB that may include at least monthly function renal tests, urine ZN smear, and *Mtb* cultures. ADN amplification tests for *Mtb* and imaging studies should be used on clinical judgment and probably performed at the end of both intensive and continues phases. Response to treatment may be difficult to assess and should be based on clinical, radiologic, and eradication of *Mtb* on subsequent cultures [94].

To maximize completion of therapy, management strategies should utilize a broad range of approaches. Among these, DOT is the practice of observing the patient swallow their anti-TB drugs and has been widely used as the standard of practice in many TB programs. DOT can be advantageous for early recognition of adverse drug reactions and treatment irregularities. DOT remains the standard of practice in the majority of TB programs in the United States [105, 106] and Europe [107].

Gastrointestinal and skin disorders adverse reactions are common; the frequency can reach up to 30% especially early in therapy. Less frequent adverse events are muscle-joints disorders, fever, headache, hepatic problems, and even death [108, 109]. Four-drug fixed-doses therapy may reduce the incidence of gastrointestinal adverse effects and the use of antacids or proton pump inhibitors for reducing gastrointestinal can contribute to better tolerance with minor impact on drugs absorption [110]. INH, RIF, and PZA can cause drug-induced liver injury that is the most frequent serious adverse event [111]. It is necessary to promote some strategies that improve the quality of patient care and to control TB safely, treating preexisting diseases or dysfunctions, such as diabetes and alcoholism. These strategies may improve the patient adherence to treatment and therapeutic outcome.

7.2. Invasive procedures

Invasive procedures or surgery are indicated in certain situations: hydronephrosis drainage (ureter dilation or percutaneous nephrostomy), abscesses and collection drainage, definitive treatment of renal TB (partial nephrectomy), superior urinary tract reconstruction, bladder dilation, ureter reconstruction and others [112]. In a study of 4298 patients with GUTB, 2364 (37%) underwent surgery: remove or preserve an organ and reconstruction surgery were the most frequent interventions. Other surgical modalities included ureteral neoimplantation using intestinal transplants (ileocystoplasty, sigmoidocystoplasty, and cecocystoplasty) [113].

Other surgical intervention can be double-J stenting use and percutaneous nephrostomy for hydronephrosis cases, drainage of abscesses, partial or polar nephrectomy, reconstruction of the upper urinary tract, and bladder augmentation with ileum replacement [114].

The standard treatment for a unilateral nonfunctional kidney secondary to renal TB is a nephrectomy combined with anti-TB therapy [16]. The patients that end up in nephrectomy have an advanced stage [13, 37]. Nephrectomy is recommended only in cases of secondary sepsis, bleeding, pain, uncontrollable hypertension, and continued positive urinary cultures for *Mtb* [38].

Radical or reconstructive surgical interventions are recommended be carried out in the first 2 months of intensive GUTB therapy [115].

7.3. Treatment of special situations

7.3.1. *Patients with HIV infection*

HIV and TB create a deadly synergy, speeding the progression of both diseases. HIV enhances the reactivation and progression of latent TB to overt TB disease. The treatment represents a challenge were the most significant concern is to avoid drug-drug interactions and the control of adverse events. Whenever possible, the use of combination formulations, both antituberculous and ARV drugs, is recommended in order to simplify the treatment.

The recommendation for HIV-infected patients receiving ARV and initial TB disease with susceptible *Mtb* is a short course of 6 months of therapy. During the first 2 months of daily regimen (initial phase), patients should be treated with INH, RIF, PZA, and EMB. This is followed by a continuation phase of 4 months of INH plus RIF thrice-weekly regimen. HIV-infected patients that still do not receive ARV; the recommendation is to extend the continuation phase with INH and RIF for additional 3 months (i.e., a continuation phase of 7 months in duration, corresponding to a total of 9 months of therapy) [9].

Once a week, TB continuation phase regimen can be safe and effective treating pulmonary TB in HIV-negative patients without cavitation on chest radiography [116]. However, relapses and rifamycin monoresistant tuberculosis occurs among HIV infected patients treated with a once-weekly isoniazid/rifapentine during continuation phase regimen [117]. A study with 169 HIV-infected patients and pulmonary TB, nine (5.3%) had failure or relapse, eight of these nine isolates were detected with acquired rifamycin resistance, low CD4 lymphocyte counts and the use of twice-weekly therapy during intensive phase were the most important factors associated [118]. Lower plasma rifabutin and INH concentrations are associated with acquiring rifamycin resistance [119].

HIV/TB co-infected patients treated during continuation phases with thrice-weekly anti-TB regimen showed a higher risk of relapse and death as well as emergence of rifamycin resistance compared with HIV-uninfected patients. ARV therapy reduces but does not eliminate the risk of these complications [120]. A prompt diagnosis of HIV, earlier ARV initiation, and avoiding intermittent TB treatment regimens could prevent relapses and drug resistance emergence. Rifabutin can be substituted for RIF to decrease drug interactions with drugs used in the treatment of HIV infection (protease inhibitors and transcriptase reverse non-nucleoside inhibitors) [9].

Immune reconstitution inflammatory syndrome (IRIS) is a paradoxical clinical worsening of a known or new condition occurring shortly after initiating ARV therapy, mainly in patients with low CD4+ cell counts [121]. *Mtb* is among the most frequently reported pathogen associated with IRIS; signs may include high fever, lymphadenopathy, worsening of respiratory symptoms, new pulmonary infiltrates, and pleural effusions. Extra-pulmonary presentations are also possible expanding to central nervous system, intra-abdominal abscesses, osteomyelitis, and others [122]. For more severe cases of IRIS, treatment with corticosteroids is effective. In a placebo-controlled trial of prednisone for patients with moderate IRIS, prednisone 1.25 mg/kg/day significantly reduced the need for hospitalization or surgical procedures [123].

7.3.2. Renal failure

Renal TB can result in acute or chronic renal failure with an incidence of 24%. If renal TB progresses to chronic kidney disease (CKD), it has effects in the immune system too. The alterations on systemic immunity included persistent systemic inflammation and acquired immunosuppression state [124]. The mechanisms associated with end-stage renal disease include obliterative endarteritis, renal amyloidosis, and obstructive uropathy [7, 93].

The patients with CKD by other etiology are at increased risk of TB than those with normal renal function. Drug-induced hepatitis and all-cause mortality are more common among TB patients with CKD [125]. One of principal factors to consider in TB treatment with CKD included drug pharmacokinetics, drugs removed by hemodialysis that should be dosed after dialysis [126]. INH, RIF, and EMB are not significantly dialyzed. However, PZA is removed by hemodialysis and should be administered after hemodialysis [127]. Other factors included co-existent illnesses, dosage adjustment, drug interactions, and drug accumulate predisposing to toxicities. Initial regimen with standard doses and no more than three times weekly for PZA, EMB, and aminoglycosides is recommended [128].

The fluoroquinolones used for TB treatment are levofloxacin, moxifloxacin, and gatifloxacin. According to degree of renal impairment, levofloxacin dosage adjustment is required. Nevertheless, neither hemodialysis nor continuous ambulatory peritoneal dialysis removed levofloxacin [129]. Moxifloxacin may be administered at the normal dosage even with severe renal failure [130].

7.3.3. Advanced age

Age over 60 years is significantly associated with serious adverse events related to INH, PZA, and RIF, with greater frequency of hepatitis episodes and gastrointestinal intolerance [131, 132]. However, the risk of hepatotoxicity in advanced age might not increase after 12 weeks with standard treatment containing INH and RIF [133]. The severity of INH-induced hepatitis has been associated with higher mortality in this patient population [131]. Dose adjustments or alternative regiments should be considered to avoid stopping the treatment, increasing the probability of failure and mortality [9, 134]. The duration of TB treatment depends of initial regimen during the intensive phase [9].

Author details

Gerardo Amaya-Tapia[1,2]* and Guadalupe Aguirre-Avalos[1,3]

*Address all correspondence to: gamaya@cencar.udg.mx

1 Centro Universitario Ciencias de la Salud at Universidad de Guadalajara, Guadalajara, Jalisco, Mexico

2 Infectious Diseases Department at Hospital General de Occidente, Guadalajara, Jalisco, Mexico

3 Intensive Care Unit at Hospital Civil de Guadalajara "Fray Antonio Alcalde", Guadalajara, Jalisco, Mexico

References

[1] Rieder HL, Snider DE Jr, Cauthen GM. Extrapulmonary tuberculosis in the United States. The American Review of Respiratory Disease. 1990;**141**:347-351

[2] Gupta NP. Genitourinary tuberculosis. Indian Journal of Urology. 2008;**24**:355

[3] Naidich DP, Garay SM, Leitman BS, McCauley DI. Radiographic manifestations of pulmonary disease in the acquired immunodeficiency syndrome (AIDS). Seminars in Roentgenology. 1987;**22**:14-30

[4] Tonkin AK, Witten DM. Genitourinary tuberculosis. Seminars in Roentgenology. 1979;**14**:305-318

[5] Wise GJ. Urinary tuberculosis: Modern issues. Current Urology Reports. 2009;**10**:313-318

[6] Merchant SA. Tuberculosis of the genitourinary system. The Indian Journal of Radiology and Imaging. 1993;**3**:253-274

[7] Daher Ede F, Silva Junior GB, Damasceno RT, Santos GM, Corsino GA, Silva SL, Gutierrez-Adrianzén OA. End-stage renal disease due to delayed diagnosis of renal tuberculosis: A fatal case report. The Brazilian Journal of Infectious Diseases. 2007;**11**:169-171

[8] Jonas V, Alden MJ, Curry JI, Kamisango K, Knott CA, Lankford R, et al. Detection and identification of *Mycobacterium tuberculosis* directly from sputum sediments by amplification of rRNA. Journal of Clinical Microbiology. 1993;**31**:2410-2441

[9] Nahid P, Dorman SE, Alipanah N, Barry PM, Brozek JL, Cattamanchi A, et al. Official American thoracic society/centers for disease control and prevention/infectious diseases society of America Clinical Practice Guidelines: Treatment of drug-susceptible tuberculosis. Clinical Infectious Diseases. 2016;**63**:853-867

[10] Global Tuberculosis Report. Geneva: World Health Organization; 2017. Licence: CC BY-NCSA 3.0 IGO; 2017

[11] Peto HM, Pratt RH, Harrington TA, LoBue PA, Lori R, Armstrong LR. Epidemiology of extrapulmonary tuberculosis in the United States, 1993-2006. CID. 2009;**49**:1350-1357

[12] Lam TB, Van der Werf MJ, Richter C, Borgdorff MW. Extrapulmonary tuberculosis by nationatily, the Netherlands. Emerging Infectious Diseases. 2006;**12**(9):1375-1382

[13] Krishnamoorthy S, Palaniyandi V, Kumaresan N, Govindaraju S, Rajasekaran J, Murugappan I, et al. Aspects of evolving genito urinary tuberculosis-A profile of genito urinary tuberculosis (GUTB) in 110 patients. Journal of Clinical and Diagnostic Research. 2017;**11**:1-5

[14] Altiparmak MR, Trabulus S, Balkan II, Yalin SF, Denizli N, Aslan G, et al. Urinary tuberculosis: A cohort of 79 adult cases. Renal Failure. 2015;**37**(7):1157-1163

[15] Wagaskar VG, Chirmade RA, Baheti VH, Tanwar HV, Patwardhan SK, Gopalakrishnan G. Urinary tuberculosis with renal failure: Challenges in management. Journal of Clinical and Diagnostic Research. 2016;**10**:1-3

[16] Zhang S, Luo Y, Wang C, Xiong H, Fu SJ, Yang L. Open surgery versus retroperitoneal laparoscopic nephrectomy for renal tuberculosis: A retrospective study of 120 patients. Peer J. 2016;**29**:e2708

[17] Gaudiano C, Tadolini M, Busato F, Vanino E, Pucci S, Corcioni B, et al. Multidetector CT urography in urogenital tuberculosis: use of reformatted images for the

assessment of the radiological findings. A pictorial essay. Abdominal Radiology. 2017;**42**:2314-2324

[18] Hartman DS, Stagg PL. Diagnosis please. Case 3: Renal tuberculosis. Radiology. 1998;**209**: 69-72

[19] Wang LJ, Wong YC, Chen CJ, Lim KE. CT features of genitourinary tuberculosis. Journal of Computer Assisted Tomography. 1997;**21**:254-258

[20] Muttarak M, ChiangMai WN, Lojanapiwat B. Tuberculosis of the genitourinary tract: Imaging features with pathological correlation. Singapore Medical Journal. 2005;**46**: 568-574

[21] Eastwood JB, Corbishley CM, Grange JM. Tuberculosis and the kidney. Journal of the American Society of Nephrology. 2001;**12**:1307-1314

[22] Engin G, Acunaş B, Acunaş G, Tunaci M. Imaging of extrapulmonary tuberculosis. Radiographics. 2000;**20**:471-488

[23] Daher Ede F, Da Silva GB Jr, Barros EJ. Review: Renal tuberculosis in the modern era. The American Journal of Tropical Medicine and Hygiene. 2013;**88**(1):54-64

[24] Merchant S, Bharati A, Merchant N. Tuberculosis of the genitourinary system-urinary tract tuberculosis: Renal tuberculosis–Part I. Indian Journal of Radiology and Imaging. 2013;**23**(1):46-63

[25] Vijayaraghavan SB, Kandasamy SV, Arul M, Prabhakar M, Dhinakaran CL, Palanisamy R. Spectrum of high-resolution sonographic features of urinary tuberculosis. Journal of Ultrasound in Medicine. 2004;**23**:585-594

[26] Pouchot J, Dreyfuss D, Gardin JP, Mier L, Rémy P, Esdaile JM, et al. Ectopic production of 1,25-dihydroxyvitamin D3 in tuberculosis. Nephrology, Dialysis, Transplantation. 1993;**8**:560-562

[27] Wise GJ, Shteynshlyuger A. An update on lower urinary tract tuberculosis. Current Urology Reports. 2008;**9**:305-313

[28] Gibson MS, Puckett ML, Shelly ME. Renal tuberculosis. Radiographics. 2004;**24**:251-256

[29] Christensen WI. Genitourinary tuberculosis: Review of 102 cases. Medicine (Baltimore). 1974;**53**:377-390

[30] Narayana A. Overview of renal tuberculosis. Urology. 1982;**19**:231-237

[31] Simon HB, Weinstein AJ, Pasternak MS, Swartz MN, Kunz LJ. Genitourinary tuberculosis. Clinical features in a general hospital population. The American Journal of Medicine. 1977;**63**:410-420

[32] Fanning A. Tuberculosis: 6. Extrapulmonary disease. CMAJ. 1999;**160**(11):1597-1603

[33] Figueiredo AA, Lucon AM. Urogenital tuberculosis: Update and review of 8961 cases from the world literature. Revista de Urología. 2008;**10**(3):207-217

[34] Wechsler H, Westfall M, Lattimer JK. The earliest signs and symptoms in 127 male patients with genitourinary tuberculosis. The Journal of Urology. 1960;**83**:801-803

[35] García-Rodríguez JA, García-Sánchez JE, Muñoz-Bedillo JL, Montes-Martínez I, Rodríguez-Hernández J, Fernández- Gorostarzu J, et al. Genitourinary tuberculosis in Spain: Review of 81 cases. CID. 1994;**18**:557-561

[36] Gokce G, Kilicarslan H, Ayan S, Tas F, Akar R, Kaya K, et al. Genitourinary tuberculosis: A review of 174 cases. Scandinavian Journal of Infectious Diseases. 2002;**34**:338-340

[37] Ye Y, Hu X, Shi Y, Zhou J, Zhou Y, Song X, et al. Clinical features and drug-resistance profile of urinary tuberculosis in south-western China: A cross-sectional study. Medicine (Baltimore). 2016;**95**:e3537

[38] Ghaleb K, Afifi M, El-Gohary M. Assessment of diagnostic techniques of urinary tuberculosis. Mediterranean Journal of Hematology and Infectious Diseases. 2013;**5**(1):e2013034

[39] Berta M, Sturm G, Juri L, Cosiansi MC, Barzón S, Barnes AI, Rojo SC. Bacteriological diagnosis of renal tuberculosis: An experience at the regional tuberculosis laboratory in Córdoba Province, Argentina. Revista Argentina de Microbiología. 2011;**43**(3):191-194

[40] Pais VM, Dionne-Odom J, von Reyn CF, Curhan G, Baron EL, Sheridan AM. Renal Disease in Tuberculosis. UpToDate. 2015. Available at: http://www.uptodate.com

[41] Hillemann D, Richter E, Rüsch-Gerdes S. Use of the BACTEC mycobacteria growth indicator tube 960 automated system for recovery of mycobacteria from 9,558 extrapulmonary specimens, including urine samples. Journal of Clinical Microbiology. 2006;**44**:4014-4017

[42] Wang SX, Tay L. Evaluation of three nucleic acid amplification methods for direct detection of *Mycobacterium tuberculosis* complex in respiratory specimens. Journal of Clinical Microbiology. 1999;**37**:1932-1934

[43] Portillo GL, Morris S, Panduro A. Rapid and efficient detection of extrapulmonary *Mycobacterium tuberculosis* by PCR analysis. The International Journal of Tuberculosis and Lung Disease. 2000;**4**:361-370

[44] Piersimoni C, Scarparo C, Piccoli C, Rigon A, Ruggiero G, Nista D, Bornigia S. Performance assessment of two commercial amplification assays for direct detection of *Mycobacterium tuberculosis* complex from respiratory and extrapulmonary specimens. Journal of Clinical Microbiology. 2002;**40**:4138-4142

[45] Van Volle HP, Heyns CF, de Beer PM, Whitaker P, van Helden PD, Victor T. Polymerase chain reaction in the diagnosis of urinary tract tuberculosis. Urological Research. 1996;**24**:107-111

[46] Missirliu A, Gasman D, Vogt B, Poveda JD, Abbou CC, Chopin D. Genito-urinary tuberculosis: Rapid diagnosis using the polymerase chain reaction. European Urology. 1996; **30**(4):523

[47] Ferrie BG, Rundle JS. Genito-urinary tuberculosis in Glasgow 1970 to 1979: A review of 230 patients. Scottish Medical Journal. 1985;**30**(1):30-34

[48] Mortier E, Pouchot J, Girard L, Boussougant Y, Vinceneux P. Assessment of urine analysis for the diagnosis of tuberculosis. BMJ. 1996;**312**(7022):27-28

[49] Moussa OM, Eraky I, El-Far MA, Osman HG, Ghoneim MA. Rapid diagnosis of genitourinary tuberculosis by polymerase chain reaction and non-radioactive DNA hybridization. The Journal of Urology. 2000;**164**(2):584-588

[50] Kafwabulula M, Ahmed K, Nagatake T, Gotoh J, Mitarai S, Oizumi K, Zumla A. Evaluation of PCR-based methods for the diagnosis of tuberculosis by identification of mycobacterial DNA in urine samples. The International Journal of Tuberculosis and Lung Disease. 2002;**6**:732-737

[51] Hemal AK, Gupta NP, Rajeev TP, Kumar R, Dar L, Seth P. Polymerase chain reaction in clinically suspected genitourinary tuberculosis: Comparison with intravenous urography, bladder biopsy, and urine acid fast bacilli culture. Urology. 2000;**56**(4):570-574

[52] Yuen KY, Yam WC, Wong LP, Seto WH. Comparison of two automated DNA amplification systems with a manual one-tube nested PCR assay for diagnosis of pulmonary tuberculosis. Journal of Clinical Microbiology. 1997;**35**:1385-1389

[53] Montenegro SH, Gilman RH, Sheen P, Cama R, Caviedes L, Hopper T, et al. Improved detection of *Mycobacterium tuberculosis* in Peruvian children by use of a heminested IS6110 polymerase chain reaction assay. Clinical Infectious Diseases. 2003;**36**:16-23

[54] Honore S, Vincensini JP, Hocqueloux L, Noguera ME, Farge D, Lagrange P, Herrmann JL. Diagnostic value of a nested polymerase chain reaction assay on peripheral blood mononuclear cells from patients with pulmonary and extra pulmonary tuberculosis. The International Journal of Tuberculosis and Lung Disease. 2001;**5**(8):754-762

[55] Pierre C, Lecossier D, Boussougant Y, Bocart D, Joly V, Yeni P, Hance AJ. Use of reamplification protocol improves sensitivity of detection of *Mycobacterium tuberculosis* in clinical samples by amplification of DNA. Journal of Clinical Microbiology. 1991;**29**:712-717

[56] Amaya-Tapia G, Portillo-Gómez L, Aguirre-Avalos G, Rodríguez-Toledo A, Sosa-Iglesias EG, Aguilar-Benavides S. DNA amplification for *M. tuberculosis* detection in patients with suspected urinary tract tuberculosis. In: 43th Annual Meeting of Infectious Diseases Society of America (IDSA) San Francisco; 2005. abstract #228

[57] Miyazaki Y, Koga H, Kohno S, Kaku M. Nested polymerase chain reaction for detection of *Mycobacterium tuberculosis* in clinical samples. Journal of Clinical Microbiology. 1993;**31**:2228-2232

[58] Caskurlu T, Resim S, Bayraktar Z, Taşçi AI, Sevin G. Urinary tuberculosis in a two-year-old boy. International Urology and Nephrology. 1998;**30**:525-528

[59] Becker JA. Renal tuberculosis. Urologic Radiology. 1988;**10**:25-30

[60] Kollins SA, Hartman GW, Carr DT, Segura JW, Hattery RR. Roentgenographic findings in urinary tract tuberculosis. A 10 year review. The American Journal of Roentgenology, Radium Therapy, and Nuclear Medicine. 1974;**121**:487-499

[61] Elkin M. Urogenital tuberculosis. In: Pollack HM, editor. Clinical Urography. Philadelphia: WB Saunders; 1990. pp. 1020-1052

[62] Pastsernak MS, Rubin RH. Urinary tract tuberculosis. In: Schrier RW, editor. Diseases of the Kidney and Urinary Tract. 7th ed. Philadelphia: Lipincott Williams and Wilkins; 2001. pp. 1017-1037

[63] Modesto A, Marty L, Suc JM, Kleinknecht D, de Frémont JF, Marsepoil T, et al. Renal complications of intravesical bacillus Calmette-Guérin therapy. American Journal of Nephrology. 1991;**11**:501-504

[64] Harisinghani MG, Mc Loud TC, Shepard JA, Ko JP, Shroff MM, Mueller PR. Tuberculosis from head to toe. Radiographics. 2000;**20**:449-470

[65] Premkumar A, Lattimer J, Newhouse JH. CT and sonography of advanced urinary tract tuberculosis. AJR. American Journal of Roentgenology. 1987;**148**:65-69

[66] Apperson JW, Wechsler H, Lattimer JK. The trequent occurrence of both renal calculi and renal calcifications in tuberculous kidneys. The Journal of Urology. 1962;**87**:643-646

[67] Kapoor R, Ansari MS, Mandhani A, Gulia A. Clinical presentation and diagnostic approach in cases of genitourinary tuberculosis. Indian Journal of Urology. 2008;**24**:401-405

[68] Navarro-Vilasaró M, Font B, Sala M, Prera A, Malet A, Mariscal D, et al. Genitourinary mycobacteriosis: Retrospective study of 45 cases in a general hospital. Enfermedades Infecciosas y Microbiología Clínica. 2008;**26**:540-545

[69] Kenney PJ. Imaging of chronic renal infections. AJR. American Journal of Roentgenology. 1990;**155**:485-494

[70] Schaffer R, Becker JA, Goodman J. Sonography of tuberculous kidney. Urology. 1983;**22**:209-211

[71] Juul N, Torp-Pedersen S, Grønvall S, Holm HH, Koch F, Larsen S. Ultrasonically guided fine needle aspiration biopsy of renal masses. The Journal of Urology. 1985;**133**:579-581

[72] Das KM, Vaidyanathan S, Rajwanshi A, Indudhara R. Renal tuberculosis: Diagnosis with sonographically guided aspiration cytology. AJR. American Journal of Roentgenology. 1992;**158**(3):571

[73] Qunibi WY, al-Sibai MB, Taher S, Harder EJ, de Vol E, al-Furayh O, et al. Mycobacterial infection after renal transplantation—Report of 14 cases and review of the literature. The Quarterly Journal of Medicine. 1990;**77**:1039-1060

[74] Rui X, Li XD, Cai S, Chen G, Cai B. Ultrasonographic diagnosis and typing of renal tuberculosis. International Journal of Urology. 2008;**15**:135-139

[75] Browne RF, Zwirewich C, Torreggiani WC. Imaging of urinary tract infection in the adult. European Radiology. 2004;**14**:E168-E183

[76] Papanicolaou N, Pfister RC. Acute renal infections. Radiologic Clinics of North America. 1996;**34**:965-995

[77] Lu P, Li C, Zhou X. Significance of the CT scan in renal tuberculosis. Zhonghua Jie He He Hu Xi Za Zhi. 2001;**24**:407-409

[78] Merchant S, Bharati A, Merchant N. Tuberculosis of the genitourinary system—Urinary tract tuberculosis: Renal tuberculosis – Part II. Indian Journal of Radiology and Imaging. 2013;**23**(1):64-77

[79] McCarthy CL, Cowan NC. Multidetector CT urography (MD-CTU) for urothelial imaging (abstr). Radiology. 2002;**225**(P):137

[80] Leder RA, Low VH. Tuberculosis of the abdomen. Radiologic Clinics of North America. 1995;**33**:691-705

[81] Goldman SM, Fishman EK, Hartman DS, Kim YC, Siegelman SS. Computed tomography of renal tuberculosis and its pathological correlates. Journal of Computer Assisted Tomography. 1985;**9**:771-776

[82] Pedrosa I, Sun MR, Spencer M, Genega EM, Olumi AF, Dewolf WC, et al. MR imaging of renal masses: Correlation with findings at surgery and pathologic analysis. Radiographics. 2008;**28**:985-1003

[83] Verswijvel G, Oyen R. Magnetic resonance imaging in the detection and characterization of renal diseases. Saudi Journal of Kidney Diseases and Transplantation. 2004;**15**:283-299

[84] Leyendecker JR, Barnes CE, Zagoria RJ. MR urography: Techniques and clinical applications. Radiographics. 2008;**28**:23-46

[85] Khanna PC, Karnik ND, Jankharia BG, Merchant SA, Joshi AR, Kukreja KU. Magnetic resonance urography (MRU) versus intravenous urography (IVU) in obstructive uropathy: A prospective study of 30 cases. The Journal of the Association of Physicians of India. 2005;**53**:527-534

[86] Buckley O, Colville J, Torreggiani WC, Leyendecker JR. Re: MR urographic techniques. Radiographics. 2008;**28**:907 author reply 907-8

[87] Kim S, Jacob JS, Kim DC, Rivera R, Lim RP, Lee VS. Time-resolved dynamic contrast-enhanced MR urography for the evaluation of ureteral peristalsis: Initial experience. Journal of Magnetic Resonance Imaging. 2008;**28**:1293-1298

[88] Sadowski EA, Bennett LK, Chan MR, Wentland AL, Garrett AL, Garrett RW, et al. Nephrogenic systemic fibrosis: Risk factors and incidence estimation. Radiology. 2007; **243**:148-157

[89] Baniel J, Manning A, Leiman G. Fine needle cytodiagnosis of renal tuberculosis. The Journal of Urology. 1991;**146**(3):689-691

[90] Porter B, Karp W, Forsberg L. Percutaneous cytodiagnosis of retroperitoneal masses by USG guided FNAB. Acta Radiologica. 1981;**22**:663-668

[91] Kedar RP, Patel VH, Merchant SA, Aggarwal V, Pandit AA. Ultrasound guided aspiration cytology—A valuable diagnostic aid. Journal of Postgraduate Medicine. 1991;**37**:84-87

[92] Mangal N, Sharma VK, Verma N, Agarwal AK, Sharma SP, Aneja S. Ultrasound guided fine needle aspiration cytology in the diagnosis of retroperitoneal masses: A study of 85 cases. Journal of Cytology. 2009;**26**:97-101

[93] Wise GJ, Marella VK. Genitourinary manifestations of tuberculosis. The Urologic Clinics of North America. 2003;**30**:111-121

[94] Centers for Disease Control and Prevention. Treatment of tuberculosis, American Thoracic Society, CDC, and Infectious Diseases Society of America. MMWR. 2003; 52(No. RR-11)

[95] Gow JG. Genito-urinary tuberculosis. A study of the disease in one unit over a period of 24 years. Annals of the Royal College of Surgeons of England. 1971;**49**:50-70

[96] Skutil V, Varsa J, Obsitnik M. Six-month chemotherapy for urogenital tuberculosis. European Urology. 1985;**11**:170-176

[97] Amaya-Tapia G, Martín-Del Campo L, Aguirre-Avalos G, Portillo-Gómez L, Covarrubias-Pinedo A, Aguilar-Benavides S. Primary and acquired resistance of *Mycobacterium tuberculosis* in westerns México. Microbial Drug Resistance. 2000;**6**:143-145

[98] LoBue PA, Moser KS. Isoniazid- and rifampin-resistant tuberculosis in San Diego County, California, United States, 1993-2002. The International Journal of Tuberculosis and Lung Disease. 2005;**9**:501-506

[99] Hoopes AJ, Kammerer JS, Harrington TA, Ijaz K, Armstrong LR. Isoniazid monoresistant tuberculosis in the United States, 1993 to 2003. Archives of Internal Medicine. 2008;**168**:1984-1992

[100] Jenkins HE, Zignol M, Cohen T. Quantifying the burden and trends of isoniazid resistant tuberculosis, 1994-2009. PLoS One. 2011;**6**(7):e22927

[101] Yuen CM, Jenkins HE, Rodriguez CA, Keshavjee S, Becerra MC. Global and regional burden of isoniazid-resistant tuberculosis. Pediatrics. 2015;**136**:e50-e59

[102] Snider DE Jr. Pyridoxine supplementation during isoniazid therapy. Tubercle. 1980;**61**: 191-196

[103] Visser ME, Texeira-Swiegelaar C, Maartens G. The short-term effects of antituberculosis therapy on plasma pyridoxine levels in patients with pulmonary tuberculosis. The International Journal of Tuberculosis and Lung Disease. 2004;**8**:260-262

[104] Wang LJ, Wu CF, Wong YC, Chuang CK, Chu SH, Chen CJ. Imaging findings of urinary tuberculosis on excretory urography and computerized tomography. The Journal of Urology. 2003;**169**(2):524-528

[105] Chaulk CP, Kazandjian VA. Directly observed therapy for treatment completion of pulmonary tuberculosis: Consensus statement of the public health tuberculosis guidelines panel. JAMA. 1998;**279**:943-948

[106] Liu SY, Li JH, Schluger NW. DOT and timely treatment completion among Asian-born immigrant tuberculosis patients. The International Journal of Tuberculosis and Lung Disease. 2005;**9**:884-889

[107] Migliori GB, Zellweger JP, Abubakar I, Ibraim E, Caminero JA, De Vries G, et al. European Union standards for tuberculosis care. The European Respiratory Journal. 2012;**39**: 807-819

[108] Gravendeel JM, Asapa AS, Becx-Bleumink M, Vrakkin HA. Preliminary results of an operational field study to compare side-effects, complaints and treatment results of a single-drug short-course regimen with a four-drug fixed-doses combination (4FDC) regimen in South Sulawesi, Republic of Indonesia. Tuberculosis (Edinburgh, Scotland). 2003;**83**:183-186

[109] Zaka-Ur-Rehman Z, Jamshaid M, Chaudhry A. Clinical evaluation and monitoring of adverse effect for fixed multidose combination against single drug therapy in pulmonary tuberculosis patiens. Pakistan Journal of Pharmaceutical Sciences. 2008;**21**:185-194

[110] Lin MY, Lin SJ, Chan LC, Lu YC. Impact of food and antacids on the pharmacokinetics of anti-tuberculosis drugs: Systematic review and meta-analysis. The International Journal of Tuberculosis and Lung Disease. 2010;**14**:806-818

[111] Navarro VJ, Senior JR. Drug-related hepatotoxicity. The New England Journal of Medicine. 2006;**354**:731-739

[112] Small PM, Fujiwara PI. Management of tuberculosis in the United States. The New England Journal of Medicine. 2001;**345**:189-200

[113] Mochalova TP, Starikova IY. Reconstructive surgery for treatment of urogenital tuberculosis: 30 years of observation. World Journal of Surgery. 1997;**21**(5):511

[114] Krishnamoorthy S, Gopalakrishnan G. Surgical management of renal tuberculosis. Indian Journal of Urology. 2008;**24**(3):369-375

[115] Cek M, Lenk S, Naber KG, Bishop MC, Johansen TE, Botto H, et al. EAU guidelines for the management of genitourinary tuberculosis. European Urology. 2005;**48**:353-362

[116] Benator D, Bhattacharya M, Bozeman L, Burman W, Cantazaro A, Chaisson C, et al. Rifapentine and isoniazid once a week versus rifampicin and isoniazid twice a week for treatment of drug-susceptible pulmonary tuberculosis in HIV-negative patients: A randomised clinical trial. Lancet. 2002;**360**:528-534

[117] Vernon A, Burman W, Benator D, Khan A, Bozeman L. Acquired rifamycin monoresistance in patients with HIV-related tuberculosis treated with once weekly rifapentine and isoniazid. Tuberculosis Trials Consortium. Lancet. 1999;**353**:1843-1847

[118] Burman W, Benator D, Vernon A, Khan A, Jones B, Silva C, et al. Acquired rifamycin resistance with twice-weekly treatment of HIV-related tuberculosis. American Journal of Respiratory and Critical Care Medicine. 2006;**173**:350-356

[119] Weiner M, Benator D, Burman W, Peloquin CA, Khan A, Vernon A, et al. Association between acquired rifamycin resistance and the pharmacokinetics of rifabutin and isoniazid among patients with HIV and tuberculosis. Clinical Infectious Diseases. 2005;**40**:1481-1491

[120] Narendran G, Menon PA, Venkatesan P, Vijay K, Padmapriyadarsini C, Ramesh Kumar S, et al. Acquired rifampicin resistance in thrice-weekly antituberculosis therapy: Impact of HIV and antiretroviral therapy. Clinical Infectious Diseases. 2014;**59**:1798-1804

[121] Luetkemeyer AF, Kendall MA, Nyirenda M, Wu X, Ive P, Benson CA, et al. Tuberculosis immune reconstitution inflammatory syndrome in A5221 STRIDE timing, severity,

and implications for HIV-TB programs. Journal of Acquired Immune Deficiency Syndromes. 2014;**65**:423-428

[122] Meintjes G, Lawn SD, Scano F, Maartens G, French MA, Worodria W, et al. Tuberculosis-associated immune reconstitution inflammatory syndrome: Case definitions for use in resource-limited settings. The Lancet Infectious Diseases. 2008;**8**:516-523

[123] Meintjes G, Wilkinson RJ, Morroni C, Pepper DJ, Rebe K, Rangaka MX, et al. Randomized placebo-controlled trial of prednisone for paradoxical tuberculosis-associated immune reconstitution inflammatory syndrome. AIDS. 2010;**24**:2381-2390

[124] Kurts C, Panzer U, Anders HJ, Rees AJ. The immune system and kidney disease: Basic concepts and clinical implications. Nature Reviews Immunology. 2013;**13**:738-753

[125] Baghaei P, Marjani M, Tabarsi P, Moniri A, Rashidfarrokhi F, Ahmadi F, et al. Impact of chronic renal failure on antituberculosis treatment outcomes. The International Journal of Tuberculosis and Lung Disease. 2014;**18**:352-356

[126] Malone RS, Fish DN, Spiegel DM, Childs JM, Peloquin CA. The effect of hemodialysis on cycloserine, ethionamide, para-aminosalicylate, and clofazimine. Chest. 1999; **116**:984-990

[127] Malone RS, Fish DN, Spiegel DM, Childs JM, Peloquin CA. The effect of hemodialysis on isoniazid, rifampin, pyrazinamide, and ethambutol. American Journal of Respiratory and Critical Care Medicine. 1999;**159**(5 pt 1):1580-1584

[128] Alsultan A, Peloquin CA. Therapeutic drug monitoring in the treatment of tuberculosis: An update. Drugs. 2014;**74**:839-854

[129] Fish DN, Chow AT. The clinical pharmacokinetics of levofloxacin. Clinical Pharmacokinetics. 1997;**32**:101-119

[130] Launay-Vacher V, Izzedine H, Deray G. Pharmacokinetic considerations in the treatment of tuberculosis in patients with renal failure. Clinical Pharmacokinetics. 2005;**44**:221-235

[131] Saukkonen JJ, Cohn DL, Jasmer RM, Schenker S, Jereb JA, Nolan CM, et al. An official ATS statement: Hepatotoxicity of antituberculosis therapy. American Journal of Respiratory and Critical Care Medicine. 2006;**174**:935-952

[132] Yee D, Valiquette C, Pelletier M, Parisien I, Rocher I, Menzies D. Incidence of serious side effects from first-line antituberculosis drugs among patients treated for active tuberculosis. American Journal of Respiratory and Critical Care Medicine. 2003;**167**:1472-1477

[133] Chang KC, Leung CC, Yew WW, Lau TY, Tam CM. Hepatotoxicity of pyrazinamide: Cohort and case-control analyses. American Journal of Respiratory and Critical Care Medicine. 2008;**177**:1391-1396

[134] Cruz-Hervert LP, García-García L, Ferreyra-Reyes L, Bobadilla-Del-Valle M, Cano-Arellano B, Canizales-Quintero S, et al. Tuberculosis in ageing: High rates, complex diagnosis and poor clinical outcomes. Age and Ageing. 2012;**41**:488-495

8

Mycobacterium tuberculosis: Macrophage Takeover and Modulation of Innate Effector Responses

Khalid Hussain Bhat and Imtiyaz Yaseen

Abstract

Macrophages mediate the first line of defense in the host against various intracellular pathogens. They are armed with several immune-effector mechanisms to detect and combat pathogens. However, intracellular pathogens have developed strategies to overcome the macrophage protective immune responses and colonize inside the macrophages. Tuberculosis (TB), both pulmonary and extrapulmonary, is an infectious disease of global concern caused by *Mycobacterium tuberculosis*. *M. tuberculosis* is a highly successful pathogen and has acquired various strategies to downregulate critical innate-effector immune responses of macrophages such as phagosome-lysosome fusion, antigen presentation, autophagy, and inhibition of reactive oxygen (ROI) and reactive nitrogen (RNI) species to ensure its longer survival inside the macrophages. In addition to these, the bacilli also modulate T cell immune response which can help the bacilli to survive inside the host for a long time. In this chapter, we focus to describe important macrophage innate defense mechanisms and the signaling that can influence T cell adaptive response and the strategies adopted by the bacilli to exploit these signaling cascades to favor its replication and persistence inside the macrophages for establishing a productive infection.

Keywords: *Mycobacterium tuberculosis*, monocytes/macrophages, macrophage effector response and signaling cascades, host responses and *M. tuberculosis* pathogenesis

1. Introduction

Macrophages mediate the first line of defense in the host against various intracellular pathogens [1]. They are armed with several immune-effector mechanisms to detect and combat pathogens [2, 3]. However, intracellular pathogens have developed strategies to overcome the macrophage protective immune responses and colonize inside the macrophages. Tuberculosis (TB), is an infectious disease caused by a extremely successful pathogen, *Mycobacterium tuberculosis*, as it has evolved numerous clever strategies over time to modulate important macrophage innate-effector immune responses such as phagosome maturation, antigen presentation, inhibition of reactive oxygen (ROI) and reactive nitrogen (RNI) species, and autophagy to ensure its survival inside the macrophages [4–6]. In addition to these, the bacilli also modulate T cell immune response which can help the bacilli to survive inside the host for a long time [7]. In this chapter, we focus to describe important macrophage innate defense mechanisms and the signaling that can influence T cell adaptive response and the strategies adopted by the bacilli to exploit these signaling cascades to favor its replication and persistence inside the macrophages for establishing a productive infection.

2. Monocytes/macrophages

2.1. History and development

Eli Metchnikoff's obsession, the "phagocyte" [phagos-to eat, cyte-cell], is a constituent of Ludwig Aschoff's reticuloendothelial system (RES) [8]; the macrophage plays a key role at almost all the stages of immune response including innate and adaptive immune responses. Macrophages provide the first line of defense against the invading pathogens. In addition to protecting the body against attacks by foreign organisms, macrophages regulate important physiological functions. Their role in homeostasis has been well established. Macrophages clear almost 2×10^{11} erythrocytes per day. This enormous metabolic turnover is crucial for iron homeostasis and to prevent formation of toxic intermediates [9]. Macrophages are equipped with scavenger receptors such as phosphatidylserine receptors, thrombospondin receptor, integrins, and complement receptors to clear the cell debris and rapidly remove the apoptotic cells to help in tissue-remodeling processes. Antigens from the engulfed cells are presented along with the MHC molecules to activate the adaptive immune responses [10]. Thus, macrophage serves as a professional scavenger of the dying cells that not only clears the corpus but also regulates the immune system.

The circulating monocytes that are considered to be the developmental intermediates between bone marrow precursors and tissue macrophages emigrate from the blood vessels and differentiate into tissue macrophages [11]. Macrophages and monocytes originate from hematopoietic stem cell-derived progenitors with myeloid-restricted differentiation potential [1]. The bone marrow progenitors, monocytes, and macrophages collectively were classified into mononuclear phagocytic system, a concept pioneered by van Furth [12]. Monocytes are initially identified by the expression of CD14 molecules and lack of CD16 expression on the surface. These monocytes are termed as "classical monocytes" with $CD14^{++}CD16^{-}$ phenotype and accounting for about 90% of human blood monocytes. However, later studies have proved the expression of CD16 on the surface of some cell populations that were termed as "non-classical monocytes" with $CD14^{+}CD16^{++}$ phenotype [13]. The replenishment of tissue macrophages with the circulating monocytes is well established, but in some instances like in microglial cells of brain, local proliferation of macrophages has been established. Owing to the adaptability and plasticity of macrophages and their responsiveness to different microenvironments in different tissues such as lung, spleen, liver, gut, and brain, a considerable heterogeneity exists among them [14]. For example, lung alveolar macrophages being constantly exposed to a variety of antigens, express a high level of pattern recognition receptors and scavenger receptors on the surface. In contrast, the macrophages of the gut exhibit high levels of phagocytic and antibacterial activities compared to other macrophages [15].

2.2. Macrophage activation

Activation is defined as the acquisition of competence to execute a complex function [16]. The factor responsible for macrophage activation was found to be the interferon-gamma (IFN-γ) produced by CD8$^+$ cytotoxic T (Tc1) cells, CD4$^+$ T helper 1 (Th1) T cells, and natural killer (NK) cells. IFN-γ activation leads to conversion of macrophages to potent phagocytotic cells with increased production of reactive oxygen intermediates and reactive nitrogen intermediates, superoxides and proinflammatory cytokines helping the cells to efficiently kill the intracellular pathogens. These macrophages have increased antigen presentation activity, thus they mount an effective immune responses in the host. The IFN-γ-mediated activation is known as "classical activation" and the macrophages are classified as "type 1 or M1 macrophages" [3, 18] (**Figure 1**). IFN-γ stimulation is not enough for the classical activation of macrophages, and may require additional stimulation by TNF-α. As TNF-α is not

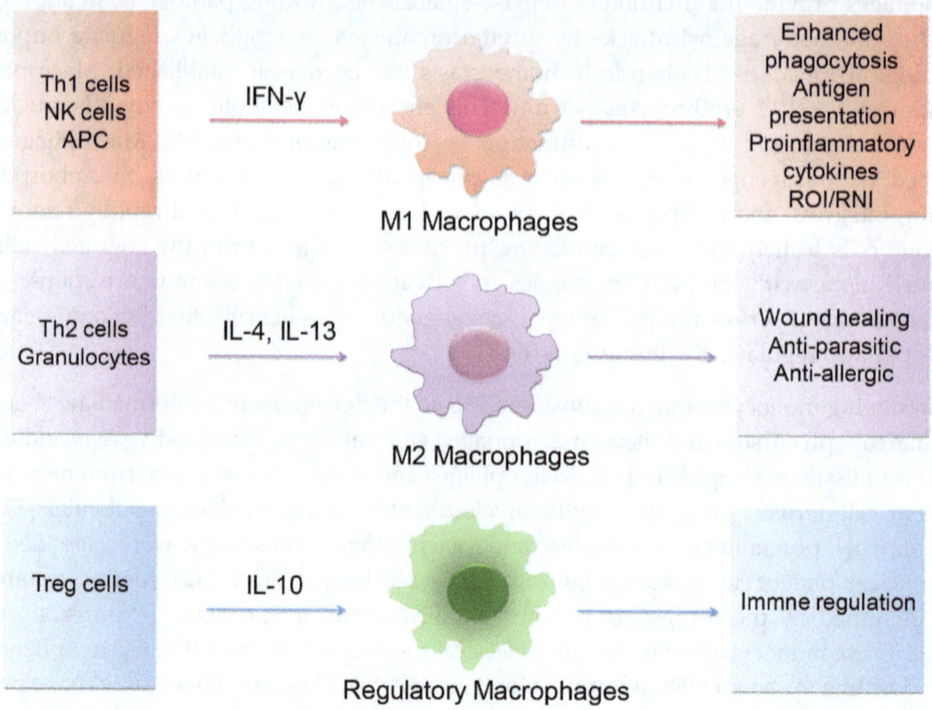

Figure 1. Schematic diagram showing different types of macrophages. Th1 cytokines primarily produced by T cells, natural killer (NK) cells and other antigen presenting cells (APC) result in the development of classically activated (M1) macrophages having microbicidal functions. While Th2 cytokines result in the development of macrophages that predominantly perform tissue repair and anti-inflammatory functions (M2), T reg cells result in the development of regulatory macrophages having immunosuppressive activities.

constitutively present in the environment, specific receptor ligands like lipopolysaccharides (LPS) and various microbial ligands may help in the induction of endogenous expression of TNF-α in macrophages [19, 20].

The T helper 2 (Th2) type of cytokines, IL-4 and IL-13, induce a response distinct from the one induced by IFN-γ with distinct set of genes being expressed and is known as "alternative activation" pathway of macrophages, and the cells are named as "alternative activated type 2 or M2 macrophages" [21]. In addition to T cells and B cells, IL-4 and IL-13 are also produced by various other cells such as mast cells, basophils, eosinophils, NK T cells, and macrophages that are involved in regulation of innate immune responses. Hence, alternative activation can be of both innate and acquired origin. Other than these two cytokines, immune complexes, IL-10, glucocorticoid, or secosteroid (vitamin D3) hormone can also contribute to the activation of M2 macrophages [22–25]. M2 macrophages are characterized by expression of scavenger, mannose [26], and galactose-type receptors, and markers such as dectin-1, arginase 1, Ym1, and FIZZ1 [27]. The M2 macrophages have anti-inflammatory properties and are associated with allergic and anti-parasite responses, and are thought to regulate humoral immunity [27, 28]. The alternatively activated macrophages are found to be recruited to wounds and other sites of tissue injury and are programmed to perform a wound healing function by expressing arginase. These macrophages are termed as "repair macrophages" or "wound healing macrophages" [19, 29, 30]. The M1 and M2 macrophages thus represent two populations of cells with different biological functions [31]. For example, the M1 macrophages, but not the M2 macrophages, produce high levels of reactive oxygen and nitrogen intermediates) and inflammatory cytokines (IL-1β, TNF-α, IL-6), and have low arginase activity, express relatively high levels of CD86, and are efficient APCs. While the M1 cells have an IL-12^{high}, IL-23^{high}, and IL-10^{low} phenotype and play an important role in inducing a dominant Th1 response and provide resistance against intracellular pathogens and tumors [17, 23, 32–34], the various forms of M2 macrophages share an IL-12^{low} and IL-23^{low} phenotype, virtually devoid of the co-stimulatory molecules and fail to mount a strong T cell proliferation [35, 36]. The innate and adaptive immune responses can also lead to the production of the "regulatory macrophages" (M reg) (**Figure 1**). The M reg cells are shown to be very stable in their phenotype and have regulatory activity. These cells are a novel type of suppressor macrophage which induces tolerance during organ transplantation. They have potent T cell suppressive function [37] and inhibit production of the IL-12 cytokine [38].

The activated macrophages exhibit a profound change in their capacities and functions. In addition to other physiological changes, there is a rapid membrane turnover found in case of macrophages even in the resting stage. This membrane flow is enormously increased in the activated state as a result of enhanced phagocytic activity and lysosomal degradation of the ingested material [39, 40]. Phagosomes undergo a series of maturation steps resulting in gradual acidification and increase in the hydrolytic activity. In addition to hydrolases, lethal superoxide generating enzyme activities become prevalent toward the end of phagosome maturation [40]. The NADPH oxidase activity of the enzyme complex leads to formation of H_2O_2 in presence of superoxide dismutase enzyme [41].

3. *M. tuberculosis*: infection and disease

Mycobacteria are rod-shaped bacteria of phylum Actinobacteria mostly found in soil or water. The *M. tuberculosis, M. bovis, M. africanum, M. microti, M. canettii, M. caprae, M. pinnipedii,* and *M. mungi* all cause TB disease and are classified as *M. tuberculosis* complex [42–44]. The *M. tuberculosis,* a facultative intracellular pathogen, was discovered by Robert Koch in 1882 as a causative agent for TB disease in human, those days commonly known as "consumption" or "white plague" [45]. Different strains of *M. tuberculosis* differ in virulence and in distribution among different human populations. *M. tuberculosis* W-Beijing strain is one of the most pathogenic strains distributed throughout the world [46, 47]. The use of chemotherapeutics against *M. tuberculosis* has resulted in the appearance of drug-resistant strains [48]. Multiple drug-resistant (MDR), extensive drug-resistant (XDR), and total drug-resistant (TDR) strains are becoming increasingly prevalent [49–52]. The *M. tuberculosis* bacteria are highly aerobic, non-sporulating, and non-motile bacteria. They have a high guanine plus cytosine (G + C) content (61–71%) in their genomic DNA, and are characterized by the presence of large hydroxylated branched-chain fatty acids called mycolic acids in their cell envelope [53, 54]. Although they have been classified with other Gram-positive actinomycetes due to their lack of an outer cell membrane, mycobacteria stain weakly with crystal violet and are resistant to decolorization with acid-alcohol solutions after staining with alkaline arylmethane dyes such as carbol fuchsin, hence called acid-fast. *M. tuberculosis* primarily infects not only lungs (pulmonary) but can also colonize other body parts (extra-pulmonary). The symptoms of TB disease include chronic cough, blood with sputum, weight loss, fever and night sweats, cavitation, and fibrosis [55, 56].

TB is a major public health burden. Despite the availability of effective short-course chemotherapy (DOTS) and *M. bovis* bacillus Calmette-Guérin (BCG) vaccine, more than 9 million new cases of *M. tuberculosis* infections are reported every year that accounts to more than 2 billion (one third of world population) being positive for the infection, resulting in 2 million deaths every year and one fifth of all adult deaths in developing countries. Developing countries are the most affected by this pandemic with 30% of the cases being reported from Africa and 55% from Asia. India and China alone are harboring 35% of the cases. With no new drug in use for a while, TB has become increasingly resistant to drugs and multi-, extensive-, and total-drug resistant TB have emerged. Interaction with other infectious diseases like HIV is making it challenging to handle the disease [57]. Other pathological conditions and risk factors associated with TB such as diabetes mellitus, renal diseases, hematological disorders and use of anti-TNF-a drugs has complicated the problem [58]. Socioeconomic factors and variable efficacy of BCG vaccination are also responsible for further aggravating the already complex problem [55, 59].

After infection with *M. tuberculosis,* an individual may not necessarily develop active disease. In case the immune system is competent enough, an individual will either clear the infection or remain latently infected with no clinical signs of disease throughout the life or can have reactivation of TB during weakening of immune system or co-infection with other pathogens like HIV [60, 61]. The molecular factors or environmental conditions that influence the progression of latent phase to active disease are not well understood. During latency, the *M. tuberculosis* bacterium remains inside the infected macrophages in granulomas. These tiny granulomas show no clinical symptoms although they may be visible in chest X-rays and give positive tuberculin skin test [62, 63]. In 5% of the cases where immune system is weakened, the microscopic primary lesion progresses to a larger primary caseous lesion. The caseation of the primary lesion may lead to hematogenous spread of bacteria causing miliary TB or extrapulmonary TB, where the infection spreads to liver, spleen, and kidneys [63]. In case the bacteria find their way into brain, they may cause tuberculous meningitis [63]. Patients with active pulmonary TB are diagnosed most commonly by sputum smear microscopy where bacteria are directly observed under microscope in the sputum samples of patients or culturing the samples to check for colony forming units and by chest X-ray. Diagnosis of extrapulmonary TB patients is carried out by tissue biopsy, urine culture, cerebrospinal fluid test, CT scan, or MRI. Latent TB has long been diagnosed by tuberculin skin test; however, its specificity has been questioned due to false positive results as a result of infection with other non-tuberculous bacteria or prior vaccination with BCG [64, 65]. Therefore, in recent years, interferon gamma release assays (IGRAs) have been used as an alternative for the diagnosis of both latent TB infection and active TB cases [66].

4. Infection of macrophages with *M. tuberculosis* and host immune responses

4.1. The host-bacilli interplay

M. tuberculosis infection is transmitted via aerosol route. Prolonged and close contacts with infected patients result in the transmission of the pathogen in healthy persons as it is known that survival of the bacterium ranges from one to few hours in the aerosol droplets, which are about 1–2 μm or less size [67, 68]. Once the pathogen enters the respiratory track, it is finally engulfed by the alveolar macrophages of lung through surface receptors. A number of studies reveal that complement receptors and complement-mediated opsonization are majorly involved in the entry of *M. tuberculosis* inside the macrophages. One of the most important receptors for mycobacteria is complement receptor 3 (CR3), while other receptors such as CR1 and CR4, mannose receptor, surfactant protein A receptor, CD14, Fcγ receptor, scavenger receptors, etc., have also been implicated in phagocytosis and internalization of the bacteria inside the macrophages [69–71]. For alveolar dendritic cells (DC), DC-specific intercellular adhesion molecule 3-grabbing nonintegrin (DC-SIGN) is the main receptor for *M. tuberculosis* [72]. Though complement receptors are found to be important for phagocytosis of both the avirulent and virulent strains of *M. tuberculosis*, the decline of mannose receptors was found to be associated with reduced binding of only the virulent strains [73]. The mycobacterial surface glycoprotein, mannose-capped lipoarabinomannan (Man-LAM) is recognized by the C-type lectins and the macrophage mannose receptor (MMR) [74, 75]. An important role of toll-receptors, mainly the TLR2, has been demonstrated for the attachment of mycobacteria to macrophages [76]. Interestingly, a large number of surface proteins of *M. tuberculosis* interact with the TLR2 receptors [76]. After binding, the bacteria are internalized and engulfed into phagosomes, where they can be killed by several defense mechanisms. Thoma-Uszynski et al., (2001) have shown a role of the TLR2-triggered signaling to induce cytotoxicity against *M. tuberculosis* in alveolar macrophages [77]. Soon after the first contact of *M. tuberculosis* with alveolar macrophages, generally a robust proinflammatory immune response is induced that confers protection against the bacilli. It is observed that dampening of the proinflammatory signaling can increase *M. tuberculosis* infection burden in mice [78]. Following intracellular infection, adaptive immunity is generated against the invading pathogen via activation of $CD4^+$ T cells and $CD8^+$ T cells. Many times this adaptive immunity fails to provide a sterilizing immunity resulting in longer persistence of the infection and reactivation of *M. tuberculosis* bacteria. The bacilli are found to inhibit the class I, class II, and cross presentation of mycobacterial antigen to T cells, thus avoiding immune recognition by T cells. It has been observed that integrity of bacterial cell wall is important for *M. tuberculosis* in evading adaptive responses. At the site of infection, proinflammatory IFNs and cytokines are secreted, which help in the recruitment of $CD4^+$ T cells, $CD8^+$ T cells, natural killer T cells, and neutrophils [79]. Many a time, the induction of acquired immune response against *M. tuberculosis* is slow and the establishment of infection wins against the induction of full-fledged response [4, 80]. The cell-mediated immune response initiated at the sites of infection is found to be modulated by the bacilli. After establishing the infection, the *M. tuberculosis* antigens move with the help of alveolar dendritic cells to the draining lymph node, which leads to the stimulation of naive $CD4^+$ T cells. The active role of $CD4^+$ T cells in fighting against *M. tuberculosis* infection was proposed in 1974 in mice. In addition, the HIV mediated depletion of $CD4^+$ T cells and a defective macrophage activation in some genetic disorders has been associated with worst TB prognosis [4, 81]. Furthermore, $CD4^{-/-}$ knockout and MHC-$II^{-/-}$ knockout mice have been found to be prone to infection by *M. tuberculosis* [82]. The inhibitory effect of stimulated Th1-type $CD4^+$ T cells is by the production proinflammatory cytokines such as IFN-γ and TNF-α, which inhibit bacillary growth [81]. In comparison, when stimulated in the context of MHC class II, Th2-type $CD4^+$ T cells proliferate and produce anti-inflammatory cytokines such as IL-4, IL-5, and IL-10, which are favorable for the bacilli to establish a productive infection [79, 81]. Many studies indicate that *M. tuberculosis* bacilli suppress the pro-inflammatory cytokines such as IL-12 and IFN-γ and activate production of anti-inflammatory cytokines like IL-10 to skew the anti-mycobacterial immune response from a protective Th1 to a non-protective Th2-type. At the early stages of infection, activation of $CD8^+$ T cells by APC leads to bacterial killing. However, the role of $CD8^+$ T cells at later stages of infection has not been established [82]. The $CD8^+$ T cells can also be activated by the cross presentation of *M. tuberculosis* antigen along with MHC class I molecules. Post infection, $CD8^+$ T cells migrate to the infected tissue and produce IFN-γ. This migration of $CD8^+$ T cells is a characteristic of the granuloma establishment [83]. Higher bacterial load was found in mice deficient in some of the components of class I presentation and $CD8^+$ T cell activation pathways like β_2 microglobulin, transporter associated with antigen processing protein (TAP), and T cell co-receptor CD8α [83].

4.2. Formation of granuloma

M. tuberculosis infection of alveolar macrophages leads to the activation of alveolar dendritic cells which migrate to lymph nodes. In the lymph nodes, $CD4^+$ T cells, $CD8^+$ T cells, and $\gamma\delta$ T cells proliferate in response to activation by the alveolar dendritic cells. At the site of infection, the resulting immune activation leads to a microenvironment of cytokines and chemokines which induces the expression of integrins, selectins, and addressins on the surfaces of lymphocytes and endothelial cells. This facilitates a mass migration of immune cells resulting in the formation of a focus of immune cells called "tubercle" or granuloma around the primary site of infection. Macrophages and giant nucleated epithelioid cells form layers around the granuloma. While the inner core of granuloma becomes necrotic, the outer surface is covered by fibrous tissue and vasculature is developed. The granuloma is formed by the immune system to contain *M. tuberculosis* to the site of infection and not allowing its spread to other normal tissues. The latent infection may persist and remain dormant for life time without proceeding to diseased condition [79, 84]. At the nascent stage of granuloma, the recruitment of uninfected and susceptible macrophages to the site of infection may lead to their infection due to apoptosis of the existing infected macrophages. This may lead to initial proliferation of the bacteria till equilibrium is attained by containment of bacteria in the granuloma and control of infection due to adaptive immune response. Some of the newly infected macrophages egress from granuloma and nucleate the formation of new granulomas at other uninfected parts of the lungs (**Figure 2**) [85]. It has been noticed that bacterial dissemination and rapid disease progression are related with larger necrotic granulomas [57], however, containment of disease is found to be associated with smaller solid granulomas [86]. Furthermore, *M. tuberculosis* contributes to the formation of granuloma by secreting pathogenic factors

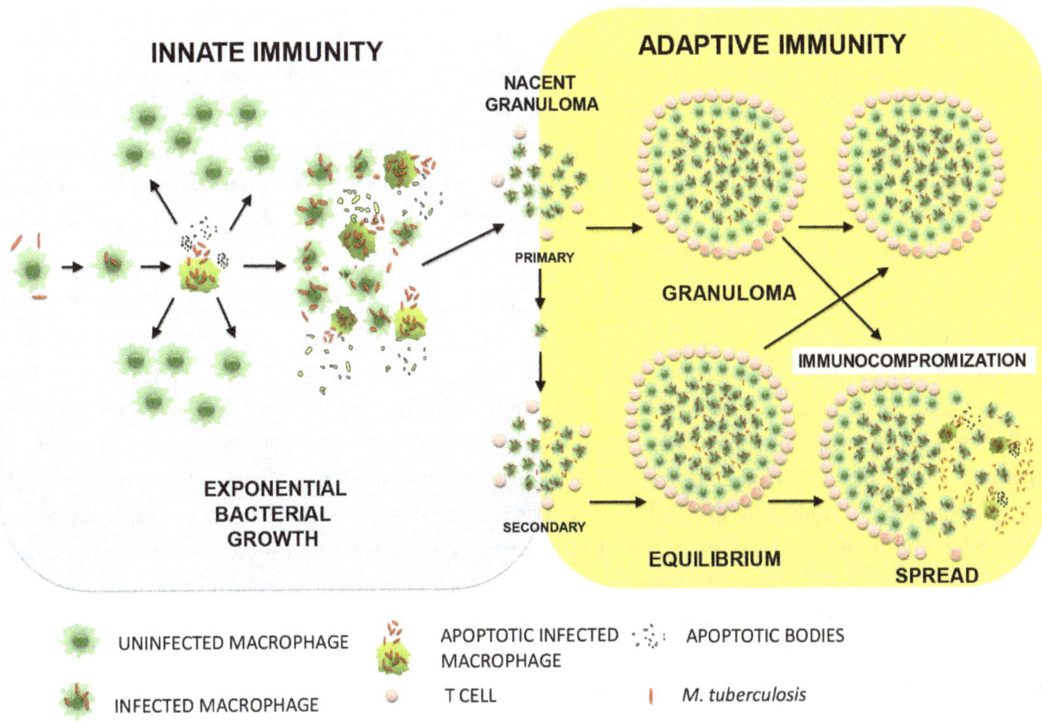

Figure 2. Development of granuloma. Immediately post infection, innate immune response is induced. The immune activation and apoptosis of infected cells lead to a microenvironment of cytokines and chemokines which attracts more uninfected macrophages. At this stage, some newly infected macrophages can migrate to uninfected areas and initiate the formation of new granulomas. This results in initial proliferation of the bacilli. Adaptive immunity although inherently slow in development, checks further spread of infection resulting in an equilibrium state. Immunocompromization of an individual at later stages can lead to caseation of the granuloma and the bacteria are rapidly disseminated.

as RD1 deficient bacteria show attenuated granuloma formation and macrophage migration to the primary site of infection in zebra fish model [85]. Studies in non-human primate, rabbit, and guinea pig models indicate hypoxic inside the environment of granuloma. In combination with nutrient deficiency, hypoxia induces a dormancy program in the bacilli which is characterized by changes in gene expression and alterations in the bacterial metabolism. Hence probably a latent infection is established which may be activated latter during immunocompromization. Thus, after entry in the human lungs, *M. tuberculosis* faces a series of host defense attacks. However, the overall outcome of infection with *M. tuberculosis* depends on the balance between (i) outgrowth and killing of *M. tuberculosis* and (ii) the extent of tissue necrosis, fibrosis, and regeneration.

4.3. Phagosome maturation response

After phagocytosis, *M. tuberculosis* bacteria reside inside the endosomes of the macrophages. Normally, endosome fuses with lysosome to degrade the pathogens, but *M. tuberculosis* bacteria are capable of inhibiting the process of phagosome maturation, as a result of which acidification of phagosome is compromised. The intracellular survival and persistence of the tubercle bacilli rests upon its ability to prevent phagosome-lysosome fusion, thus avoiding degradation, antigen processing, and cidal properties of the phagolysosome. Lipoarabinomannan capped with mannose (Man-LAM), a cell wall component of *M. tuberculosis* and SapM, a phosphatidylinositol 3-phosphate (PI3P) phosphatase secreted by the bacilli, are found to interfere with phosphoinositide metabolism of macrophages by depleting PI3P in phagosome [87, 88]. The latter is used as a docking molecule by peripheral proteins of lysosomes [7]. *M. tuberculosis* also possess protein phosphatases (Ptp A and B) that may interfere with host trafficking process possibly by modulating vacuolar sorting proteins [89].

The transport of *M. tuberculosis* containing vacuoles to lysosomes is mediated by a class of GTPases called Rab GTPases. A phagosome, when it normally matures into the phagolysosome, undergoes a transition between the stages marked by early endocytic Rabs (e.g., Rab5) and late endocytic GTPases (e.g., Rab7). Under normal circumstances, Rab proteins are actively recruited to the vesicles and assembled resulting in fusion of different vesicular compartments. In case of *M. tuberculosis* infection, it was observed that recruitment of Rab7 to the vacuole containing *M. tuberculosis* was inhibited while Rab5 was recruited normally indicating a maturation block between a Rab5 and Rab7 stage in infected macrophages that causes inhibition of phagosome-lysosome fusion. The exchange of Rab5 protein with Rab7 was later named as Rab conversion [90, 91]. Rab5 interacts with early endosomal autoantigen 1 (EEA1), which in turn interacts with phosphatidylinositol 3-phosphate (PI3P). Thus, inhibition of PI3P production by *M. tuberculosis* appears to be also critical for the inhibition of maturation of endolysosomes [91]. A series of Rab proteins are bind to phagosomes to ensure its acidification and recruitment of cathepsin D, while the process is severely inhibited in case of *M. tuberculosis* infection. A soluble eukaryotic-like protein kinase PknG of pathogenic *M. tuberculosis* is shown to be crucial for the prevention of phagosome-lysosome fusion [92]. A recent study has also shown that the *M. tuberculosis* secretory proteins, ESAT-6 and CFP-10 encoded by RD1 region play crucial roles in preventing phagolysosomal fusion [93]. Genetic screens using comprehensive mutant libraries of *M.*

tuberculosis and BCG suggest that additional mycobacterial products directly or indirectly can influence trafficking processes which probably are important for intracellular survival [94, 95]. Coronin1, exclusively recruited to *M. tuberculosis* containing phagosome, is an important host factor that specifically prevents the lysosomal delivery and death of mycobacteria inside macrophage [96]. Coronin1 prevents phagosome-lysosome fusion by regulating Ca^{2+}-dependent signaling processes when macrophages are infected with *M. tuberculosis* [97]. The *Nramp1* (natural-resistance-associated macrophage protein 1) gene involved in macrophage activation and mycobacterial killing [98] becomes part of the phagosome following phagocytosis and displays reduced phagosomal maturation and acidification [99].

A family of IFN-γ-inducible GTPases, also called immunity-related GTPases (IRGs), was found to play a critical role in host innate immunity against intracellular pathogens [100–102]. A member of IRG family, 47 kDa Irgm1 (also called LRG-47) protein (which is strongly inducible by IFN-γ and *M. tuberculosis* infection in mice) is an important anti-*M. tuberculosis* protein [100]. The anti-mycobacterial role of Irgm1 is due to its interaction with phosphatidylinositol-3,4-bisphosphate (PtdIns (3,4)P2) and PtdIns(3,4,5)P3 present on the phagosomal surface harboring *M. tuberculosis*. Irgm1 also increases phosphorylation of lipids by augmenting the PI3K activity. Normally, Irgm1 interacts with a membrane trafficking protein Snapin, which interacts with SNARE to ensure the fusion of phagosomes with lysosomes resulting in the elimination of bacilli. *M. tuberculosis* has developed a way to counter Irgm1 effect by exploiting a natural pathway of Irgm1 inhibition by Rab14 protein that is critical for phagosome-lysosome fusion. It has been shown that the mycobacterial phagosomes recruit and retain Rab14 [103]. Rab 14 is inhibited by unphosphorylated form of AS160 protein. Manipulation of Rab14-pathway by *M. tuberculosis* is mediated by the activation of Akt1 that phosphorylates AS160. Phosphorylated AS160 is unable to inhibit Rab14 hence leaving it free to inhibit Irgm1 recruitment to phagolysosomal compartment resulting in the failure of phagolysosome maturation (**Figure 3**) [103–105]. The fusion of phagosomes with lysosomes has been shown to be dependent on Ca^{2+} ions. Ca^{2+} ions and Ca-binding protein calmodulin are critical for the delivery of lysosomal components to phagosomes using PI3P-dependent pathways. Blockade of Ca^{2+}/calmodulin pathway by *M. tuberculosis* is also found to be one of the ways to block phagosomal maturation [70].

4.4. Autophagy

Autophagy (also called xenophagy) is an evolutionary conserved basic homeostatic mechanism of a cell to digest intracellular organelles and large protein aggregates that are difficult to digest by normal proteasomal pathway. The engagement of TLRs with mycobacterial ligands induces autophagy using both MyD88-dependent and TRIF-dependent pathways [106, 107]. This suggests that autophagy is an effector of innate immune response. The IFN-γ induces IRG proteins that are mainly involved in induction of autophagy and elimination of *M. tuberculosis* bacilli [108] and polymorphism at IRG locus is shown to be associated with resistance to *M. tuberculosis* [109]. Many autophagy-associated proteins are shown to be involved in phagosome-lysosome fusion process [110]. Expression of a number of host genes involved in autophagy is shown to be modulated at the onset of *M. tuberculosis* infection. The pathogen has therefore acquired

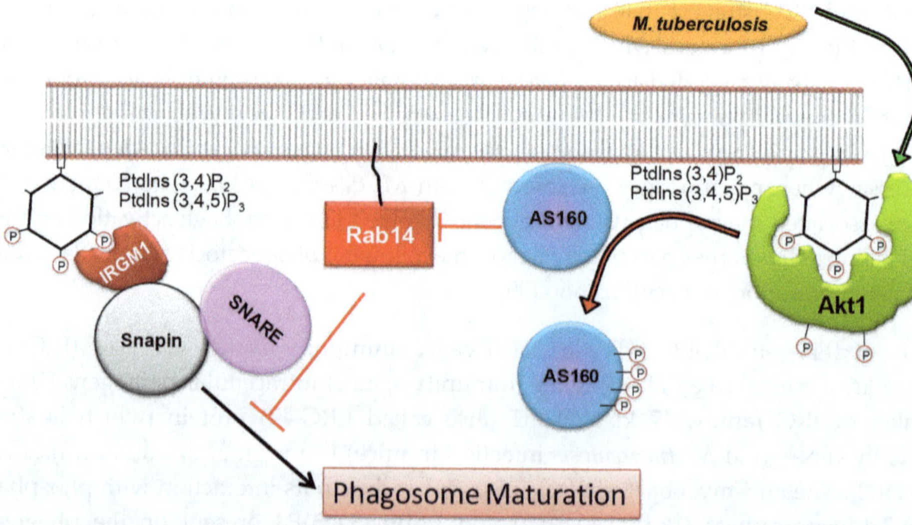

Figure 3. Critical balance between Rab14 and Irgm1 is important to counter *M. tuberculosis* infection. Pathogen results in the production of phosphatidylinositol-3,4-bisphosphate (PtdIns(3,4)P_2) and PtdIns(3,4,5)P_3 which act as a docking site for Akt1. The phosphorylated Akt1 phosphorylates AS160 which is inactive and is unable to deactivate Rab14. The active Rab14 blocks the phagosome maturation. PdlIns also recruit Irgm1 which along with Snapin protein may help in maturation of phagosomes and elimination of intracellular bacteria.

mechanisms to subvert the autophagy to induce a favorable condition for its persistence inside the host [111]. *M. tuberculosis* can also inhibit autophagy by skewing the immune response toward the Th2-type. While proinflammatory cytokines such as TNF-α and IFN-γ promote autophagy, Th2 cytokines such as IL-4 and IL-13 inhibit autophagy in human and murine macrophages, and this is dependent on the Akt-STAT6-signaling pathway [112]. Autophagy is known to help in antigen presentation via both MHC class I and class II pathways and, by inhibiting autophagy, *M. tuberculosis* also achieves the goal of suppression of MHC class I- and class II-mediated antigen presentation [112]. Vaccines that are designed to elicit a strong autophagic response can prove to be effective against latent TB infection and also drugs designed to modulate autophagy can be effective against the drug-resistant strain of *M. tuberculosis* [113].

4.5. Apoptosis

Macrophages use apoptosis as an effector mechanism to eliminate *M. tuberculosis* and to constrain the spreading of infection [114]. The apoptotic vesicles are readily engulfed by the neighboring dendritic cells. The dendritic cells in turn activate CD8$^+$ T cells by cross-presenting the processed antigens in the context of MHC class I. This results in an effective immune response against the bacilli. Necrosis, however, is favorable for the dissemination of bacteria and spread of infection. Hence, *M. tuberculosis* has developed mechanisms to suppress apoptosis and favor necrosis during active infection state [6, 63, 115, 116]. Inhibition of host cell apoptosis by *M. tuberculosis* has been implicated as a potential virulence mechanism. In fact, an inverse correlation between virulence of mycobacterial strains and their capacity to induce apoptosis has been reported [114]. Infection with virulent *M. tuberculosis* strain H37Rv is found to be associated with reduced expression of several pro-apoptotic genes and increased expression of the anti-apoptotic gene as compared to uninfected macrophages [117]. Studies using H37Rv and H37Ra strains of *M. tuberculosis* to infect alveolar macrophages have indicated that although both could induce apoptosis, the virulent H37Rv induce less apoptosis than the avirulent H37Ra by upregulating expression of the anti-apoptotic gene Bcl-2 in macrophages [118]. TNF-α is shown to play important role in host cell apoptosis infected with avirulent H37Ra strain [114, 119]. Also, the role of Bfl-1/A1 is realized in inhibition of apoptosis by *M. tuberculosis*, as decreased intracellular H37Rv growth was observed in Bfl-1/A1 siRNA-treated macrophages [120]. These cells show enhancement of phagosome-lysosome fusion and Caspase-3 activity indicating that expression of Bfl-1/A1 in H37Rv-infected macrophages provides the bacteria a survival strategy to overcome host defense. Nuclear factor-kappaB (NF-κB) activation is shown to play an essential role in the inhibition of host cell apoptosis by *M. tuberculosis* H37Rv [119]. Infection of macrophages with virulent *M. tuberculosis* confers resistance to apoptotic stimuli like Fas ligand (FasL) or TNF-α by reducing the cell surface expression of Fas receptors or secreting soluble TNF-α-receptor, respectively [121, 122]. Interestingly, Divangahi et al. have shown that virulent *M. tuberculosis* strains inhibit the production of prostaglandin E_2 by interfering with lipoxigenase pathway leading to inhibition of apoptosis and promotion of necrosis [115]. The other mechanism by which *M. tuberculosis* could possibly inhibit apoptotic process is via the *nuoG* gene, which can neutralize the NOX-2-mediated increase in ROS and TNF-α production in phagosomes containing *M. tuberculosis* thereby inhibiting apoptosis [123, 124]. Also, secA2 and pknE play roles in resistance against apoptosis as mutants of these genes induce more apoptosis in macrophages as compared to the wild-type *M. tuberculosis* strains [124–126].

4.6. Reactive oxygen and nitrogen intermediates (ROIs and RNIs)

ROIs and RNIs are produced in cells like macrophages in response to proinflammatory cytokines [127, 128]. ROIs and RNIs being small molecules defuse easily through the membranes and have a detrimental effect on the pathogens been engulfed in phagocytic vacuoles [129]. Studies have indicated that these molecules are important in providing innate host defense against *M. tuberculosis* [4, 129]. ROIs are produced by phagocytes, particularly the polymorphonuclear leukocytes and the activated macrophages, while RNIs are produced mainly by the activated macrophages. ROIs ($O^{2}\bullet^{-}$, H_2O_2, $OH^{\bullet}$,) are generated through the action of phagocyte oxidase (also called NADPH-oxidase). They further react with halides and amines to generate more reactive species (**Figure 4**). The important role of NADPH-oxidase in defense against *M. tuberculosis* and other pathogens is proven by the susceptibility of mice deficient in NADPH oxidase [129–131]. Children carrying mutations in gp91phox subunit of phagocyte oxidase enzyme are found to be more susceptible to TB infection than normal population [132]. In macrophages, IFN-γ in synergy with the TNF-α induces production of nitric oxide (•NO) with the help of inducible nitric oxide synthase (iNOS) (**Figure 4**). Not only does NO exert its effects on its own but also reacts with ROIs and the reaction products like peroxynitrite $^{(OONO-)}$ and other reaction intermediates can be even more toxic [127, 133]. After production, NO is not restricted to the area but readily defuses to other areas by using S-nitrosothiols, S-nitrosylated proteins, and nitrosyl-metal complexes as transport vehicles. NO produces heterogenous and diverse effects owing to its non-specific reactivity with a number of regulatory proteins [129,

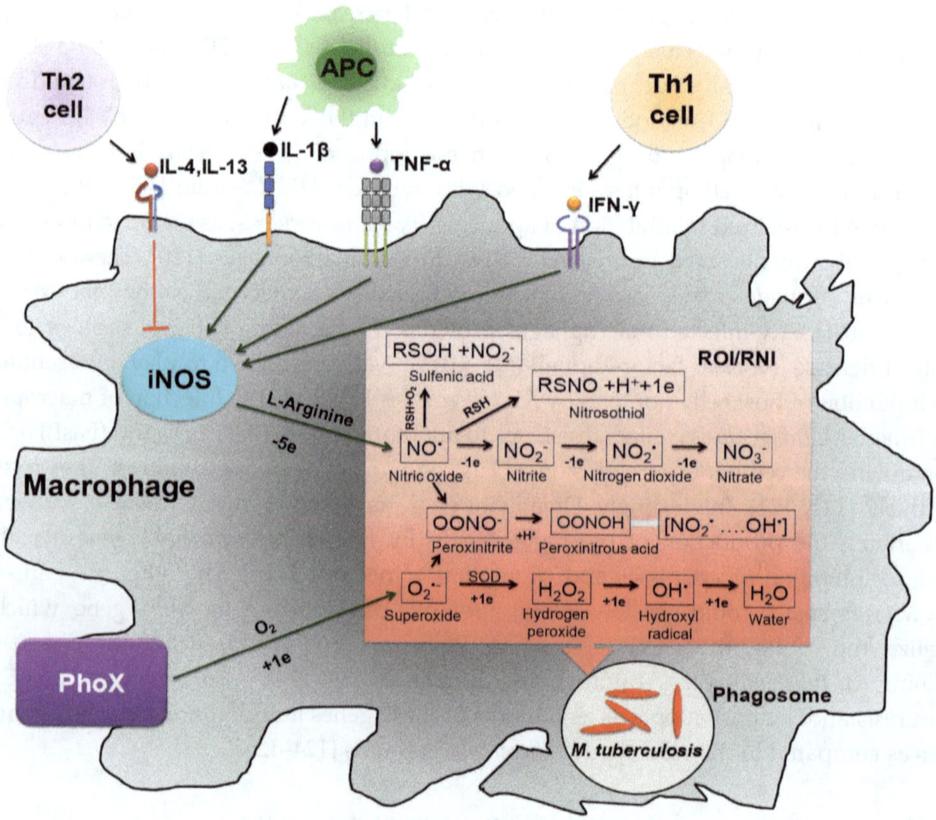

Figure 4. Regulation and function of iNOS during *M. tuberculosis* infection: Th1 cytokines like IFN-γ, TNF-α and IL-1β produced by Th1 T cells or antigen-presenting cells (APC) induce nitric oxide synthase (iNOS) enzyme. IL-4 and IL-13 secreted by Th2 cells negatively regulate iNOS expression. The products of phagocyte oxidase (Phox) and iNOS react and produce even more toxic intermediates like peroxynitrite against *M. tuberculosis*. NO also gives rise to sulfenic acid and nitrosothiols on reaction with sulfhydryl groups.

134]. In mouse macrophages, activation of TLR2 by various bacterial ligands induces iNOS promoter activity, production of NO, and killing of intracellular *M. tuberculosis*. However, protective role of NO in human TB is controversial. An essential role of NO/iNOS in anti-mycobacterial immunity was established by infection studies using iNOS knock-out mice [135, 136]. Mouse homozygous for knock-out allele for iNOS gene $^{(iNOS-/-)}$ when challenged with *M. tuberculosis* showed a very high susceptibility to infection [135]. Although most of the studies were conducted in mouse model, recent studies reveal that NO/iNOS is also important in killing the bacteria in human TB [134, 137, 138]. The iNOS activation through TLR2 pathway was found to enhance the killing of intracellular *M. tuberculosis* [77, 139]. All these studies indicate that probably iNOS also plays crucial role in anti-mycobacterial immunity in human. A comparative study of mice deficient either in phagocyte oxidase or in iNOS showed higher anti-mycobacterial activities by RNIs as compared to ROIs [131]. ROIs and RNIs damage the DNA and react with variety of other chemical moieties such as Fe-S clusters, tyrosyl radicals, hemes, sulfhydryls, thioethers, and alkenes to inactivate important components of the invading pathogens to compromise its survival inside the host.

Like other effector mechanisms, *M. tuberculosis* has evolved effective strategies to counter RNIs- and ROIs-mediated toxicity. The inhibition of the recruitment of iNOS to the infected phagosome would be one of the ideal strategies used by the bacilli [140]. EBP50, a scaffold protein in activated macrophages, targets iNOS to phagosomes [141]. *M. tuberculosis* downregulate EBP50 in the infected macrophages thereby reducing the transport of iNOS to the infected phagosome [141]. The bacteria also induce various genes to protect them from intracellular oxidative stress [109]. For example, mycobacterial catalase peroxidase (*katG*) and alkyl hydroperoxide reductase (*ahpC*) have role in antioxidant defenses, defend bacteria from intracellular oxidative stress [142, 143], and play roles in the virulence of *M. tuberculosis* [144, 145]. It has been shown that virulence of different clinical as well as recombinant strains of *M. tuberculosis* is correlated with varying expression levels of the peroxidase enzymes [143, 144]. NO induces a low oxygen state (hypoxia) in mycobacteria resulting in the overexpression of *katG* and *ahpC* [129, 146]. These genes were also reported to be overexpressed *in vivo* during infection with mycobacteria and studies indicate that these responses are abrogated in the phagosomal environment of $NOS2^{-/-}$ mice [147–149]. Oxidative stress has been established to induce a two-component system called DosR/DosS, consisting of a sensor histidine kinase DosS/DosT and a response regulator DosR [150–152]. The system helps the bacilli to cope oxidative and other stress (S-nitrosoglutathione, ethanol, etc.) conditions by initiating a complex response.

The DosR is characterized as a transcription factor responsible for transcription of the genes in response to oxidative stress. Genes expressed during the stress response, like α-crystallin was shown to carry sequences in the regulatory regions for DosR binding. In response to upstream activation signals, DosR is phosphorylated at Asp54 that results in its binding to DNA via its C-terminal domain and subsequent activation of DosR responsive genes. The sensor kinases, DosS and DosT, respond to redox environment and hypoxia, respectively. Both the proteins contain two GAF domains at N-terminal harboring a heme prosthetic group which interacts with O_2, NO or CO to induce autophosphorylation of the kinases and induce transcription of genes by activating DosR (**Figure 5**). CO is produced by heme oxygenase (HO) enzyme of macrophages. The enzyme is significantly upregulated during *M. tuberculosis* infection, oxidative stress, hypoxia, and stimulation with various cytokines. The enzyme catalyzes degradation of heme to biliverdin, free iron, and produces sufficient physiological amount of CO to induce dormancy program via binding primarily to DosS while DosT plays a little role in CO sensing. Although CO is sufficient to induce dormancy regulon, it was established that iNOS is required for optimal induction of response. Under aerobic condition, both the sensors are blocked and maintain a basal level of DosR responsive genes, while in anaerobic condition, they respond to the ligands and upregulate the DosR responsive genes to help the pathogen to survive in the stress caused by ROIs and RNIs (**Figure 5**) [153–155].

4.7. Vitamin D3

Vitamin D has long been known to be one of the nutritional therapeutic agents with a capacity to modulate the immune system in the case of an *M. tuberculosis* infection [156]. There has been a greater incidence of TB during the spring/summer months in temperate countries like UK [157], which can be correlated to a decrease in Vitamin D production on account of lower sun

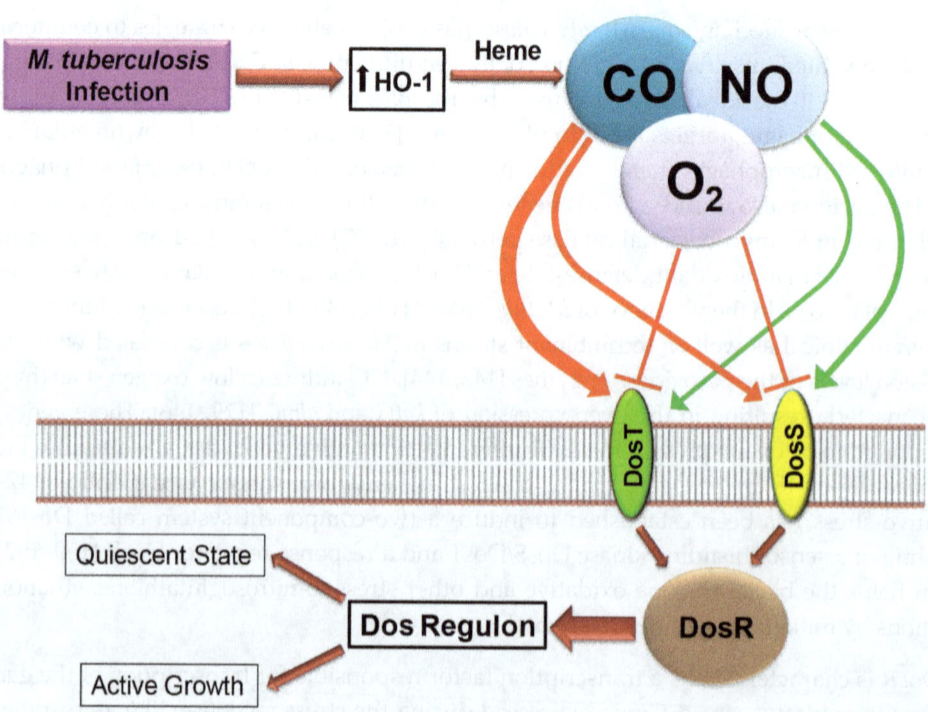

Figure 5. Role of NO, O_2 and CO in regulation of DosR/S/T regulon: NO, O_2, and CO are recognized in conjunction by DosS and DosT in a concentration gradient-dependent manner. CO mostly signals via DosS than DosT, while O_2 inhibits both DosS and DosT. *M. tuberculosis* infection upregulates the production of heme oxygenase-1(HO-1) which metabolizes heme to produce CO.

exposure in the winter months. Dietary composition also seemed to have a bearing with a predisposition toward TB, since a study conducted on an immigrant Gujarati Indian population in UK showed a marked increase in TB cases. It must be mentioned here that this population is a vegetarian one and hence dietary intake of Vitamin D is markedly less [158]. The genetic reason for this preponderance has been worked out to be an association with the VDR polymorphisms associated with the Gujarati Asian population concerned and Vitamin D deficiency [159]. Various studies indicate that Vitamin D can help the body fight against *M. tuberculosis* infections [160]. In a recent study, it has been found that patients administered with Vitamin D in combination with antibiotics recovered from TB more quickly than the patients administered with only antibiotics [161].

The mechanisms for a correlation of Vitamin D and TB are unknown, but it could be the antimicrobial peptides in association of Vitamin D generated by the pattern receptor stimulation in lieu of an infection with *M. tuberculosis* [162]. This stimulation then induces expression of cathelicidin [162] and β-defensin 2 (DEFB4) [163]. Cathelicidin induces phagolysosomal fusion which is necessary for killing of *M. tuberculosis*. In addition, 1,25(OH)2D, which is another downstream biochemical produced in Vitamin D biosynthetic pathway, induces autophagy [160, 164] and downregulates metalloproteinases (MMPs) [165]. All these processes help in the formation of phagolysosomes and the subsequent killing of *M. tuberculosis*. Vitamin D also seems to affect the adaptive immune system albeit in a regulatory manner. This is ensued as the downstream product 1,25(OH)2D upregulates regulatory responses with a skew toward the Th2-phenotype pattern. This can be ascertained by the anti-proliferative effects of 1,25(OH)2D on $CD4^+$ T cells [166]. It also seems to inhibit Th1 cytokine production [167, 168], while promoting T regulatory function at the same time [169]. It also seemingly upregulates Th2 cytokine production [170]. Studies using 1α,25-dihydroxyvitamin D3 indicate that vitamin D3 increases generation of oxygen intermediates via NADPH-dependent phagocyte oxidase involving the phosphatidylinositol 3-kinase [171]. In addition to this, Vitamin D3 can downregulate transcription of tryptophan-aspartate containing coat protein [172], which is important for the entry and survival of *M. tuberculosis* in human macrophages [173]. Thus, the role of proper nutrition in the control of *M. tuberculosis* is evident. Vitamin D which has otherwise been associated as the "anti-cold" Vitamin seems to have critical roles in the control of *M. tuberculosis* infection at the innate and the adaptive levels of the immune system of the host.

5. Conclusion

TB remains a global pandemic and despite thorough and constructive measures to eradicate TB, it has flourished and continues killing people. It has evolved into various MDR, XDR, and TDR strains, notwithstanding the best healthcare available, which are resistant to the obsolete group of drugs. This necessitates the need to find new drug targets as well as drugs to counter the menace of TB. Therefore, it becomes imperative to understand the biology of *M. tuberculosis* and the host response modulation mechanisms it has evolved. The same can be achieved by dissecting the biochemical processes throughout the life cycle of the pathogen and by understanding the host-pathogen interaction mechanisms in TB, both of which are prerequisites for the development of effective anti-TB vaccines/drugs. More importantly, the processes associated with the so-called "dormant stage" needs to be identified since this stays the biggest challenge in identifying asymptomatic TB patients, and understanding this Trojan can therefore escalate our steps to eradicate this menace by eons. In this chapter, we have attempted to address various host processes that are subverted by *M. tuberculosis* to survive inside its host as well as launch an assault when the host immune defenses are weakened. Right from when *M. tuberculosis* enters inside the body, it counters the host innate defenses by downregulating the oxidative burst inside the macrophages. It also subverts other macrophage effector functions like inhibition of phagolysosomal fusion which is critical for the action of lytic enzymes and therefore forms an important block where it escapes the host defenses. Most importantly, it modulates the host signaling targeting the PAMP receptors, more importantly the TLR2 or to downregulate the proinflammatory signaling cascade known to be detrimental for its intracellular survival. The adaptive responses are similarly affected as one of the major mechanisms, viz. antigen presentation seems to be downregulated. Both MHC class I and class II and even cross presentation are affected. This results in a very less or delayed outcome of protective adaptive immune response which again helps the pathogen to survive very efficiently inside the macrophages. It also affects critical host processes like apoptosis which could clear the pathogen in a controlled manner without allowing it to spread. Downregulating the proinflammatory signaling cascade also involves skewing the macrophage responses from a protective Th1- to a non-protective Th2-type. This involves most importantly a shift in the cytokine secretion pattern which subverts the host favorable macrophage signaling and effector functions in favor of the host. We have described important pathophysiological events during *M. tuberculosis* infection and the virulence processes by which the bacilli can escape the macrophage surveillance mechanisms, and use it as their safe refuge which may help in designing suitable interventions against *M. tuberculosis* infection.

Author details

Khalid Hussain Bhat[1]* and Imtiyaz Yaseen[2]

*Address all correspondence to: khalidbio@gmail.com

1 Department of Microbiology and Immunology, University of Illinois College of Medicine, Chicago, USA

2 Welcome Trust Center for Cell Biology, Scotland, UK

References

[1] Geissmann F, Manz MG, Jung S, Sieweke MH, Merad M, Ley K. Development of monocytes, macrophages, and dendritic cells. Science. 2010;**327**(5966):656-661

[2] Mackaness GB. The immunological basis of acquired cellular resistance. The Journal of Experimental Medicine. 1964;**120**:105-120

[3] Martinez FO, Sica A, Mantovani A, Locati M. Macrophage activation and polarization. Frontiers in Bioscience: a Journal and Virtual Library. 2008;**13**:453

[4] Flynn JL, Chan J. Immunology of tuberculosis. Annual Review of Immunology. 2001;**19**: 93-129

[5] Flynn JL, Chan J. Immune evasion by *Mycobacterium tuberculosis*: Living with the enemy. Current Opinion in Immunology. 2003;**15**(4):450-455

[6] Behar SM, Divangahi M, Remold HG. Evasion of innate immunity by *Mycobacterium tuberculosis*: Is death an exit strategy? Nature Reviews Microbiology. 2010;**8**(9):668-674

[7] Jozefowski S, Sobota A, Kwiatkowska K. How *Mycobacterium tuberculosis* subverts host immune responses. BioEssays. 2008;**30**(10):943-954

[8] Tauber AI. Metchnikoff and the phagocytosis theory. Nature Reviews Molecular Cell Biology. 2003;**4**(11):897-901

[9] De Domenico I, McVey Ward D, Kaplan J. Regulation of iron acquisition and storage: Consequences for iron-linked disorders. Nature Reviews Molecular Cell Biology. 2008; **9**(1):72-81

[10] Savill J, Fadok V. Corpse clearance defines the meaning of cell death. Nature. 2000; **407**(6805):784-788

[11] Ebert R, Florey H. The extravascular development of the monocyte observed in vivo. British Journal of Experimental Pathology. 1939;**20**(4):342

[12] van Furth R, Cohn ZA. The origin and kinetics of mononuclear phagocytes. The Journal of Experimental Medicine. 1968;**128**(3):415-435

[13] Wong KL, Tai JJ, Wong WC, Han H, Sem X, Yeap WH, et al. Gene expression profiling reveals the defining features of the classical, intermediate, and nonclassical human monocyte subsets. Blood. 2011;**118**(5):e16-e31

[14] Geissmann F, Gordon S, Hume DA, Mowat AM, Randolph GJ. Unravelling mononuclear phagocyte heterogeneity. Nature Reviews Immunology. 2010;**10**(6):453-460

[15] Smythies LE, Sellers M, Clements RH, Mosteller-Barnum M, Meng G, Benjamin WH, et al. Human intestinal macrophages display profound inflammatory anergy despite avid phagocytic and bacteriocidal activity. The Journal of Clinical Investigation. 2005; **115**(1):66-75

[16] Adams DO. Molecular interactions in macrophage activation. Immunology Today. 1989; **10**(2):33-35

[17] Nathan CF, Murray HW, Wiebe ME, Rubin BY. Identification of interferon-γ as the lymphokine that activates human macrophage oxidative metabolism and antimicrobial activity. The Journal of Experimental Medicine. 1983;**158**(3):670-689

[18] O'Shea JJ, Murray PJ. Cytokine signaling modules in inflammatory responses. Immunity. 2008;**28**(4):477-487

[19] Mosser DM, Edwards JP. Exploring the full spectrum of macrophage activation. Nature Reviews Immunology. 2008;**8**(12):958-969

[20] Schroder K, Sweet MJ, Hume DA. Signal integration between IFNγ and TLR signalling pathways in macrophages. Immunobiology. 2006;**211**(6–8):511-524

[21] Gordon S, Martinez FO. Alternative activation of macrophages: Mechanism and functions. Immunity. 2010;**32**(5):593-604

[22] Gordon S. Alternative activation of macrophages. Nature Reviews Immunology. 2003; **3**(1):23-35

[23] Goerdt S, Politz O, Schledzewski K, Birk R, Gratchev A, Guillot P, et al. Alternative versus classical activation of macrophages. Pathobiology. 1999;**67**(5–6):222-226

[24] Mantovani A, Sozzani S, Locati M, Allavena P, Sica A. Macrophage polarization: Tumor-associated macrophages as a paradigm for polarized M2 mononuclear phagocytes. Trends in Immunology. 2002;**23**(11):549-555

[25] Satoh T, Takeuchi O, Vandenbon A, Yasuda K, Tanaka Y, Kumagai Y, et al. The Jmjd3-Irf4 axis regulates M2 macrophage polarization and host responses against helminth infection. Nature Immunology. 2010;**11**(10):936-944

[26] Stein M, Keshav S, Harris N, Gordon S. Interleukin 4 potently enhances murine macrophage mannose receptor activity: A marker of alternative immunologic macrophage activation. The Journal of Experimental Medicine. 1992;**176**(1):287-292

[27] Raes G, De Baetselier P, Noel W, Beschin A, Brombacher F, Hassanzadeh Gh G. Differential expression of FIZZ1 and Ym1 in alternatively versus classically activated macrophages. Journal of Leukocyte Biology. 2002;**71**(4):597-602

[28] Reese TA, Liang HE, Tager AM, Luster AD, Van Rooijen N, Voehringer D, et al. Chitin induces accumulation in tissue of innate immune cells associated with allergy. Nature. 2007;**447**(7140):92-96

[29] Raes G, Beschin A, Ghassabeh GH, De Baetselier P. Alternatively activated macrophages in protozoan infections. Current Opinion in Immunology. 2007;**19**(4):454-459

[30] Daley JM, Brancato SK, Thomay AA, Reichner JS, Albina JE. The phenotype of murine wound macrophages. Journal of Leukocyte Biology. 2010;**87**(1):59-67

[31] Edwards JP, Zhang X, Frauwirth KA, Mosser DM. Biochemical and functional characterization of three activated macrophage populations. Journal of Leukocyte Biology. 2006;**80**(6):1298-1307

[32] Dalton DK, Pitts-Meek S, Keshav S, Figari IS, Bradley A, Stewart TA. Multiple defects of immune cell function in mice with disrupted interferon-γ genes. Science. 1993;**259**(5102): 1739-1742

[33] Mills CD, Kincaid K, Alt JM, Heilman MJ, Hill AM. M-1/M-2 macrophages and the Th1/Th2 paradigm. Journal of Immunology. 2000;**164**(12):6166-6173

[34] Mosser DM. The many faces of macrophage activation. Journal of Leukocyte Biology. 2003;**73**(2):209-212

[35] Munder M, Eichmann K, Modolell M. Alternative metabolic states in murine macrophages reflected by the nitric oxide synthase/arginase balance: Competitive regulation by CD4+ T cells correlates with Th1/Th2 phenotype. Journal of Immunology. 1998;**160**(11): 5347-5354

[36] Martinez FO, Gordon S, Locati M, Mantovani A. Transcriptional profiling of the human monocyte-to-macrophage differentiation and polarization: New molecules and patterns of gene expression. Journal of Immunology. 2006;**177**(10):7303-7311

[37] Hutchinson JA, Riquelme P, Geissler EK, Fandrich F. Human regulatory macrophages. Methods in Molecular Biology. 2011;**677**:181-192

[38] Gerber JS, Mosser DM. Reversing lipopolysaccharide toxicity by ligating the macrophage Fcγ receptors. Journal of Immunology. 2001;**166**(11):6861-6868

[39] Ogmundsdottir HM, Weir DM. Stimulation of phosphatidylinositol turnover in the macrophage plasma membrane: A possible mechanism for signal transmission. Immunology. 1979;**37**(3):689-696

[40] Adams DO, Hamilton TA. The cell biology of macrophage activation. Annual Review of Immunology. 1984;**2**(1):283-318

[41] Russell DG, Vanderven BC, Glennie S, Mwandumba H, Heyderman RS. The macrophage marches on its phagosome: Dynamic assays of phagosome function. Nature Reviews Immunology. 2009;**9**(8):594-600

[42] Huard RC, Fabre M, De Haas P, Lazzarini LCO, van Soolingen D, Cousins D, et al. Novel genetic polymorphisms that further delineate the phylogeny of the *Mycobacterium tuberculosis* complex. Journal of Bacteriology. 2006;**188**(12):4271-4287

[43] Brosch R, Gordon SV, Marmiesse M, Brodin P, Buchrieser C, Eiglmeier K, et al. A new evolutionary scenario for the *Mycobacterium tuberculosis* complex. Proceedings of the National Academy of Sciences. 2002;**99**(6):3684-3689

[44] Alexander KA, Laver PN, Michel AL, Williams M, van Helden PD, Warren RM, et al. Novel *Mycobacterium tuberculosis* complex pathogen, *M. mungi*. Emerging Infectious Diseases. 2010;**16**(8):1296

[45] Murray JF. *Mycobacterium tuberculosis* and the cause of consumption from discovery to fact. American Journal of Respiratory and Critical Care Medicine. 2004;**169**(10):1086-1088

[46] Bifani PJ, Mathema B, Kurepina NE, Kreiswirth BN. Global dissemination of the *Mycobacterium tuberculosis* W-Beijing family strains. Trends in Microbiology. 2002; **10**(1):45-52

[47] Glynn JR, Whiteley J, Bifani PJ, Kremer K, Van Soolingen D. Worldwide occurrence of Beijing/W strains of *Mycobacterium tuberculosis*: A systematic review. Emerging Infectious Diseases. 2002;**8**(8):843

[48] Johnson R, Streicher EM, Louw GE, Warren RM, van Helden PD, Victor TC. Drug resistance in *Mycobacterium tuberculosis*. Current Issues in Molecular Biology. 2006;**8**(2): 97-111

[49] Udwadia ZF, Amale RA, Ajbani KK, Rodrigues C. Totally drug-resistant tuberculosis in India. Clinical Infectious Diseases. 2012;**54**(4):579-581

[50] Gillespie SH. Evolution of drug resistance in *Mycobacterium tuberculosis*: Clinical and molecular perspective. Antimicrobial Agents and Chemotherapy. 2002;**46**(2):267-274

[51] Zumla A, Abubakar I, Raviglione M, Hoelscher M, Ditiu L, McHugh TD, et al. Drug-resistant tuberculosis-current dilemmas, unanswered questions, challenges, and priority needs. Journal of Infectious Diseases. 2012;**205**(Suppl 2):S228-S240

[52] Raviglione M. XDR-TB: Entering the post-antibiotic era? The International Journal of Tuberculosis and Lung Disease: the official journal of the International Union against Tuberculosis and Lung Disease. 2006;**10**(11):1185

[53] Sutcliffe IC. Cell envelope composition and organisation in the genus Rhodococcus. Antonie Van Leeuwenhoek. 1998;**74**(1–3):49-58

[54] Minnikin DE, Kremer L, Dover LG, Besra GS. The methyl-branched fortifications of *Mycobacterium tuberculosis*. Chemistry & Biology. 2002;**9**(5):545-553

[55] Smith I. *Mycobacterium tuberculosis* pathogenesis and molecular determinants of virulence. Clinical Microbiology Reviews. 2003;**16**(3):463-496

[56] Rook GA, Dheda K, Zumla A. Immune responses to tuberculosis in developing countries: Implications for new vaccines. Nature Reviews Immunology. 2005;**5**(8):661-667

[57] Bloom BR, editor. Tuberculosis: Pathogenesis, Protection and Control. N. W: American Society for Microbiology; 1994

[58] Tatar D, Senol G, Alptekin S, Karakurum C, Aydin M, Coskunol I. Tuberculosis in diabetics: Features in an endemic area. Japanese Journal of Infectious Diseases. 2009;**62**(6):423-427

[59] Fatkenheuer G, Taelman H, Lepage P, Schwenk A, Wenzel R. The return of tuberculosis. Diagnostic Microbiology and Infectious Disease. 1999;**34**(2):139-146

[60] Lawn SD, Wood R, Wilkinson RJ. Changing concepts of "latent tuberculosis infection" in patients living with HIV infection. Clinical and Developmental Immunology. 2011;**2011**

[61] Narain JP, Raviglione MC, Kochi A. HIV-associated tuberculosis in developing countries: Epidemiology and strategies for prevention. Tubercle and Lung Disease. 1992; **73**(6):311-321

[62] Kaufmann SH. Recent findings in immunology give tuberculosis vaccines a new boost. Trends in Immunology. 2005;**26**(12):660-667

[63] Dannenberg AM. Pathogenesis of Human Pulmonary Tuberculosis: Insights from the Rabbit Model. N. W: American Society for Microbiology; 2006

[64] Nienhaus A, Schablon A, Diel R. Interferon-γ release assay for the diagnosis of latent TB infection–analysis of discordant results, when compared to the tuberculin skin test. PLoS One. 2008;**3**(7):e2665

[65] Miranda C, Tomford JW, Gordon SM. Interferon-γ-release assays: Better than tuberculin skin testing? Cleveland Clinic Journal of Medicine. 2010;**77**(9):606-611

[66] Pai M, Zwerling A, Menzies D. Systematic review: T-cell–based assays for the diagnosis of latent tuberculosis infection: An update. Annals of Internal Medicine. 2008;**149**(3):177

[67] Gannon BW, Hayes CM, Roe JM. Survival rate of airborne *Mycobacterium bovis*. Research in Veterinary Science. 2007;**82**(2):169-172

[68] Hickman C, MacDonald KL, Osterholm MT. Exposure of passengers and flight crew to *Mycobacterium tuberculosis* on commercial aircraft, 1992-1995. Morbidity and Mortality Weekly Report. 1995;**44**(8):137-140

[69] Ernst JD. Macrophage receptors for *Mycobacterium tuberculosis*. Infection and Immunity. 1998;**66**(4):1277-1281

[70] Vergne I, Chua J, Singh SB, Deretic V. Cell biology of *Mycobacterium tuberculosis* phagosome. Annual Review of Cell and Developmental Biology. 2004;**20**:367-394

[71] Pasula R, Downing JF, Wright JR, Kachel DL, Davis Jr TE, Martin W 2nd. Surfactant protein a (SP-A) mediates attachment of *Mycobacterium tuberculosis* to murine alveolar macrophages. American Journal of Respiratory and Critical Care Medicine. 1997;**17**(2):209

[72] Tailleux L, Schwartz O, Herrmann JL, Pivert E, Jackson M, Amara A, et al. DC-SIGN is the major *Mycobacterium tuberculosis* receptor on human dendritic cells. The Journal of Experimental Medicine. 2003;**197**(1):121-127

[73] Schlesinger LS. Macrophage phagocytosis of virulent but not attenuated strains of *Mycobacterium tuberculosis* is mediated by mannose receptors in addition to complement receptors. Journal of Immunology. 1993;**150**(7):2920-2930

[74] Schlesinger LS, Hull SR, Kaufman TM. Binding of the terminal mannosyl units of lipoarabinomannan from a virulent strain of *Mycobacterium tuberculosis* to human macrophages. Journal of Immunology. 1994;**152**(8):4070-4079

[75] Geijtenbeek TBH, Van Vliet SJ, Koppel EA, Sanchez-Hernandez M, Vandenbroucke-Grauls CMJE, Appelmelk B, et al. Mycobacteria target DC-SIGN to suppress dendritic cell function. The Journal of Experimental Medicine. 2003;**197**(1):7-17

[76] Mukhopadhyay S, Nair S, Ghosh S. Pathogenesis in tuberculosis: Transcriptomic approaches to unraveling virulence mechanisms and finding new drug targets. FEMS Microbiology Reviews. 2012;**36**(2):463-485

[77] Thoma-Uszynski S, Stenger S, Takeuchi O, Ochoa MT, Engele M, Sieling PA, et al. Induction of direct antimicrobial activity through mammalian toll-like receptors. Science. 2001;**291**(5508):1544-1547

[78] Court N, Vasseur V, Vacher R, Fremond C, Shebzukhov Y, Yeremeev VV, et al. Partial redundancy of the pattern recognition receptors, scavenger receptors, and C-type lectins for the long-term control of *Mycobacterium tuberculosis* infection. Journal of Immunology. 2010;**184**(12):7057-7070

[79] Russell DG. Who puts the tubercle in tuberculosis? Nature Reviews Microbiology. 2007; **5**(1):39-47

[80] Schluger NW, Rom WN. The host immune response to tuberculosis. American Journal of Respiratory and Critical Care Medicine. 1998;**157**(3 Pt 1):679-691

[81] Cooper AM. Cell-mediated immune responses in tuberculosis. Annual Review of Immunology. 2009;**27**:393-422

[82] Mogues T, Goodrich ME, Ryan L, LaCourse R, North RJ. The relative importance of T cell subsets in immunity and immunopathology of airborne *Mycobacterium tuberculosis* infection in mice. The Journal of Experimental Medicine. 2001;**193**(3):271-280

[83] Grotzke JE, Lewinsohn DM. Role of CD8+ T lymphocytes in control of *Mycobacterium tuberculosis* infection. Microbes and Infection. 2005;**7**(4):776-788

[84] Ulrichs T, Kaufmann SH. New insights into the function of granulomas in human tuberculosis. The Journal of Pathology. 2006;**208**(2):261-269

[85] Davis JM, Ramakrishnan L. The role of the granuloma in expansion and dissemination of early tuberculous infection. Cell. 2009;**136**(1):37-49

[86] Capuano SV, Croix DA, Pawar S, Zinovik A, Myers A, Lin PL, et al. Experimental *Mycobacterium tuberculosis* infection of cynomolgus macaques closely resembles the various manifestations of human *M. tuberculosis* infection. Infection and Immunity. 2003; **71**(10):5831-5844

[87] Vergne I, Chua J, Lee HH, Lucas M, Belisle J, Deretic V. Mechanism of phagolysosome biogenesis block by viable *Mycobacterium tuberculosis*. Proceedings of the National Academy of Sciences. 2005;**102**(11):4033-4038

[88] Festjens N, Bogaert P, Batni A, Houthuys E, Plets E, Vanderschaeghe D, et al. Disruption of the SapM locus in Mycobacterium bovis BCG improves its protective efficacy as a vaccine against *M. tuberculosis*. EMBO Molecular Medicine. 2011;**3**(4):222-234

[89] Grundner C, Ng HL, Alber T. *Mycobacterium tuberculosis* protein tyrosine phosphatase PtpB structure reveals a diverged fold and a buried active site. Structure. 2005;**13**(11): 1625-1634

[90] Via LE, Deretic D, Ulmer RJ, Hibler NS, Huber LA, Deretic V. Arrest of mycobacterial phagosome maturation is caused by a block in vesicle fusion between stages controlled by rab5 and rab7. Journal of Biological Chemistry. 1997;**272**(20):13326-13331

[91] Deretic V, Singh S, Master S, Harris J, Roberts E, Kyei G, et al. *Mycobacterium tuberculosis* inhibition of phagolysosome biogenesis and autophagy as a host defence mechanism. Cellular Microbiology. 2006;**8**(5):719-727

[92] Pieters J. *Mycobacterium tuberculosis* and the macrophage: Maintaining a balance. Cell Host & Microbe. 2008;**3**(6):399-407

[93] Tan T, Lee WL, Alexander DC, Grinstein S, Liu J. The ESAT-6/CFP-10 secretion system of *Mycobacterium marinum* modulates phagosome maturation. Cellular Microbiology. 2006; **8**(9):1417-1429

[94] Pethe K, Swenson DL, Alonso S, Anderson J, Wang C, Russell DG. Isolation of *Mycobacterium tuberculosis* mutants defective in the arrest of phagosome maturation. Proceedings of the National Academy of Sciences. 2004;**101**(37):13642-13647

[95] Stewart GR, Patel J, Robertson BD, Rae A, Young DB. Mycobacterial mutants with defective control of phagosomal acidification. PLoS Pathogens. 2005;**1**(3):269-278

[96] Ferrari G, Langen H, Naito M, Pieters J. A coat protein on phagosomes involved in the intracellular survival of mycobacteria. Cell. 1999;**97**(4):435-447

[97] Jayachandran R, Sundaramurthy V, Combaluzier B, Mueller P, Korf H, Huygen K, et al. Survival of mycobacteria in macrophages is mediated by coronin 1-dependent activation of calcineurin. Cell. 2007;**130**(1):37-50

[98] Blackwell JM, Searle S, Goswami T, Miller EN. Understanding the multiple functions of Nramp1. Microbes and Infection. 2000;**2**(3):317-321

[99] Hackam DJ, Rotstein OD, Zhang W, Gruenheid S, Gros P, Grinstein S. Host resistance to intracellular infection: Mutation of natural resistance-associated macrophage protein 1 (Nramp1) impairs phagosomal acidification. The Journal of Experimental Medicine. 1998;**188**(2):351-364

[100] MacMicking JD, Taylor GA, McKinney JD. Immune control of tuberculosis by IFN-γ-inducible LRG-47. Science. 2003;**302**(5645):654-659

[101] Taylor GA, Feng CG, Sher A. p47 GTPases: Regulators of immunity to intracellular pathogens. Nature Reviews Immunology. 2004;**4**(2):100-109

[102] Taylor GA. IRG proteins: Key mediators of interferon-regulated host resistance to intracellular pathogens. Cellular Microbiology. 2007;**9**(5):1099-1107

[103] Kyei GB, Vergne I, Chua J, Roberts E, Harris J, Junutula JR, et al. Rab14 is critical for maintenance of *Mycobacterium tuberculosis* phagosome maturation arrest. The EMBO Journal. 2006;**25**(22):5250-5259

[104] Tiwari S, Choi HP, Matsuzawa T, Pypaert M, MacMicking JD. Targeting of the GTPase Irgm1 to the phagosomal membrane via PtdIns(3,4)P(2) and PtdIns(3,4,5)P(3) promotes immunity to mycobacteria. Nature Immunology. 2009;**10**(8):907-917

[105] Kuijl C, Neefjes J. New insight into the everlasting host-pathogen arms race. Nature Immunology. 2009;**10**(8):808-809

[106] Deretic V. Autophagy in immunity and cell-autonomous defense against intracellular microbes. Immunological Reviews. 2011;**240**(1):92-104

[107] Harris J, Hope J, Lavelle E. Autophagy and the immune response to TB. Transboundary and Emerging Diseases. 2009;**56**(6–7):248-254

[108] Singh SB, Davis AS, Taylor GA, Deretic V. Human IRGM induces autophagy to eliminate intracellular mycobacteria. Science. 2006;**313**(5792):1438-1441

[109] King KY, Lew JD, Ha NP, Lin JS, Ma X, Graviss EA, et al. Polymorphic allele of human IRGM1 is associated with susceptibility to tuberculosis in African Americans. PLoS One. 2011;**6**(1):e16317

[110] Levine B, Mizushima N, Virgin HW. Autophagy in immunity and inflammation. Nature. 2011;**469**(7330):323-335

[111] Kumar D, Nath L, Kamal MA, Varshney A, Jain A, Singh S, et al. Genome-wide analysis of the host intracellular network that regulates survival of *Mycobacterium tuberculosis*. Cell. 2010;**140**(5):731-743

[112] Harris J, De Haro SA, Master SS, Keane J, Roberts EA, Delgado M, et al. T helper 2 cytokines inhibit autophagic control of intracellular *Mycobacterium tuberculosis*. Immunity. 2007;**27**(3):505-517

[113] Ni Cheallaigh C, Keane J, Lavelle E, Hope J, Harris J. Autophagy in the immune response to tuberculosis: Clinical perspectives. Clinical and Experimental Immunology. 2011;**164**(3):291-300

[114] Keane J, Remold HG, Kornfeld H. Virulent *Mycobacterium tuberculosis* strains evade apoptosis of infected alveolar macrophages. Journal of Immunology. 2000;**164**(4):2016-2020

[115] Divangahi M, Desjardins D, Nunes-Alves C, Remold HG, Behar SM. Eicosanoid pathways regulate adaptive immunity to *Mycobacterium tuberculosis*. Nature Immunology. 2010;**11**(8):751-758

[116] Behar S, Martin C, Booty M, Nishimura T, Zhao X, Gan H, et al. Apoptosis is an innate defense function of macrophages against *Mycobacterium tuberculosis*. Mucosal Immunology. 2011;**4**(3):279-287

[117] Spira A, Carroll JD, Liu G, Aziz Z, Shah V, Kornfeld H, et al. Apoptosis genes in human alveolar macrophages infected with virulent or attenuated *Mycobacterium tuberculosis*: A pivotal role for tumor necrosis factor. American Journal of Respiratory and Critical Care Medicine. 2003;**29**(5):545-551

[118] Sly LM, Hingley-Wilson SM, Reiner NE, McMaster WR. Survival of *Mycobacterium tuberculosis* in host macrophages involves resistance to apoptosis dependent upon induction of antiapoptotic Bcl-2 family member Mcl-1. Journal of Immunology. 2003;**170**(1): 430-437

[119] Dhiman R, Raje M, Majumdar S. Differential expression of NF-κB in mycobacteria infected THP-1 affects apoptosis. Biochimica et Biophysica Acta. 2007;**1770**(4):649-658

[120] Dhiman R, Kathania M, Raje M, Majumdar S. Inhibition of bfl-1/A1 by siRNA inhibits mycobacterial growth in THP-1 cells by enhancing phagosomal acidification. Biochimica et Biophysica Acta. 2008;**1780**(4):733-742

[121] Oddo M, Renno T, Attinger A, Bakker T, MacDonald HR, Meylan PR. Fas ligand-induced apoptosis of infected human macrophages reduces the viability of intracellular *Mycobacterium tuberculosis*. Journal of Immunology. 1998;**160**(11):5448-5454

[122] Balcewicz-Sablinska MK, Keane J, Kornfeld H, Remold HG. Pathogenic *Mycobacterium tuberculosis* evades apoptosis of host macrophages by release of TNF-R2, resulting in inactivation of TNF-α. Journal of Immunology. 1998;**161**(5):2636-2641

[123] Velmurugan K, Chen B, Miller JL, Azogue S, Gurses S, Hsu T, et al. *Mycobacterium tuberculosis* nuoG is a virulence gene that inhibits apoptosis of infected host cells. PLoS Pathogens. 2007;**3**(7):e110

[124] Miller JL, Velmurugan K, Cowan MJ, Briken V. The type I NADH dehydrogenase of *Mycobacterium tuberculosis* counters phagosomal NOX2 activity to inhibit TNF-α-mediated host cell apoptosis. PLoS Pathogens. 2010;**6**(4):e1000864

[125] Jayakumar D, Jacobs WR Jr, Narayanan S. Protein kinase E of *Mycobacterium tuberculosis* has a role in the nitric oxide stress response and apoptosis in a human macrophage model of infection. Cellular Microbiology. 2008;**10**(2):365-374

[126] Hinchey J, Jeon BY, Alley H, Chen B, Goldberg M, Derrick S, et al. Lysine auxotrophy combined with deletion of the SecA2 gene results in a safe and highly immunogenic candidate live attenuated vaccine for tuberculosis. PLoS One. 2011;**6**(1): e15857

[127] Ding AH, Nathan CF, Stuehr DJ. Release of reactive nitrogen intermediates and reactive oxygen intermediates from mouse peritoneal macrophages. Comparison of activating cytokines and evidence for independent production. Journal of Immunology. 1988; **141**(7):2407-2412

[128] Sato K, Akaki T, Tomioka H. Differential potentiation of anti-mycobacterial activity and reactive nitrogen intermediate-producing ability of murine peritoneal macrophages activated by interferon-γ (IFN-γ) and tumour necrosis factor-α (TNF-α). Clinical and Experimental Immunology. 1998;**112**(1):63-68

[129] Nathan C, Shiloh MU. Reactive oxygen and nitrogen intermediates in the relationship between mammalian hosts and microbial pathogens. Proceedings of the National Academy of Sciences. 2000;**97**(16):8841-8848

[130] Jackson SH, Gallin JI, Holland SM. The p47phox mouse knock-out model of chronic granulomatous disease. The Journal of Experimental Medicine. 1995;**182**(3):751-758

[131] Adams L, Dinauer M, Morgenstern D, Krahenbuhl J. Comparison of the roles of reactive oxygen and nitrogen intermediates in the host response to *Mycobacterium tuberculosis* using transgenic mice. Tubercle and Lung Disease. 1997;**78**(5):237-246

[132] Lau Y, Chan G, Ha S, Hui Y, Yuen K. The role of phagocytic respiratory burst in host defense. Clinical Infectious Diseases. 1998;**26**(1):226-227

[133] Shiloh MU, Nathan CF. Reactive nitrogen intermediates and the pathogenesis of salmonella and mycobacteria. Current Opinion in Microbiology. 2000;**3**(1):35-42

[134] Chan ED, Chan J, Schluger NW. What is the role of nitric oxide in murine and human host defense against tuberculosis? Current knowledge. American Journal of Respiratory and Critical Care Medicine. 2001;**25**(5):606

[135] MacMicking JD, North RJ, LaCourse R, Mudgett JS, Shah SK, Nathan CF. Identification of nitric oxide synthase as a protective locus against tuberculosis. Proceedings of the National Academy of Sciences. 1997;**94**(10):5243-5248

[136] MacMicking J, Xie QW, Nathan C. Nitric oxide and macrophage function. Annual Review of Immunology. 1997;**15**:323-350

[137] Nicholson S, Bonecini-Almeida Mda G, Lapa e Silva JR, Nathan C, Xie QW, Mumford R, et al. Inducible nitric oxide synthase in pulmonary alveolar macrophages from patients with tuberculosis. The Journal of Experimental Medicine. 1996;**183**(5):2293-2302

[138] Wang CH, Lin HC, Liu CY, Huang KH, Huang TT, Yu CT, et al. Upregulation of inducible nitric oxide synthase and cytokine secretion in peripheral blood monocytes from pulmonary tuberculosis patients. The International Journal of Tuberculosis and Lung Disease: the official journal of the International Union against Tuberculosis and Lung Disease. 2001;**5**(3):283-291

[139] Brightbill HD, Libraty DH, Krutzik SR, Yang RB, Belisle JT, Bleharski JR, et al. Host defense mechanisms triggered by microbial lipoproteins through toll-like receptors. Science. 1999;**285**(5428):732-736

[140] Miller BH, Fratti RA, Poschet JF, Timmins GS, Master SS, Burgos M, et al. Mycobacteria inhibit nitric oxide synthase recruitment to phagosomes during macrophage infection. Infection and Immunity. 2004;**72**(5):2872-2878

[141] Davis AS, Vergne I, Master SS, Kyei GB, Chua J, Deretic V. Mechanism of inducible nitric oxide synthase exclusion from mycobacterial phagosomes. PLoS Pathogens. 2007;**3**(12):e186

[142] Master SS, Springer B, Sander P, Boettger EC, Deretic V, Timmins GS. Oxidative stress response genes in *Mycobacterium tuberculosis*: Role of ahpC in resistance to peroxynitrite and stage-specific survival in macrophages. Microbiology. 2002;**148**(Pt 10):3139-3144

[143] Heym B, Zhang Y, Poulet S, Young D, Cole ST. Characterization of the katG gene encoding a catalase-peroxidase required for the isoniazid susceptibility of *Mycobacterium tuberculosis*. Journal of Bacteriology. 1993;**175**(13):4255-4259

[144] Manca C, Paul S, Barry CE 3rd, Freedman VH, Kaplan G. *Mycobacterium tuberculosis* catalase and peroxidase activities and resistance to oxidative killing in human monocytes in vitro. Infection and Immunity. 1999;**67**(1):74-79

[145] Li Z, Kelley C, Collins F, Rouse D, Morris S. Expression of katG in *Mycobacterium tuberculosis* is associated with its growth and persistence in mice and Guinea pigs. Journal of Infectious Diseases. 1998;**177**(4):1030-1035

[146] Hu Y, Butcher PD, Mangan JA, Rajandream MA, Coates AR. Regulation of hmp gene transcription in *Mycobacterium tuberculosis*: Effects of oxygen limitation and nitrosative and oxidative stress. Journal of Bacteriology. 1999;**181**(11):3486-3493

[147] Schnappinger D, Ehrt S, Voskuil MI, Liu Y, Mangan JA, Monahan IM, et al. Transcriptional adaptation of *Mycobacterium tuberculosis* within macrophages: Insights into the Phagosomal environment. The Journal of Experimental Medicine. 2003;**198**(5):693-704

[148] Voskuil MI, Schnappinger D, Visconti KC, Harrell MI, Dolganov GM, Sherman DR, et al. Inhibition of respiration by nitric oxide induces a *Mycobacterium tuberculosis* dormancy program. The Journal of Experimental Medicine. 2003;**198**(5):705-713

[149] Ohno H, Zhu G, Mohan VP, Chu D, Kohno S, Jacobs WR Jr, et al. The effects of reactive nitrogen intermediates on gene expression in *Mycobacterium tuberculosis*. Cellular Microbiology. 2003;**5**(9):637-648

[150] Dasgupta N, Kapur V, Singh KK, Das TK, Sachdeva S, Jyothisri K, et al. Characterization of a two-component system, devR-devS, of *Mycobacterium tuberculosis*. Tubercle and Lung Disease. 2000;**80**(3):141-159

[151] Sherman DR, Voskuil M, Schnappinger D, Liao R, Harrell MI, Schoolnik GK. Regulation of the *Mycobacterium tuberculosis* hypoxic response gene encoding α-crystallin. Proceedings of the National Academy of Sciences. 2001;**98**(13):7534-7539

[152] Kendall SL, Movahedzadeh F, Rison SC, Wernisch L, Parish T, Duncan K, et al. The *Mycobacterium tuberculosis* dosRS two-component system is induced by multiple stresses. Tuberculosis (Edinburgh, Scotland). 2004;**84**(3–4):247-255

[153] Kumar A, Toledo JC, Patel RP, Lancaster JR Jr, Steyn AJ. *Mycobacterium tuberculosis* DosS is a redox sensor and DosT is a hypoxia sensor. Proceedings of the National Academy of Sciences. 2007;**104**(28):11568-11573

[154] Kumar A, Deshane JS, Crossman DK, Bolisetty S, Yan BS, Kramnik I, et al. Heme oxygenase-1-derived carbon monoxide induces the *Mycobacterium tuberculosis* dormancy regulon. Journal of Biological Chemistry. 2008;**283**(26):18032-18039

[155] Shiloh MU, Manzanillo P, Cox JS. *Mycobacterium tuberculosis* senses host-derived carbon monoxide during macrophage infection. Cell Host & Microbe. 2008;**3**(5):323-330

[156] Nnoaham KE, Clarke A. Low serum vitamin D levels and tuberculosis: A systematic review and meta-analysis. International Journal of Epidemiology. 2008;**37**(1):113-119

[157] Douglas AS, Strachan DP, Maxwell JD. Seasonality of tuberculosis: The reverse of other respiratory diseases in the UK. Thorax. 1996;**51**(9):944-946

[158] Strachan DP, Powell KJ, Thaker A, Millard FJ, Maxwell JD. Vegetarian diet as a risk factor for tuberculosis in immigrant south London Asians. Thorax. 1995;**50**(2):175-180

[159] Wilkinson RJ, Llewelyn M, Toossi Z, Patel P, Pasvol G, Lalvani A, et al. Influence of vitamin D deficiency and vitamin D receptor polymorphisms on tuberculosis among Gujarati Asians in West London: A case-control study. Lancet. 2000;**355**(9204):618-621

[160] Liu PT, Stenger S, Tang DH, Modlin RL. Cutting edge: Vitamin D-mediated human antimicrobial activity against *Mycobacterium tuberculosis* is dependent on the induction of cathelicidin. Journal of Immunology. 2007;**179**(4):2060-2063

[161] Coussens AK, Wilkinson RJ, Hanifa Y, Nikolayevskyy V, Elkington PT, Islam K, et al. Vitamin D accelerates resolution of inflammatory responses during tuberculosis treatment. Proceedings of the National Academy of Sciences. 2012;**109**(38):15449-15454

[162] Liu PT, Stenger S, Li H, Wenzel L, Tan BH, Krutzik SR, et al. Toll-like receptor triggering of a vitamin D-mediated human antimicrobial response. Science. 2006;**311**(5768):1770-1773

[163] Liu PT, Schenk M, Walker VP, Dempsey PW, Kanchanapoomi M, Wheelwright M, et al. Convergence of IL-1β and VDR activation pathways in human TLR2/1-induced antimicrobial responses. PLoS One. 2009;**4**(6):e5810

[164] Yuk JM, Shin DM, Lee HM, Yang CS, Jin HS, Kim KK, et al. Vitamin D3 induces autophagy in human monocytes/macrophages via cathelicidin. Cell Host & Microbe. 2009;**6**(3):231-243

[165] Anand SP, Selvaraj P. Effect of 1, 25 dihydroxyvitamin D(3) on matrix metalloproteinases MMP-7, MMP-9 and the inhibitor TIMP-1 in pulmonary tuberculosis. Clinical Immunology. 2009;**133**(1):126-131

[166] Mahon BD, Wittke A, Weaver V, Cantorna MT. The targets of vitamin D depend on the differentiation and activation status of CD4 positive T cells. Journal of Cellular Biochemistry. 2003;**89**(5):922-932

[167] Vidyarani M, Selvaraj P, Jawahar MS, Narayanan PR. 1, 25 Dihydroxyvitamin D3 modulated cytokine response in pulmonary tuberculosis. Cytokine. 2007;**40**(2):128-134

[168] Imazeki I, Matsuzaki J, Tsuji K, Nishimura T. Immunomodulating effect of vitamin D3 derivatives on type-1 cellular immunity. Biomedical Research. 2006;**27**(1):1-9

[169] Daniel C, Sartory NA, Zahn N, Radeke HH, Stein JM. Immune modulatory treatment of trinitrobenzene sulfonic acid colitis with calcitriol is associated with a change of a T helper (Th) 1/Th17 to a Th2 and regulatory T cell profile. Journal of Pharmacology and Experimental Therapeutics. 2008;**324**(1):23-33

[170] Cantorna MT, Humpal-Winter J, DeLuca HF. In vivo upregulation of interleukin-4 is one mechanism underlying the immunoregulatory effects of 1,25-dihydroxyvitamin D(3). Archives of Biochemistry and Biophysics. 2000;**377**(1):135-138

[171] Sly LM, Lopez M, Nauseef WM, Reiner NE. 1α,25-Dihydroxyvitamin D3-induced monocyte antimycobacterial activity is regulated by phosphatidylinositol 3-kinase and mediated by the NADPH-dependent phagocyte oxidase. Journal of Biological Chemistry. 2001;**276**(38):35482-35493

[172] Anand PK, Kaul D. Vitamin D3-dependent pathway regulates TACO gene transcription. Biochemical and Biophysical Research Communications. 2003;**310**(3):876-877

[173] Anand PK, Kaul D. Downregulation of TACO gene transcription restricts mycobacterial entry/survival within human macrophages. FEMS Microbiology Letters. 2005;**250**(1): 137-144

9

Tuberculosis: A Risk Factor Approach

Leonardo F. Jurado and Diana M. Palacios

Abstract

One in three people in the world is infected with *Mycobacterium tuberculosis*, and 10% of infected individuals will develop the disease at any time in their lifetime. Today, despite the advances in diagnosis and treatment, tuberculosis (TB) remains as one of the biggest challenges in global public health, and low and middle-income countries are the most affected. The risk for developing the disease depends on endogenous, exogenous, and environmental factors. Among the most relevant conditions that could precipitate TB development are those that affect the host-immune response. HIV infection increase about 20 times the risk of TB, and other more common conditions, such as diabetes mellitus, malnutrition, and smoking, also contribute in a big way to the TB pandemic. Global TB control programs in order to achieve the disease control objectives must integrate strategies that have a direct impact on risk factors, not only at an individual level but also on a public health policy level. Here, we review some of the most important risk factors for the development of TB, as one of the most relevant ways for TB control.

Keywords: tuberculosis, risk factor, epidemiology, prevention, control

1. Introduction

Tuberculosis (TB) is a bacterial infectious disease caused by *Mycobacterium tuberculosis* complex organisms, it is an airborne-transmitted condition pathologically characterized by a necrotizing granulomatous response (**Figure 1**) that involves the lungs in 80% of cases, however any organ can be affected [1]. This disease probably emerged about 70,000 years ago, along with the modern-human being's migration from Africa [2]. An estimated of 1 billion people have died of TB in the last two centuries, and now represents one of the biggest public health problems worldwide [3].

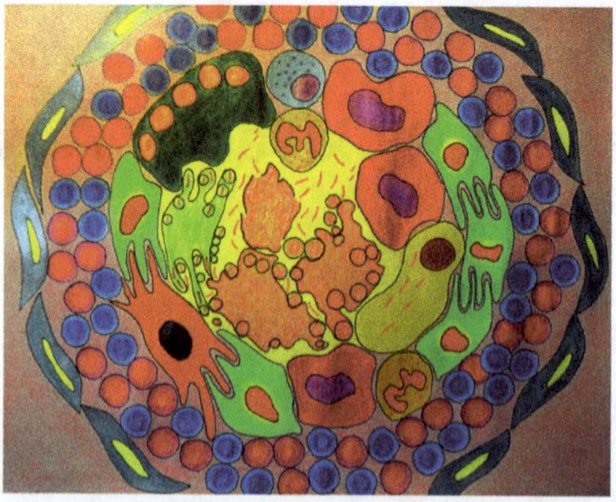

Figure 1. This illustration represents a tuberculous granuloma at its most basic way. It is a compact, dynamic and organized aggregate of epithelioid macrophages, and these cells usually fuse into multinucleated giant cells or differentiate into foam cells characterized by lipid accumulation. *M. tuberculosis* is usually present in the central necrotic area in which dead and dying cells are present. Many other cell types are also infiltrating the granuloma (neutrophils, dendritic cells, B and T lymphocytes, natural killer cells and fibroblasts) (original illustration by Jurado LF).

One third of world population is latently infected with *M. tuberculosis*, but only 10% of infected people will develop active disease during their live, half during the first 2 years after infection, and the remainder at any moment of their lifetime [4]. In most infected individuals, the progression is contained by the immune system. In 2013, an estimated 9 million new TB cases were reported globally, equivalent to 126 cases per 100,000 population, with more than 60% of the ill people living in 22 countries (considered as high-burden countries). However, according to WHO estimations during the same year around 3.3 million cases were missed (not reported or undiagnosed), accounting for a detection rate of only around 64%. The global HIV-coinfection proportion was 13% (1.1 million people), and HIV-associated TB deaths accounted for 25% of the total number of TB deaths [5].

The pathogenic mechanisms that determine active-TB progression are a multiple-stage game before and after the infection event, where the host-immune response integrity is one of the most relevant performers [6]. The infected individual may either rapidly progress to disease (primary progressive disease), may develop a particular status called latent TB infection, or may be able to kill the organism [7]. The occurrence of one of these scenarios depends on the determinants of host-immune response and the infection-stage in each individual. Most of the immune determinants that drive this pandemic constitute risk factors, which could be modified in order to impact positively on global TB control.

Among the relevant risk factors for TB, HIV infection is the most important, however, at the population level, diabetes mellitus (DM), malnutrition, tobacco smoking, and even immunosuppressive drugs, which are present in a larger section of the population than HIV infection, can represent a bigger impact on TB epidemiology [8, 9]. This chapter aims to summarize some of the most relevant risk factors for TB, focusing on general interventions for disease control.

2. Human immunodeficiency virus and TB coinfection

HIV coinfection is the most important immunosuppressive condition for developing active TB [10]. HIV infection substantially increases the possibility of TB reactivation from latent infection [11], and in the same way contributes to rapid TB progression after infection with *M. tuberculosis* [12, 13]. According to WHO estimations, people living with HIV (PLWHIV) latently TB-infected, have a 26-fold-higher risk of disease progression than those with no HIV [14]. Thus, HIV and TB coinfection configure a lethal synergy, where HIV markedly increases susceptibility for TB and exacerbates the severity of the disease, while TB accelerates HIV replication and its associated morbidity and mortality outcomes [10, 15].

In 2012, 34.5 million people were living with HIV worldwide [16]. This epidemic affects every country in the world, but the disease burden is highest in developing countries, among which the sub-Saharan Africa region is the most affected, where 69% of worldwide infected people live [16]. Due to the advances on therapy and prevention strategies, deaths related to HIV have decreased substantially over the past years, but reductions in TB-related deaths have not kept pace, a sample of this, in 2014 TB overpasses HIV as the leading cause of global infectious-related mortality [10].

Among 9.6 million new TB cases reported worldwide in 2014, 12% (1.2 million) were also HIV positive, and of the 1.5 million who died from TB, 33% (4,00,000) were HIV coinfected, thus TB constitutes main mortality cause in PLWHIV [14]. Evidently, the TB incidence and TB-related mortality are strengthened by HIV burden and represent a real public health challenge in areas where HIV and poverty coexist [10].

It is clear that antiretroviral therapy (ART) reduces rapidly and substantially TB incidence in PLWHIV, and this is true both in high and low endemic TB areas [17–19]. Nevertheless, even in people under ART, the risk of TB remains high compared with the general population. For HIV-negative people with latent TB infection (LTBI), the lifetime risk of developing TB rounds 5–10% [20, 21], but in the case of PLWHIV the annual risk of reactivation is 3–16% [22], with the higher risk of TB disease almost immediately after HIV infection, even with normal CD4 cell levels [10].

The immunologic control of TB is an intricate phenomenon that involves multiple pathways, cellular lines, and host-pathogen interactions [6]. In PLWHIV, macrophages present a phenotype with altered activity of molecules like iNOS and TNFα, which is reflected as incapacity for *M. tuberculosis* killing [23]. The histopathologic features in PLWHIV who develop TB, correlate and depend on the level of immunosuppression, individuals with apparently normal immune response present typical granulomas (**Figure 1**), these well-structured aggregates may break down, giving way to cavitary disease and bacilli expectoration, but as the immunodeficiency advance, granulomas are poorly formed or even absent, so the cavitary form is less frequent, with sputum smears likely negative [24].

In like manner that HIV infection increases the TB risk and its related complications, TB also affects HIV infection outcomes. In a study conducted by Lawn et al. [25], HIV patients on

ART who develop TB, presented more alterations on CD4 counts than individuals who never developed TB. Studies have shown that TB associates with rapid progression to AIDS and higher death risk [26, 27] and TB also appears to induce viral replication and viral diversity via up regulating the host-immune response [15, 28].

As we previously exposed, PLWHIV have the higher risk of progression from latent to active TB disease, this possibility can be reduced using two fundamental strategies: adequate ART and prophylactic LTBI treatment [19, 29], studies support the use of both strategies even in patients with high CD4 counts [33]. Thus, it is highly recommended to provide ART to all HIV-infected people irrespective of CD4 count [17].

Considering the risk, all PLWHIV should be screened using TST for LTBI at the time of HIV diagnosis [30]. Once a patient has a positive result for LTBI, active disease must be ruled out, and preventive therapy offered. Among the preventive therapy options, two of the most accepted are: daily isoniazid 5 mg/kg (maximum 300 mg) for 9 months plus pyridoxine supplementation or once a week rifapentine plus isoniazid (900/900 mg) for 3 months (12 total doses) [31, 32]. These regimens can be used with nucleoside reverse transcriptase inhibitors and efavirenz [33], rifapentine cannot be administered together with protease inhibitors, but it could be offered with raltegravir [34].

3. Diabetes mellitus and TB comorbidity

The worldwide rising in type II diabetes mellitus prevalence constitutes one of the biggest challenges for TB control [35]; in fact, nowadays there are more individuals living with DM-TB comorbidity that HIV-TB coinfection [36]. This association has been recognized historically [37]; however, it became less evident in the 1950s, in part due to the development of insulin therapy for a DM and antibiotics for TB [35]. Since 1980 as the DM pandemic (prevalence increasing >20% in three decades) was more evident, many papers on the DM-TB association began to reemerge [35].

As a result of a sedentary lifestyle, changes in diet, population aging, and urbanization, the global DM prevalence by 2000 was 171 million people, and is predicted that this number reaches 642 million in 2040, considering that 80% of DM population live in low- and middle-income countries, where the TB situation is worst [38].

Biological evidence supports that DM induces a direct impairment on innate and adaptive immune responses, increasing TB susceptibility [8]. However, the DM case differs from other causes of immunological impairment like HIV infection or malnutrition, because DM response is more dysfunctional rather than dismissing, characterized by excessive and/or delayed responses against *M. tuberculosis* [39]. Investigations in humans and animals have shown altered production of cytokines as INF-γ and IL-17 that affects the T-cell immune response [40] and reduced chemotaxis of neutrophils [41].

According to multiple studies, at an individual level, people with DM have three times more risk of developing TB, and two-fold increase in adverse TB therapy outcomes [8]. A systematic review of 13 studies reported that DM increases three times the risk of developing TB, (relative risk 3.11; 95% IC 2.27 – 4.26) [42], notwithstanding, this epidemiological aspect is the best characterized in the DM-TB association, a wide variation between studies is observed, with risk ratios around 0.99 and 7.83 [39], which evidences the difficulty of studying DM-TB relation, in part due the heterogeneity in the prevalence and other sociodemographic and cultural features of DM and TB in each part of the world. Besides, in the case of DM, the presence of other host characteristics as smoking, malnutrition, micro- and macrovascular compromise, can synergize and increase the TB risk [43].

The relevance of the DM-TB comorbidity is higher in low and middle-income countries, where both diseases are more prevalent. In fact, as reported by the WHO, of the 10 countries with more DM patients worldwide, six are also classified as high burden countries for TB (China, India, Brazil, Bangladesh, Indonesia, and Russia) [44]. During the last years, studies have marked differences in DM's frequency among patients with TB, from 36% in Mexico to 40 and 56% in the Pacific Islands and India, respectively [45–48].

Talking about the impact of DM in TB control, at the population level, the general attributable risk is 10–20%, and also a variation between different populations is observed, even in the same country, for example, in the United Kingdom, the general population risk rounds 10%, but rises 20% for Asian males [49], in countries like Mexico, where DM is endemic the general attributable risk is about 20% [50], and in the EU – Mexico border, 51% of the TB patients who are 35–60 years-old also have DM [45]. And even though the DM confers a notably lower risk compared with HIV, in certain populations where the HIV prevalence is low, the contribution of DM is more important than HIV infection [51].

Recently, an elegant study by Pan et al. [52], using models of dynamic TB transmission, estimated the potential effects of DM on TB epidemiology in 13 high burden countries, found that interrupting the rise in DM incidence, could prevent 6 million cases and 1.1 million deaths due TB in 2 decades. These findings show how beneficial for TB control would be an integral intervention on DM occurrence.

It is known that DM modifies the clinical presentation, disease-course and TB prognosis, and represents a risk factor for treatment-failure [35]. DM-TB patients (versus TB patients without DM) are more prone to develop sputum smear-positive TB, pulmonary TB (versus extrapulmonary), cavitary (versus noncavitary) at the moment of diagnosis, and in DM-TB patients the sputum smear conversion takes more time [53]. *Mycobacterium tuberculosis* infection induces a strong cell-mediated immune response that triggers a granulomatous response, which, according to recent investigations is a double-edged sword for the host [54], because although this phenomenon initially limits bacilli replication, the growing and rupture of these structures into the airways, facilitates not only the cavitary form of the disease but also, its sputum smear-positive presentation [44]. These findings, allows to postulate that DM-TB patients would be more infectious that TB-only patients.

Evidence from observational studies, have shown that DM comorbidity is related to adverse TB outcomes, as delays in sputum conversion, increased risk for treatment failures, relapse, death, and even reinfection [55]. Baker et al. [56] in a meta-analysis of recent DM-TB association studies found that the odds of dying of TB, or any other reason, was 2-fold higher [RR, 1.89; 95% CI, 1.52–2.36], and this risk rise to 4.95, when data was adjusted for age and potential confounders, the same study also calculated a 4-fold risk of relapse for DM-TB individuals versus TB-only patients.

Considering this, the World Health Organization has argued that DM is a reemerging and an important risk factor for TB, which needs programmatically routed efforts to positively impact on TB control [57].

4. Malnutrition and TB

For centuries, the association between malnutrition and TB has been recognized. Nutritional supplementation with protein-rich foods for sick people was reported since the ancient Greece [58]. A classic report from Denmark reports high TB rates during the First World War, once food supplies were restored, TB rates were drastically reduced, while persisting high in neighboring countries where shortages persisted [59].

During the pre-chemotherapy era, the only treatment offered to TB patients consisted in a nutritional plan, resting, and sun therapy. The pharmacological advances of the past century, with the development of streptomycin and isoniazid, replaced nutritional therapy as the focus of anti-TB treatment, however, considering the high rates of TB in areas where malnutrition is endemic, in the last decades, an interest in this association has reemerged [60].

According to estimations of the United Nations, by 2015 there were 795 million undernourished, comprising around 13% of the population of low- and middle-income countries, with the highest prevalence in Sub-Saharan Africa and Southern Asia [61]. In the developing countries, protein-calorie malnutrition is the most frequent form of under nutrition; however, specific micronutrient deficiencies are also common [60]. In addition, the advent of climate change, population growth, the HIV pandemic, and economic inequality, have originated a negative impact on food and nutritional insecurity, and malnutrition rates, constituting one of the most challenging public health problems worldwide [43]. The general way to epidemiologically defining malnutrition is the body mass index (BMI), and malnutrition constitutes a well-known risk factor not only for TB development, but also for poor response to antibiotic treatment and TB-related complications [59].

A biologically plausible association between TB and malnutrition clearly exist; animal studies have shown that PCM affects the immune mechanisms for TB control, among the impaired processes are the TNF, iNOS, and interferon γ production; it is also known that this phenomenon can be reversed thought protein supplementation [59, 62]. Active TB and HIV infection induce a 14 and 30% increment in the resting metabolic rate, respectively, which reflects the physiological cost of the immunologic mechanisms that are activated during these diseases [63]. These conditions aggravate even more the patient-immune impairment in the malnutrition setting [64].

Considering this, is essential that all newly diagnosed individuals with TB have a complete nutritional evaluation, and in the cases with a BMI under 18.8 a micro and macronutrients supplementation at least for the first 2 months of treatment, is strongly recommended [65]. Historical evidence supports the beneficial impact of social interventions, such as improving housing conditions and nutritional interventions on TB epidemiology, therefore a well-planned wide intervention would impact positively on TB control.

5. Anti-TNF treatment and TB

People with immune-mediated inflammatory diseases, such as rheumatoid arthritis, systemic erythematous lupus, ankylosing spondylitis, inflammatory bowel disease, etc., also represent a high-risk group for developing TB, and this risk is even higher when they are treated with tumor necrosis factor α (TNF α) – antagonist [66, 67].

Different cells produce TNF, including macrophages, T cells, fibroblast, and keratinocytes. TNF is a molecule with a wide functional spectrum, plays a key role in immune response to infections, cancer etiology, and the physiopathology of many immune-mediated disorders [67]. It is also known that is important in the immune response against intracellular bacteria, and the physiology and integrity of granulomatous (**Figure 1**) TB-related response during LTBI, therefore its antagonism associates with TB progression [6].

During the past two decades, TNF antagonists have been successfully used for the treatment of inflammatory diseases, when patients do not respond to conventional therapy [67]. In the United States, using national surveillance data, found that TB incidence in AR patients increased from 6.2 per 100,000 people to 144 per 100,000 in who received infliximab and 35 per 100,000 for etanercept-treated individuals [69]. A Spanish study collected data from 71 information centers, with a total of 1540 patients receiving infliximab, estimated a TB incidence in 1893 per 100,000 people, compared with a previous reports incidence of 21 per 100,000 in the general population and 95 per 100,000 in AR patients without TNF treatment [70]. An important proportion of extrapulmonary TB is observed, and several reports have attributed differential risk for each TNF antagonist [68].

Most of the active TB cases in individuals treated with TNF antagonist correspond to reactivation from LTBI, when this occurs, generally happen concomitantly with the initiation of the TNF antagonist, nevertheless, also cases with long treatment periods, have been reported [67]. Therefore, screening for LTBI before any TNF inhibitor treatment initiation is mandatory, here, as in the case of other immunosuppressive conditions, such as HIV infection, both TST and IGRAs assays could be used, nowadays, there is not sufficient evidence to recommend one method over another, and considering this, an expert consensus, suggest using IGRAs or TST in people without history of BCG vaccination [71].

Once a patient has a positive result for LTBI, active disease must be ruled out, and preventive therapy offered. Among the preventive therapy options, two of the most accepted are: daily isoniazid 5 mg/kg (maximum 300 mg) for 9 months plus pyridoxine supplementation or a combined regimen with isoniazid and rifampicin for 3 months [69]. Multiple recommendations on delay periods between LTBI preventive chemotherapy and TNF antagonist have been proposed, ranging from starting both concurrently, to waiting even a month after finishing LTBI prophylaxis [67, 68], these decisions must always consider the patients clinical status.

In the cases when active TB is diagnosed during TNF antagonist treatment, there is no evidence that the length of anti-TB therapy needs to be prolonged, and evidence regarding the time for restarting TNF antagonist therapy is limited [72]; however, some international guidelines recommends starting TNF inhibitor at least when initial anti-TB phase is completed, while others recommend waiting until completing all TB treatment [68].

6. Smoking, alcoholism and TB

Globally, there are more than 1.5 billion smokers, the majority live in low- and middle-income countries, where, in addition, the per capita tobacco consumption is increasing continuously [73]. The prolonged exposure to tobacco smoke may directly affect the respiratory and systemic immune function, which can impair alveolar macrophage function by decreasing its TNF production [74]. Therefore, it is considered that smoking has an impact upon the susceptibility to TB development.

There is growing evidence that correlates smoking with TB disease; a cross-sectional study in Shanghai compared heavy smokers with nonsmokers and found that the odds of smokers were 2.2 times higher than nonsmokers [75]. The risk also seemed to be influenced by the amount smoked, and a study from the United States found that the greatest risk was for people who smoked for more than 30 years [76].

At a population level, exposure to tobacco smoke has a relevant impact on TB epidemiology; a Chinese modeling-study suggested that a complete cessation of smoking in that country would reduce the estimated TB incidence between 14 and 52% [77]. Considering this situation, smoking cessation as a public health strategy is a global priority.

Alcohol is one of the most abused substances in the world. By 2005 among people aged 15 years and older, the annual *per capita* consumption was 6 l [78] with the highest rates in high-income countries. Alcohol abuse is an important cause of immunological impairment, often associated with smoking and malnutrition, increasing its impact on public health [8].

There is considerable evidence to support the association between alcohol abuse and TB, even if it is independent of smoking [79]. Studies have shown that excessive alcohol consumption increases the risk of active TB development and other respiratory infections, a meta-analysis estimated a combined risk of 2.9 for active TB developing [25]. Studies have also shown higher rates of MDR-TB, TB relapse, and treatment failure in alcohol abusers [8].

7. Genetic susceptibility

Historically, infectious disease research has considered TB as a purely infectious condition. During the last decades, increasing evidence suggest that TB reflects the human genetic vulnerability [80]. Nevertheless, the precise significance and behavior of the genetic factors involved remains widely unknown, in part due to the complex game of infection, latency, and disease, which characterizes TB.

Recent findings have exposed two major principles: there is a main locus that controls most of the TB-resistance phenotypes, and there is evidence that severe forms of childhood TB are directly related with single-gene inborn errors (Mendelian Inheritance), meanwhile genetic association studies of adulthood-TB has shown limited success and reproducibility [81]. Clinical and epidemiological studies conducted since the past century has provided evidence that each step during infection and disease is strongly influenced by host genetic factors [82].

Familial studies aimed to investigate the human susceptibility to *M. tuberculosis* infection, have used TST and IGRAs responses as quantitative traits of resistance. Its results suggest that the initial infection-related events mostly depend on the IFNγ and TNF1 and its related cellular functions [83]. In regard to severe primary TB forms, during the last two decades, germ line mutations in seven autosomal and in two X-linked genes have been discovered in particular patients, further analysis have shown that these mutations result in an impairment of IFNγ- and IL12-related immunity [80, 84, 85].

Many questions of this field remain unanswered, the identification of the genetic variants underling the stages and forms of TB is critical for understanding TB pathogenesis. These findings could represent a formidable opportunity in the definition of prevention strategies, optimization of vaccines, the development of novel treatments and therefore TB control.

8. Final considerations

After this short review, it makes evident that a risk factor approach for TB control would have a huge impact on disease burden worldwide. Identification of LTBI along with prophylactic therapy and active disease surveillance constitute the most important tools for reducing the risk of TB and achieve favorable outcomes, especially in the high-risk groups previously described.

Over the last decades, the understanding of TB epidemiology behavior in the country, and at global level, has changed from an "exposure to bacteria" vision to a phenomenon where the host susceptibility plays a crucial role. Even although, HIV coinfection is the most potent risk factor, globally the most frequent conditions impacting on people immune function include malnutrition, Diabetes, smoking, and immunosuppressive drugs, and while at the individual level, these factors cause an apparently mild immunological impairment, its cumulative importance in a community needs much more attention. So, it is imperative for clinicians, researchers and policy makers, a better consideration, and understanding of these conditions as drivers of TB epidemiology, developing in this way more integrative strategies that could have a bigger impact on TB control.

Conflict of interest

The authors have no conflict of interest to declare.

Author details

Leonardo F. Jurado[1,3*] and Diana M. Palacios[1,2,3]

*Address all correspondence to: lfjuradoz@unal.edu.co

1 Pathology and Laboratories Department, Fundación Santa Fe de Bogotá University Hospital, Bogotá D.C., Colombia

2 School of Medicine, Los Andes University, Bogotá D.C., Colombia

3 Pathology Department, School of Medicine, National University of Colombia, Bogotá D.C., Colombia

References

[1] Dheda K, Barry CE 3rd, Maartens G. Tuberculosis. Lancet. 2016;**387**:1211-1226. DOI: 10.1016/ S0140-6736(15)00151-8

[2] Comas I, Coscolla M, Luo T, et al. Out-of-Africa migration and Neolithic co-expansion of mycobacterium tuberculosis in modern humans. Nature Genetics. 2013;**45**:1176-1182. DOI: 10.1038/ng. 2744

[3] Ryan F. The Forgotten Plague: How the Battle against Tuberculosis Was Won—And Lost. Boston, MA: Back Bay Books; 1994

[4] Vynnycky E, Fine PE. The natural history of tuberculosis: The implications of age-dependent risks of disease and the role of reinfection. Epidemiology and Infection. 1997;**119**:183-201

[5] Global tuberculosis Report WHO. Geneva, Switzerland: World Health Organization, 2014. Available from: http://apps.who.int/iris/bitstream/10665/137094/1/9789241564809_eng.pdf [Accessed: 2017-11-29]

[6] O'Garra A, Redford PS, McNab F, Bloom C, Wilkinson R, Berry MP. The immune response in tuberculosis. Annual Review of Immunology. 2013;**31**:475-527. DOI: 10.1146/annurev-immunol-032712-095939

[7] Mack U, Migliori GB, Sester M, Rieder HL, Ehlers S, Goletti D, et al. LTBI: Latent tuberculosis infection or lasting immune responses to M. Tuberculosis? A TBNET consensus statement. The European Respiratory Journal 2009;**33**:956-973 DOI: 10.1183/09031936.00120908

[8] Fox GJ, Menzies D. Epidemiology of tuberculosis immunology. In: Divangahi M, editor. The New Paradigm of Immunity to Tuberculosis, Advances in Experimental Medicine and Biology. New York: Springer; 2013. DOI: 10.1007/978-1-4614-6111-1_1

[9] Narasimhan P, Wood J, MacIntyre CR, Mathai D. Risk factors for tuberculosis. Pulmonary Medicine. 2013; Article ID 828939. DOI: 10.1155/2013/828939. https://www.hindawi.com/journals/pm/2013/828939/

[10] Tornheim JA, Dooley KE. Tuberculosis associated with HIV infection. Microbiology Spectrum. 2017;**5**:TNMI7-0028-2016. DOI: 10.1128/microbiolspec.TNMI7-0028-2016

[11] Bucher HC, Griffith LE, Guyatt GH. Isoniazid prophylaxis for tuberculosis in HIV infection: A meta-analysis of randomized controlled trials. AIDS. 1999;**13**:501-507

[12] Daley CL, Small PM, Schecter GF. An outbreak of tuberculosis with accelerated progression among persons infected with the human immunodeficiency virus: An analysis using restriction-fragment-length polymorphisms, The New England Journal of Medicine. 1991;**326**:231-235

[13] Shafer RS, Singh SP, Larkin C, Small PM. Exogenous reinfection with multidrug-resistant mycobacterium tuberculosis in an immunocompetent patient. Tubercle and Lung Disease. 1995;**76**:575-577

[14] World Health Organization, Geneva, Switzerland. TB/HIV facts 2015. Available from: http://www.who.int/hiv/topics/tb/tbhiv_facts_2015/en/ [Accessed: 2017-11-29]

[15] Collins KR, Quiñones-Mateu ME, Toossi Z, Arts AJ. Impact of tuberculosis on HIV-1 replication, diversity, and disease progression. AIDS Reviews. 2002;**4**:165-176

[16] Bruchfeld J, Correia-Neves M, Tuberculosis KG, Coinfection HIV. Cold Spring Harbor Perspectives in Medicine. 2015;**26**:a017871. DOI: 10.1101/cshperspect.a017871

[17] Jones JL, Hanson DL, Dworkin MS, DeCock KM, Adult/adolescent Spectrum of HIV disease group. HIV-associated tuberculosis in the era of highly active antiretroviral therapy. The International Journal of Tuberculosis and Lung Disease. 2000;**4**:1026-1031

[18] Badri M, Wilson D, Wood R. Effect of highly active anti- retroviral therapy on incidence of tuberculosis in South Africa: A cohort study. Lancet 2002;**359**:2059-2064. DOI: 10.1016/S0140-6736(02)08904-3

[19] Severe P, Juste MA, Ambroise A, Eliacin L, Marchand C, Apollon S, et al. Early versus standard antiretroviral therapy for HIV-infected adults in Haiti. The New England Journal of Medicine. 2010;**363**:257-265. DOI: 10.1056/NEJMoa0910370

[20] Recent SI. Studies in the epidemiology of tuberculosis, based on the risk of being infected with tubercle bacilli. Advances in Tuberculosis Research. 1976;**19**:1-63

[21] Comstock GW, Livesay VT, Woolpert SF. The prognosis of a positive tuberculin reaction in childhood and adolescence. American Journal of Epidemiology. 1974;**99**:131-138

[22] Sonnenberg P, Glynn JR, Fielding K, Murray J, Godfrey-Faussett P, Shearer S. How soon after infection with HIV does the risk of tuberculosis start to increase? A retrospective cohort study in south African gold miners. The Journal of Infectious Diseases. 2005;**191**:150-158. DOI: 10.1086/426827

[23] Patel NR, Zhu J, Tachado SD, Zhang J, Wan Z, Saukkonen J, Koziel H. HIV impairs TNF-alpha mediated macrophage apoptotic response to mycobacterium tuberculosis. Journal of Immunology. 2007;**179**:6973-6980. DOI: 10.4049/jimmunol. 179.10.6973

[24] Diedrich CR, O'Hern J, Wilkinson RJ. HIV-1 and the mycobacterium tuberculosis granuloma: A systematic review and meta-analysis. Tuberculosis (Edinburgh, Scotland). 2016;**98**:62-76. DOI: 10.1016/j.tube.2016.02.010

[25] Lawn SD, Badri M, Wood R. Tuberculosis among HIV-infected patients receiving HAART: Long term incidence, and risk factors in a south African cohort. AIDS 2005;**19**: 2109-2116

[26] Whalen C, Horsburgh CR, Hom D, Lahart C, Simberkoff M, Ellner J. Accelerated course of human immunodeficiency virus infection after tuberculosis. American Journal of Respiratory and Critical Care Medicine. 1995;**151**:129-135

[27] Whalen CC, Nsubuga P, Okwera A, Johnson JL, Hom DL, Michael NL, Mugerwa RD, Ellner JJ. Impact of pulmonary tuberculosis on survival of HIV-infected adults: A prospective epidemiological study in Uganda. AIDS. 2000;**14**:1219-1228

[28] Jurado LF, Murcia MI, Hidalgo P, Leguizamón JE, González LR. Phenotypic and genotypic diagnosis of bone and miliary tuberculosis in an HIV+ patient in Bogotá, Colombia. Biomédica. 2015;**35**:8-15. DOI: 10.1590/S0120-41572015000100002

[29] Briggs MA, Emerson C, Modi S, Taylor NK, Date A. Use of isoniazid preventive therapy for tuberculosis prophylaxis among people living with HIV/AIDS: A review of the literature. Journal of Acquired Immune Deficiency Syndromes. 2015;**68**(Suppl 3):S297-S305. DOI: 10.1097/QAI.0000000000000497

[30] Fisk TL, Hon HM, Lennox JL, Fordham von Reyn C, Horsburgh CR Jr. Detection of latent tuberculosis among HIV-infected patients after initiation of highly active antiretroviral therapy. AIDS. 2003;**17**:1102-1104

[31] Sterling TR, Villarino ME, Borisov AS, Shang N, Gordin F, Bliven-Sizemore E, TB Trials Consortium PREVENT TB Study Team. Three months of rifapentine and isoniazid for latent tuberculosis infection. The New England Journal of Medicine. 2011;**365**:2155-2166

[32] World Health Organization. Guidelines on the Management of Latent Tuberculosis Infection. World Health Organization, Geneva, Switzerland 2015. Available from: http://apps.who.int/iris/bitstream/10665/136471/1/9789241548908_eng.pdf?ua=1&ua=1 [Accessed: 2017-11-29]

[33] Podany AT, Bao Y, Swindells S, Chaisson RE, Andersen JW, Mwelase T. AIDS Clinical Trials Group A5279 study team. Efavirenz pharmacokinetics and pharmacodynamics in HIV-infected persons receiving rifapentine, and isoniazid for tuberculosis prevention. Clinical Infectious Diseases. 2015;**61**:1322-1327. DOI: 10.1093/cid/civ46

[34] Weiner M, Egelund EF, Engle M, Kiser M, Prihoda TJ, Gelfond JA, et al. Pharmacokinetic interaction of rifapentine and raltegravir in healthy volunteers. The Journal of Antimicrobial Chemotherapy 2014;**69**:1079-1085. DOI: 10.1093/jac/dkt483

[35] Restrepo BI. Diabetes and tuberculosis. Microbiology Spectrum. 2016;**4**(6):TNMI7-0023-2016. DOI: 10.1128/microbiolspec

[36] Ronacher K, Joosten SA, van Crevel R, Dockrell HM, Walzl G, Ottenhoff TH. Acquired immunodeficiencies and tuberculosis: Focus on HIV/AIDS and diabetes mellitus. Immunological Reviews. 2015;**264**:121-137. DOI: 10.1111/imr. 12257

[37] Root H. The association of diabetes and tuberculosis. The New England Journal of Medicine. 1934;**210**:1-13

[38] International Diabetes Federation. IDF Diabetes Atlas, 7th Ed. International Diabetes Federation, Brussels, Belgium, 2015. Available from: http://www.idf.org/diabetesatlas [Accessed: 2017-11-29]

[39] Restrepo BI, Schlesinger LS. Host-pathogen interactions in tuberculosis patients with type 2 diabetes mellitus. Tuberculosis (Edinburgh, Scotland). 2013;**93**(Suppl):S10-S14. DOI: 10.1016/S1472-9792(13)70004-0

[40] Stalenhoef JE, Alisjahbana B, Nelwan EJ. The role of interferon-gamma in the increased tuberculosis risk in type 2 diabetes mellitus. European Journal of Clinical Microbiology and Infectious Diseases. 2008;**27**:97-103. DOI: 10.1007/s10096-007-0395-0

[41] Delamaire M, Maugendre M, Moreno M, Le Goff MC, Allannic H, Genetet B. Impaired leukocyte functions in diabetic patients. Diabetic Medicine. 1997;**14**:29-34

[42] Jeon CY, Murray MB. Diabetes mellitus increases the risk of active tuberculosis: A systematic review of 13 observational studies. PLoS Medicine. 2008;**5**:e152. DOI: 10.1371/journal.pmed. 0050152

[43] Lönnroth K, Jaramillo E, Williams BG, Dye C, Raviglione M. Drivers of tuberculosis epidemics: The role of risk factors and social determinants. Social Science & Medicine. 2009;**68**:2240-2246. DOI: 10.1016/j.socscimed. 2009.03.041

[44] Restrepo BI. Convergence of the tuberculosis and diabetes epidemics: Renewal of old acquaintances. Clinical Infectious Diseases. 2007;**45**:436-438. DOI: 10.1086/519939

[45] Restrepo BI, Fisher-Hoch SP, Crespo JG, Whitney E, Perez A, Smith B, McCormick JB, Nuevo Santander Tuberculosis Trackers. Type 2 diabetes and tuberculosis in a dynamic bi-national border population. Epidemiol Infect. 2007;**135**:483-91. DOI: DOI: 10.1017/S0950268806006935

[46] Restrepo BI, Camerlin AJ, Rahbar MH, Wang W, Restrepo MA, Zarate I, Mora-Guzmán F, Crespo-Solis JG, Briggs J, McCormick JB, Fisher-Hoch SP. Cross-sectional assessment reveals high diabetes prevalence among newly-diagnosed tuberculosis cases. Bulletin of the World Health Organization. 2011;**89**:352-359. DOI: 10.2471/BLT.10.085738

[47] Viney K, Brostrom R, Nasa J, Defang R, Kienene T. Diabetes and tuberculosis in the Pacific Islands region. The Lancet Diabetes and Endocrinology. 2014;**2**:932. DOI: 10.1016/S2213-8587(14)70230-X

[48] Kornfeld H, West K, Kane K, Kumpatla S, Zacharias RR, Martinez- Balzano C, et al. High prevalence and heterogeneity of diabetes in patients with TB in South India: A report from the effects of diabetes on tuberculosis severity (EDOTS) study. Chest. 2016;**149**:1501-1508. DOI: 10.1016/j. Chest. 2016.02.675

[49] Walker C, Unwin N. Estimates of the impact of diabetes on the incidence of pulmonary tuberculosis in different ethnic groups in England. Thorax. 2010;**65**:578-581. DOI: 10.1136/thx. 2009.128223

[50] Ponce-De-Leon A, Garcia-Garcia Md ML, Garcia-Sancho MC, Gomez-Perez FJ, Valdespino-Gomez JL, Olaiz-Fernandez G, et al. Tuberculosis and diabetes in southern Mexico. Diabetes Care. 2004;**27**:1584-90. 1590. DOI: 10.2337/diacare.27.7.1584

[51] Getahun H, Gunneberg C, Granich R, Nunn P. HIV infection- associated tuberculosis: The epidemiology and the response. Clinical Infectious Diseases. 2010;**50**(Suppl 3): S201-S207. DOI: 10.1086/651492

[52] Pan SC, Ku CC, Kao D, Ezzati M, Fang CT, Lin HH. Effect of diabetes on tuberculosis control in 13 countries with high tuberculosis: A modelling study. The Lancet Diabetes and Endocrinology. 2015;**3**:323-330. DOI: 10.1016/S2213-8587 (15)00042-X

[53] Reis-Santos B, Locatelli R, Horta BL, Faerstein E, Sanchez MN, Riley LW, Maciel EL. Socio-demographic and clinical differences in subjects with tuberculosis with and without diabetes mellitus in Brazil—A multivariate analysis. PLoS One. 2013;**8**:e62604. DOI: 10.1371/journal.pone. 0062604

[54] Davis MJ, Ramakrishnan L. The role of the granuloma in expansion and dissemination of early tuberculous infection. Cell. 2009;**136**:37-49. DOI: 10.1016/j. cell. 2008.11.014

[55] Jeon CY, Murray MB, Baker MA. Managing tuberculosis in patients with diabetes mellitus: Why we care and what we know. Expert Review of Anti-Infective Therapy. 2012;**10**:863-868. DOI: 10.1586/eri.12.75

[56] Baker MA, Harries AD, Jeon CY, Hart JE, Kapur A, Lönnroth K, et al. The impact of diabetes on tuberculosis treatment outcomes: A systematic review. BMC Medicine 2011;**9**:81. DOI: 10.1186/1741-7015-9-81

[57] Ottmani SE, Murray MB, Jeon CY, Baker MA, Kapur A, Lönnroth K, Harries AD. Consultation meeting on tuberculosis and diabetes mellitus: Meeting summary and recommendations. The International Journal of Tuberculosis and Lung Disease. 2010;**14**:1513-1517

[58] van Lettow M, Whalen C. Tuberculosis. In: Semba R D, Bloem M W, editors. Nutrition and Health: Nutrition and Health in Developing Countries. 2nd Ed. Totowa, NJ, USA: Humana Press, 2008

[59] Cegielski JP, DN MM. The relationship between malnutrition and tuberculosis: Evidence from studies in humans and experimental animals. The International Journal of Tuberculosis and Lung Disease. 2004;**8**:286-298

[60] Koethe JR, von Reyn CF. Protein-calorie malnutrition, macronutrient supplements, and tuberculosis. The International Journal of Tuberculosis and Lung Disease. **20**:857-863. DOI: 10.5588/ijtld.15.0936

[61] Food and Agriculture Organization of the United Nations. The state of food insecurity in the world. Rome, Italy, 2015. Available from: http://www.fao.org/3/a-i4646e.pdf [Accessed: 2017-11-30]

[62] Chan J, Tian Y, Tanaka KE, Tsang MS, Yu K, Salgame P, et al. Effects of protein calorie malnutrition on tuberculosis in mice. Proceedings of the National Academy of Sciences. 1996;**93**:14857-14861

[63] Melchior JC, Raguin G, Boulier A, et al. Resting energy expenditure in human immunodeficiency virus-infected patients: Comparison between patients with and without secondary infections. The American Journal of Clinical Nutrition. 1993;**57**:614-619

[64] Macallan DC, McNurlan MA, Kurpad AV, et al. Whole body protein metabolism in human pulmonary tuberculosis and undernutrition: Evidence for anabolic block in tuberculosis. Clinical Science (London, England) 1998;**94**:321-331

[65] World Health Organization. Guideline: nutritional care and support for patients with tuberculosis. Geneva, Switzerland: WHO, 2013. Avaliable from: http://apps.who.int/iris/bitstream/10665/94836/1/9789241506410_eng.pdf [Accessed: 2017-11-30]

[66] Smith R, Cattamanchi A, Steingart KR, Denkinger C, Dheda K, Winthrop KL, et al. Interferon-gamma release assays for diagnosis of latent tuberculosis infection: Evidence in immune-mediated inflammatory disorders. Current Opinion in Rheumatology. 2001;**23**:377-384

[67] Galvis L, Sánchez AY, Jurado LF, Murcia MI. Tuberculosis associated with tumor necrosis factor α – Antagonist, case description and analysis of reported cases in Colombia. Biomédica. 2018;**38**. DOI: 10.7705/Biomedica.v38i0. 3273

[68] Salgado E, Gómez-Reino JJ. The risk of tuberculosis in patients treated with TNF antagonists. Expert Review of Clinical Immunology. 2011;**7**:329-340. DOI: 10.1586/eci.11.6

[69] Wallis RS, Broder MS, Wong JY, Hanson ME, Beenhouwer DO. Granulomatous infectious diseases associated with tumor necrosis factor antagonists. Clinical Infectious Diseases. 2004;**38**:1261-1265. DOI: 10.1086/383317

[70] Gómez-Reino JJ, Carmona L, Valverde VR, Mola EM, Montero MD, BIOBADASER Group. Treatment of rheumatoid arthritis with tumor necrosis factor inhibitors may predispose to significant increase in tuberculosis risk: A multicenter active-surveillance report. Arthritis and Rheumatism. 2003;**48**:2122-2127. DOI: 10.1002/art.11137

[71] Solovic I, Sester M, Gomez-Reino JJ, Rieder HL, Ehlers S, Milburn HJ, et al. The risk of tuberculosis related to TNF antagonist therapies: A TBNET consensus statement. The European Respiratory Journal. 2010;**36**:1185-1206 DOI: 10.1183/09031936.00028510

[72] Denis B, Lefort A, Flipo RM. Long-term follow-up of patients with tuberculosis as a complication of tumor necrosis factor (TNF) -an antagonist therapy: Safe re-initiation of TNF-a blocker after appropriate anti-tuberculous treatment. Clinical Microbiology Infection. 2008;**14**:183-186. DOI: 10.1111/j. 1469-0691.2007.01891.x

[73] Guindon GE, Boisclair D. Past, Current and Future Trends in Tobacco Use. Washington, DC: World Bank; 2003. Available from: https://openknowledge.worldbank.org/handle/10986/13726 Accessed: 2017-11-30

[74] Sopori M. Effects of cigarette smoke on the immune system. Nature Reviews. Immunology. 2002;**2**:372-377. DOI: 10.1038/nri803

[75] Yu GP, Hsieh CC, Peng J. Risk factors associated with the prevalence of pulmonary tuberculosis among sanitary workers in shanghai. Tubercle. 1988;**69**:105-112

[76] Buskin SE, Gale JL, Weiss NS, Nolan CM. Tuberculosis risk factors in adults in King County, Washington, 1988 through 1990. American Journal of Public Health. 1994;**84**: 1750-1756

[77] Lin HH, Murray M, Cohen T, Colijn C, Ezzati M. Effects of smoking and solid-fuel use on COPD, lung cancer, and tuberculosis in China: A time-based, multiple risk factor, modelling study. Lancet. 2008;**372**:1473-1483. DOI: 10.1016/S0140-6736(08)61345-8

[78] World Health Organization. Global status report on alcohol and health. World Health Organization, Geneva 2014. Available from: http://apps.who.int/iris/bitstream/10665/112736/1/9789240692763_eng.pdf [Accessed: 2017-11-30]

[79] Rehm J, Samokhvalov AV, Neuman MG, Room R, Parry C, Lonnroth K, et al. The association between alcohol use, alcohol use disorders and tuberculosis (TB): A systematic review. BMC Public Health. 2009;**9**:450. DOI: 10.1186/1471-2458-9-450

[80] Abel L, Fellay J, Haas DW, Schurr E, Srikrishna G, Urbanowski M, et al. Genetics of human susceptibility to active and latent tuberculosis: Present knowledge and future perspectives. The Lancet Infectious Diseases. 2017. DOI: 10.1016/ S1473-3099(17)30623-0

[81] Abel L, El-Baghdadi J, Bousfiha AA, Casanova J-L, Schurr E. 2014 Human genetics of tuberculosis: A long and winding road. Philosophical Transactions of Royal Society B. 2014;**369**:20130428. DOI: 10.1098/rstb.2013.0428

[82] Casanova JL, Abel L. Genetic dissection of immunity to mycobacteria: The human model. Annual Review of Immunology. 2002;**20**:581-620. DOI: 10.1146/annurev.immunol.20.081501.125851

[83] Stein CM, Guwatudde D, Nakakeeto M. Heritability analysis of cytokines as intermediate phenotypes of tuberculosis. The Journal of Infectious Diseases. 2003;**187**:1679-1685. DOI: 10.1086/375249

[84] Sasaki Y, Nomura A, Kusuhara K. Genetic basis of patients with bacille Calmette-Guerin osteomyelitis in Japan: Identification of dominant partial interferon-gamma receptor 1 deficiency as a predominant type. The Journal of Infectious Diseases. 2002;**185**:706-709. DOI: 10.1086/339011

[85] Picard C, Fieschi C, Altare F. Inherited interleukin-12 deficiency: IL12B genotype and clinical phenotype of 13 patients from six kindreds. American Journal of Human Genetics. 2002;**70**:336-348. DOI: 10.1086/338625

10

Common Strategies, Different Mechanisms to Infect the Host: *Anaplasma* and *Mycobacterium*

Vladimir López, Pilar Alberdi and José de la Fuente

Abstract

Intracellular bacteria such as *Anaplasma* spp. and *Mycobacterium* spp. pose a risk to human and animal populations worldwide. The main function of immune response cells is to eliminate invading pathogens. However, pathogens can deregulate host cell function and turn defense cells into suitable hosts. Intracellular bacterial have a smaller genome, compared to the host cell, thus requiring efficient mechanisms for survival and persistence within the host by inducing sustained changes in cell function and immune response. Bacterial epigenetic regulation of host cell gene transcription appears to be a general mechanism that enhances pathogen survival while altering host cell function and facilitating infection. *Anaplasma phagocytophilum* leads to modified host cell gene transcription and phenotype by epigenetically altering host chromatin. Mycobacterial infection of human cells also results in host gene silencing using a mechanism that involves HDAC complex formation and histone deacetylation. Membrane proteins are essential for cell invasion in both pathogens, and can regulate and protect the pathogen against the host response. Understanding the mechanisms employed by these bacteria to infect the host could contribute to develop effective interventions for the control of tuberculosis and anaplasmosis. This review focuses on the common strategies employed by two zoonotic pathogens, *Anaplasma* and *Mycobacterium* spp., highlighting also the different mechanisms used to infect host cells.

Keywords: *Anaplasma, Mycobacteria,* immunology, infection, tuberculosis

1. Introduction

Ticks and tick-borne diseases represent a growing problem for human and animal health worldwide whereas tuberculosis continues to be a global burden in both human and animal populations [1, 2]. Pathogenic organisms have evolved host mimicking properties and manipulate host responses for their own survival and propagation. To successfully establish and maintain a bacterial infection, the pathogens subvert the host cells defense response to survive, proliferate, and persist within the infected cell. To evade host defense systems, bacterial pathogens produce a variety of virulence factors that stimulate bacterial adherence and invasion and subvert host cell signaling cascades that regulate intracellular microbial survival and trafficking. Some of these mechanisms are mediated by factors released by the bacteria, whereas others rely on hijacking host components to prevent the production of an effective immune response thus promoting their survival within the host cell [2, 3]. Intracellular bacteria from *Anaplasma* and *Mycobacterium* genera produce similar genes expression patterns in infected ruminants [4]. Pathogen and host-specific differences could contribute to disease diagnosis and treatment of tuberculosis and anaplasmosis in ruminants.

In this review, we provide an overview of some of the mechanisms employed by *Anaplasma* and *Mycobacterium* to infect the host cell and the impact on their pathogenesis.

2. *Anaplasma phagocytophilum*, an intracellular bacterium with unusual tropism

The emergence of tick-borne pathogens has been promoted by the exploitation of environmental resources and the increase in human outdoor activities, allowing the contact with tick vectors normally present in the field [5]. *Anaplasma phagocytophilum* is an obligate intracellular rickettsial pathogen transmitted mainly by *Ixodes* spp. ticks causing human granulocytic anaplasmosis (HGA), equine, and canine granulocytic anaplasmosis, and tick-borne fever (TBF) in ruminants [6]. In the vertebrate host, *A. phagocytophilum* infects neutrophils where the pathogen multiplies within a parasitophorous vacuole or morula in the cytoplasm of tick and vertebrate host cells [7, 8]. These gram-negative bacteria are grouped within the family Anaplasmataceae [3]. Complications and fatality are rare but more common in the elderly, the immunocompromised, or if proper diagnosis and/or antibiotic therapy are delayed. Fatalities are usually not directly attributed to the infection itself; pathological findings suggest defects in host defense and the presence of secondary infections [9]. However, the severity of illness and fatality rates could also be due to underlying immunosuppression.

Anaplasma is a highly antigenically variant bacterial pathogen that displays a diversity of mechanisms to create the structural and antigenic variation necessary to escape the immune response and allows long-term persistence in the host thus being able to act as a reservoir for transmission. *A. phagocytophilum* strategies to infect vertebrate host cells include, among others, remodeling of the cytoskeleton, inhibition of cell apoptosis, manipulation of the immune response and modification of cell epigenetics and metabolism [10]. Hosts respond to infection by activating alternative pathways to regulate cell apoptosis, immunity, metabolism and stress response mediated by heat-shock proteins (Hsps) [1]. Unlike other bacteria, *A. phagocytophilum* is aflagellated and does not have a type III secretion system (T3SS) [11, 12].

Pathogens subvert cellular immune response to favor infection and multiplication. Host cell transcriptome and proteome studies have demonstrated an effect of *A. phagocytophilum* infection on the inhibition of cell innate immunity [13–15]. They employ a variety of mechanisms to create the structural and antigenic variation needed to subvert the host immune system and long-term persistence [3]. *A. phagocytophilum* also employs a type IV secretion system (T4SS) to deliver proteins or DNA into eukaryotic cells [16]. It also inhibits host cell apoptosis to allow the bacteria sufficient time to develop morulae [17].

Adaptation to a life in eukaryotic cells and transmission between hosts has been assisted by the deletion of many genes that are present in the genomes of free-living bacteria, including genes required for the biosynthesis of lipopolysaccharide and peptidoglycan that are involved in the activation of host leukocytes [18].

P44 (also known as MSP2) is a highly variable immunodominant surface protein that facilitates adherence to granulocytes [19]. The genome of *Anaplasma* consists of more than 100 *msp2(p44)* paralogs [20]. Antibodies specific to P44 inhibit *A. phagocytophilum* infection in mice and HL-60 cells, which suggests that antigenic variation of P44 proteins may help *A. phagocytophilum* to escape host immune surveillance [3]. Some *Anaplasma* strains are naturally persistent in lambs and can be used to analyze the mechanisms of persistence in the vertebrate host. Variation of the outer membrane protein MSP2(P44) is believed to play a key role in persistence of the organism [21].

A. phagocytophilum can avoid killing by innate immunity but it also induces some innate immune responses, such as the production of IFN-γ, that contribute to tissue injury and disease [22]. Signal transducer and activator of transcription 1 (Stat1) is important in host innate and adaptive immune responses to intracellular pathogens, including intracellular bacteria [23]. It mediates most of the biological functions of both type I interferon (IFNα/β) and type II IFN (IFNγ). *A. phagocytophilum* infection-induced IFNγ signaling leads to phosphorylation of Stat1 in mice and is critical for the generation of protection [24]. Experimental infections with mice have demonstrated that the absence of Stat1 converts the subclinical infection to a severe one [22] suggesting that Stat1 plays an important role in controlling the response to bacterial infections. Stat1 also participates in the IFN-γ signaling of mycobacterial immunity. IFN-γ signaling provides positive feedback to both macrophages and CD4+ T-cells, which amplifies the Th1 response [25]. Suppressor of cytokine signaling (SOCS) expression has been implicated in intracellular survival of *A. phagocytophilum* in neutrophils where expression of IFN-γ receptor alpha-chain CD119 is diminished leading to reduced Stat1 dimerization and signaling [26].

In neutrophils, the genes most downregulated in response to *A. phagocytophilum* infection include those coding for proteins involved in bacterial killing such as myeloperoxidase, transferrin, bactericidal/permeability-increasing protein and cell protection (mucin 12). Immune-system-related genes encoding interferons, cytokines, chemokines, and their receptors are upregulated in response to infection [13–15]. This suggests that pathogens have developed mechanisms to subvert the innate immune protective mechanisms in vertebrate hosts. However, some species can activate innate immune protective mechanisms to control infection and appear to play a minor role as reservoir hosts for the pathogen [27]. For instance, pigs naturally and experimentally infected with *A. phagocytophilum* control bacterial infection through activation of innate immune responses, phagocytosis, and autophagy [28] resulting in low infection levels or infection clearance.

A. phagocytophilum, a pathogen lacking the T3SS and flagellin, activates the NLRC4 inflammasome (a component of the innate immune system) and secretion of IL-1β [29]. IL-18 release mediated by the NLRC4 inflammasome regulates IFN-γ production by $CD4^+$ T cells upon *A. phagocytophilum* infection [30]. The receptor-interacting serine/threonine-protein kinase 2 (RIPK2) appears to be a major regulator of the immune response against *A. phagocytophilum*. *Ripk2–/–* immune cells exhibit a defect in activation for the nuclear factor (NF)-κB and the NLRC4 inflammasome pathways [29]. Furthermore, experimental mice lacking *COX2* (*cyclooxygenase* 2) are more susceptible to *A. phagocytophilum*, they do not secrete IL-18 and exhibit splenomegaly and damage to the splenic architecture [29].

A. phagocytophilum transiently infects bone-marrow derived macrophages (BMDMs) [31] and clinical features in animal models and infected patients suggest classical macrophage activation [32]. Deep sequencing analysis of experimentally infected macrophages indicated that the transcription of genes that encode for phospholipase A2 (*pla2g12a, pla2g5* and *pla2g2e*), *COX2* and *PGE* synthase (ptges) was increased upon *A. phagocytophilum* infection [29].

A. phagocytophilum use heat shock proteins (Hsps) for infection of vertebrate host cells [33, 34]. Host cells can also activate Hsps in response to infection [35–37]. The mammalian immune response against pathogen Hsps to control infection may trigger a detrimental autoimmune response to host Hsps [35, 36, 38]. However, recent evidence suggests that hosts may benefit from induction of Hsps in response to pathogen infection [1]. A mutant strain of *Mycobacterium tuberculosis*, that constitutively over produced Hsp70 proteins, was fully virulent in the initial stage of infection, but its survival was reduced in the chronic phase. This suggests that induction of microbial genes encoding Hsps might provide a novel strategy to boost the immune response of individuals with latent infections [39].

How *A. phagocytophilum* interacts with the mammalian immune system is still unclear. Both T and B cells have been shown to play important roles in the control and clearance of *A. phagocytophilum* [40, 41]. CD4+ T cells and T-helper 1 (Th1) play a key role in the immune response to the infection of *A. phagocytophilum* [30, 42]. IFNγ, IL-12, and IL-18 also play important roles in the early clearance of *A. phagocytophilum* [30, 43]. Well-known anti-bacterial innate immune detection system such as TLR2, TLR4, and their adaptor MyD88 appear to play no role in the immune response to *A. phagocytophilum* infection [41]. Some studies suggest that signaling through the Nod Like Receptor (NLR) family member IPAF (NLRC4), its adaptor ASC, and Caspase-1 is critical for the control of *A. phagocytophilum* infection during the early phase of infection [30].

Rip2 has been previously shown to play an essential role in the immunity against various intracellular pathogens including *Mycobacterium tuberculosis* [44]. Rip2 also plays an important role in the control of *A. phagocytophilum* infection [44]. *A. phagocytophilum* infection upregulates Rip2, the adaptor molecule of the cytoplasmic pattern recognition receptor Nod1 and 2 in immune cells [45]. Following peptidoglycan detection, Nod1/Nod2 recruit and associate with the adaptor protein Rip2, triggering proinflammatory signaling pathways via NF-κB and the mitogen-activated protein (MAP) kinases p38, JNK, and ERK [46]. IL-8, a major inflammatory chemokine, is heavily induced during *A. phagocytophilum* infection in humans [47]. Trafficking of neutrophils to the sites of infection is induced by this chemokine and Rip2, which appears to play an important role in neutrophil recruitment *in vivo* [48]. IFN-γ, another inflammatory cytokine, plays a major role in the immune pathology and early clearance of *A. phagocytophilum* infection [43]. It is also known that an adaptive CD4+ T cell mediated response is critical for the complete clearance of *A. phagocytophilum* infection [42]. Previous reports have shown the importance of natural killer (NK) cells, NKT cells [49] and CD4 + T cells [42] in the IFNγ production and host defense to *A. phagocytophilum* infection (**Figure 1**).

Using oligonucleotide array technology [50], it was observed that genes involved in the immune response were modulated in neutrophils infected with *A. phagocytophilum*. Among the genes that were most upregulated in the early transcriptional response to infection in neutrophils were cytokines, chemokines, and their receptors (e.g., *CCL3, CCL3L3, IL-8, IL-1β,* and *CXCR4*).

The major adipocyte lipid droplet-associated phosphoprotein perilipin (PLIN) is upregulated in HL60 infected cells. Both protein and mRNA levels were higher in infected cells and the over expression of *PLIN* was parallel with bacterial infection levels [51]. Furthermore, *PLIN* knockdown resulted in a reduction of *A. phagocytophilum* infection in HL60 cells, suggesting the bacteria modulate host lipid metabolism to infect and multiply in the host cell [51].

In THP-1 cells, *A, phagocytophilum* infection displays an upregulation of histone deacetylates 1 and 2 (*HDAC1* and *HDAC2),* while protein levels exhibit a similar kinetic pattern for both HDACs. Moreover, pharmacological inhibition of HDAC and *HDAC1* silencing reduced the level of bacterial infection in THP-1 cells [52]. Mycobacterial infection of THP-1 cells specifically inhibits HLA-DR gene expression by a pathway involving HDAC complex formation at the HLA-DR promoter, resulting in histone deacetylation and gene silencing [53].

Proteins secreted by bacteria are involved in many important tasks and they account for many of the virulence factors of pathogens. Outer membrane protein A (OmpA), also known as peptidoglycan-associated lipoprotein, is conserved among most Gram-negative bacteria and interacts with peptidoglycan to maintain outer membrane integrity [54]. The expression of *OmpA* increases in the early stages of infection. OmpA is presented on the pathogen's surface and is upregulated during invasion of HL-60 cells. Sera from HGA patients and experimentally infected mice recognize recombinant OmpA. Pretreatment of *A. phagocytophilum* organisms with OmpA antiserum reduces their ability to infect HL-60 cells [54].

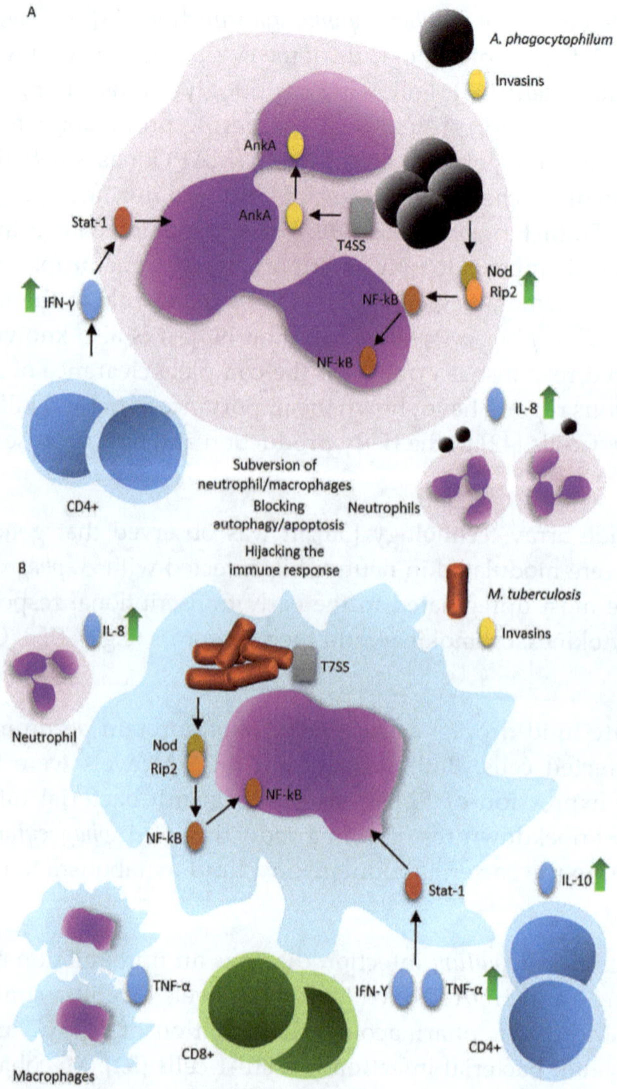

Figure 1. *A. phagocytophilum* and *M. tuberculosis* employ common strategies but different mechanisms to infect host cells: Nod proteins activate NF-κB through the serine–threonine kinase Rip2. NF-κB is translocated to the nucleus and stimulates cytokine expression. Secretion of IL-8 stimulates neutrophil and T cell migration. Stat1 participates in the IFN-γ signaling of intracellular bacteria. (A). Neutrophil infected with *A. phagocytophilum*: IFN-γ contributes to tissue injury and disease. AnkA is secreted by the bacteria and translocates to the nucleus of infected cells regulating host cell transcription facilitating intracellular bacterial survival and growth. (B). Macrophage infected with *M. tuberculosis*: IFN-γ activates macrophage phagocytosis killing intracellular bacteria. TNF-α attracts macrophages and lymphocytes at the site of infection and promotes granuloma formation thus resulting in limited antigen presentation.

A. phagocytophilum uses surface proteins invasins OmpA, Asp14, and AipA to bind and infect mammalian hosts [55, 56]. OmpA interacts with α1,3-fucose, which is critical for the bacteria to bind host cell surfaces and invade them. OmpA, Asp14, and AipA play essential roles in the *A. phagocytophilum* lifecycle [54, 55, 57]. Directing the immune response to their binding domains could enhance protective efficacy. It has been observed that an antibody cocktail specific for the OmpA, Asp14, and AipA binding domains blocked *A. phagocytophilum* infection of host cells [56]. This finding could help the development of an anti-multi-invasin vaccine to protect against human and veterinary granulocytic anaplasmosis or even against other obligate intracellular pathogens such as *Mycobacterium* spp. since they also use multiple invasins to enter host cells [58].

MSP1a and MSP1b from *Anaplasma marginale* have been shown to be adhesins for host cells [59]. Studies on the immunogenicity of recombinant BCG expressing the MSP1a antigen suggested that the immune responses were influenced by the level of antigen expression [60]. These results indicated that recombinant *M. bovis* BCG expressing MSP1a could be used to test for protective antibody production for the control of anaplasmosis.

The *A. phagocytophilum* genome encodes a type four secretion system (T4SS) that may facilitate intracellular survival by translocation of virulence factors that appear to be important for the manipulation of the host cell. Ankirin A (AnkA) is a translocated virulence factor that is tyrosine-phosphorylated by host cell kinases upon translocation into the host cell early during infection [16, 61].

Anaplasma translocation substrate 1 (Ats-1) protein belongs to T4SS of *Anaplasma*, which is secreted and localizes into the mitochondria of human neutrophils and HL60 cells. Ats-1 translocates to the host cell mitochondria matrix via the translocase of the outer mitochondrial membrane (TOM) complex. Transfection assays with RF/6A and yeast cells demonstrated that Ats-1 inhibits etoposide and Bax-induced apoptosis respectively [62] thus facilitating pathogen survival.

In mammalian cells, *A. phagocytophilum* activates extracellular signal-regulated kinase (Erk)1/2, a key protein of the MAP kinase pathway [50, 63]. AptA (*Anaplasma phagocytophilum* toxin A, formerly named APH_0233) stimulates Erk1/2 phosphorylation in HL60 and HEK293 cells [64]. Furthermore, AptA interacts with vimentin, and gene silencing and inhibitory enzymatic assays in HL60 cells and neutrophils respectively, demonstrated that vimentin is necessary for Erk1/2 activation and *Anaplasma* infection [64].

Anaplasma inclusions have a double-lipid bilayer membrane, and induce autophagosome formation in the host cell. Also, beclin 1 and light chain 3 (LC3) proteins that play a central role in autophagy are colocalized bacterial replicative inclusions. Furthermore, assays of inhibition and induction of this catabolic mechanism in HL60 infected cells demonstrated that autophagy benefits infection, rather than elimination [65]. Ref. [66] described that induction of autophagy in host cells is mediated trough beclin 1 (Becn1) that binds Ats-1 to supply nutrients for pathogen growth. Additionally, gene silencing of *Becn1* inhibits infection in mammalian cells [66].

3. The *Mycobacterium tuberculosis* complex, a global burden for human and animal health

Macrophages play a central role in the first line of defense against pathogenic microorganisms, however, they are also the key target cells for mycobacteria. The bacteria can live and replicate inside the macrophages, thus evading the innate immune response against infection of the host through immunosuppression and immune evasion [53]. Co-evolution of *M. tuberculosis* with its hosts has enabled the pathogen to develop host immune evasion strategies that interfere with both innate and adaptive immunity. These include the manipulation of their phagosome within host macrophages, the avoidance of pattern recognition receptors, the modulation of host cytokine production, and the manipulation of antigen presentation to prevent or alter the quality of T-cell responses [67]. Other mechanisms include interference with phagosomal acidification and trafficking, blocking autophagy and apoptosis-mediated killing, perturbing calcium signaling, and inhibiting the inflammasome activation in order to modulate the host immune responses. Manipulation of these host pathways is achieved by bacterial components such as cell wall lipids, serine threonine kinases, phosphatases and proteases, and using specialized secretion systems.

The outcome of infection with *Mycobacterium tuberculosis* depends on the ability of the immune response to clear or contain the infection. When this fails, the bacterium replicates, disseminates within the host, and elicits a pathologic inflammatory response. Individuals infected with *M. tuberculosis* develop mainly CD4 T cell responses to protein components of *M. tuberculosis*, an immune response that can persist for years. Infections with mycobacteria are characterized by their chronic course and, even with an adequate immune response, they can persist inside macrophages. Progression to active disease is possible even decades after exposure [68] and is typically triggered by immune compromise. Although the bacteria are concealed within the infected macrophage, B cells and antibodies also play a role on the immune response to intracellular bacteria and are likely to be important in the control of *M. tuberculosis* [69]. In addition, B cells are a major cellular component of the granuloma (an important mechanism of host defense against tuberculosis) where they can process and present antigen to T cells, secrete antibodies, and modulate inflammation through the production of IL-10 [70]. *In vitro* human B cells have been shown to ingest mycobacteria, produce IgM, and upregulate the expression of the costimulatory molecules *CD80* and *CD86* and the chemokine *CXCL10* [71]. The human CD4 T cell response exhibits Th1-response characteristics [72].

Mycobacteria have a distinct secretion system, named type VII (T7SS or ESX), which is associated with virulence and pathogenesis, including growth in macrophages [73] and antigen presentation. This system is encoded by a locus that is deleted in attenuated strains of *M. bovis* (bacille Calmette–Guérin (BCG) strains), which are used to vaccinate against tuberculosis [74].

IL-8 is a chemokine with a significant role in regulating leukocyte influx in TB. *In vivo* studies have shown that pre-treatment with anti-IL-8 alone inhibits mycobacterial granuloma formation [75]. IL-8 is involved in attracting neutrophils and T cells and in monocyte recruitment [76]. Targeting IL-8 secretion during inflammation could be the subject for new therapeutic approaches [77].

Mycobacterial components can activate MAP kinase signaling cascades but this activation varies depending on the species of *Mycobacterium*. For instance, it appears to be diminished in macrophages infected with pathogenic strains of *M. avium* [78].

IFN-γ is a Th1 cytokine that plays a vital role in the protective immune response against *M. tuberculosis* infection [2]. In cattle, IFN-γ is produced predominately by activated CD4 T cells following presentation of *M. bovis* antigens on the surface of antigen presenting cells (APCs) [79]. IL-10 is released following phagocytosis of pathogenic mycobacteria [80] and has been shown to inhibit the pro-inflammatory cytokine response through down regulation of IL-12 and IFN-γ [81, 82]. Increased IL-10 levels appear to correlate with progression of infection in a bovine tuberculosis model [83] (**Figure 1**).

Nod proteins and their adaptor molecule Rip2 are key components of a family of cytosolic innate immune pattern recognition receptors [84]. Nod2 triggers cytokine production by dendritic cells in response to live *M. tuberculosis,* but is not essential to control infection [85].

M. tuberculosis can use the TLR2 pathway to modify the host environment [86]. The adaptor molecule myeloid differentiation factor-88 (MyD88) appears to play a significant role in the pathogenesis of *Mycobacterium*. Mice lacking MyD88 are highly susceptible to *M. tuberculosis* infection, with a mean time to death of approximately 42 days.

Glycolipids are one of the most common cell surface components of macrophages and dendritic cells. They interact with intracellular bacteria, estimulating the host immune response [87]. LprG (Rv1411c), a cell membrane lipoprotein essential for *M. tuberculosis* virulence, binds to the acyl groups of lipoglycan [88]. In murine macrophage cells (RAW 264.7), LprG is essential for macrophage entry and inhibition of phagosome—lysosome fusion. Also, it has been described that LprG has a significant role in the production of lipoglycan lipoarabinomannan (LAM), one of the major cell surface components of *M. tuberculosis* [87, 89]. LprI is another lipoprotein used by *M. tuberculosis* to bind and inhibit the lytic activity of lysosomes [90].

Mycolic acids are major components of the outer membrane of *M. tuberculosis*. HadC (Rv0637) contributes to mycolic acids biosynthesis and its mutation or silencing is directly related to the loss of *M. tuberculosis* virulence [91].

M. tuberculosis encodes the serine protease Rv2224c (Hip1) that is present on the cellular membrane [92]. In primary macrophages, silencing of *Hip1* notably decreased mycobacterial growth compared to the wild type bacteria. Moreover, levels of cytokines (TNF-α, IL-1β, IL-6) were increased in macrophages infected with wild-type *M. tuberculosis* compared to the mutant *Hip1 M. tuberculosis* [93]. The stress-induced protein GroEL2 is a substrate for Hip1 [92]. Hip1 appears to limits dendritic cells cytokine secretion and through under modulation of CD40 and CD86, it could affect dendritic cell maturation, and decrease antigen presentation to CD4 T cells [94].

Transcriptional assays have shown that *M. tuberculosis* infection of human monocytes activate the MAPK pathway to promote over expression of IL-23, that is involved in the modulation of Th1/Th17 cells [95]. In addition, it has been reported that the bacteria may suppress the differentiation of monocytes into dendritic cells through the release of IL-10 [96].

Intracellular bacteria can manipulate host gene expression through epigenetic modifications to help infection and survival inside the host cell. Ghorpade et al. [97] described that *M. bovis* bacillus Calmette-Guérin (BCG) modify epigenetically nitric oxide and KLF4 to restrain the class II transactivator (CIITA) and MHC-II expression thereby eluding immune surveillance. Evidence supports that *M. tuberculosis* infection in THP1 cells induces overexpression of *HDAC1*, which is implicated in the downregulation of IL-12B that plays a key role in the Th1 response [98].

Lsr2 is a *M. tuberculosis* protein with histone-like features, including the ability to regulate a variety of transcriptional responses in mycobacteria. Lsr2 protects mycobacteria against reactive oxygen intermediates (ROI) *in vitro* and during macrophage infection shielding bacterial DNA by binding to it [99] suggesting it could be a good candidate as a drug target.

4. Conclusions

Intracellular bacteria such as *Anaplasma* and *Mycobacterium* use similar mechanisms to infect vertebrate host cells. These strategies include manipulation of the immune response, subversion of phagocyte cells and the use of proteins for infection and manipulation of host gene expression. Nevertheless, different pathogens have evolved specific strategies when infecting their hosts. Abundantly expressed proteins are often the primary targets of research, however, less prominently expressed antigens may have equally good or even superior vaccine potential. Research into the antigen catalog available for immune recognition of infected cells could provide new directions for antigen discovery and vaccine development.

Acknowledgements

VL was funded by a grant of the Universidad Autónoma de Sinaloa, Mexico.

Author details

Vladimir López[1], Pilar Alberdi[1] and José de la Fuente[1,2]*

*Address all correspondence to: jose_delafuente@yahoo.com

1 SaBio, Instituto de Investigación en Recursos Cinegéticos IREC (CSIC-UCLM-JCCM), Ciudad Real, Spain

2 Department of Veterinary Pathobiology, Center for Veterinary Health Sciences, Oklahoma State University, Stillwater, OK, USA

References

[1] de la Fuente J, Villar M, Cabezas-Cruz A, Estrada-Peña A, Ayllón N, Alberdi P. Tick-host-pathogen interactions: Conflict and cooperation. PLoS Pathogens. 2016;**12**(4):e1005488. DOI: 10.1371/journal.ppat.1005488

[2] Scriba TJ, Coussens AK, Fletcher HA. Human immunology of tuberculosis. Microbiology Spectrum. 2016;**4**(4):1-23

[3] Rikihisa Y. *Anaplasma phagocytophilum* and *Ehrlichia chaffeensis*: Subversive manipulators of host cells. Nature Reviews. Microbiology. 2010;**8**(5):328-339 Available from: http://dx.doi.org/10.1038/nrmicro2318%5Cnhttp://www.nature.com/doifinder/10.1038/nrmicro2318

[4] Galindo RC, Ayllón N, Carta T, Vicente J, Kocan KM, Gortazar C, et al. Characterization of pathogen-specific expression of host immune response genes in *Anaplasma* and *Mycobacterium* species infected ruminants. Comparative Immunology, Microbiology and Infectious Diseases. 2010;**33**(6):e133-e142

[5] Jongejan F, Uilenberg G. The global importance of ticks. Parasitology. 2005;**129**(7):S3. Available from: http://www.journals.cambridge.org/abstract_S0031182004005967; [cited 2014 Jul 11]

[6] de la Fuente J. Overview: Ticks as vectors of pathogens that cause disease in humans and animals. Frontiers in Bioscience. 2008;**13**:6938. Available from: http://www.bioscience.org/2008/v13/af/3200/list.htm

[7] Ayllón N, Villar M, Galindo RC, Kocan KM, Šíma R, López JA, et al. Systems biology of tissue-specific response to *Anaplasma phagocytophilum* reveals differentiated apoptosis in the tick vector *Ixodes scapularis*. PLoS Genetics. 2015;**11**(3):1-29

[8] Severo MS, Pedra JHF, Ayllón N, Kocan KM, de la Fuente J. Anaplasma. Molecular Medical Microbiology. 2015;**3**:2033-2042. Available from: http://linkinghub.elsevier.com/retrieve/pii/B9780123971692001104

[9] Dumler JS, Bakken JS. Erhlichial diseases of humans: Emerging tick-borne infections. Clinical Infectious Diseases. 1995;**20**:1102-1110

[10] de la Fuente J, Estrada-Peña A, Cabezas-Cruz A, Kocan KM. *Anaplasma phagocytophilum* uses common strategies for infection of ticks and vertebrate hosts. Trends in Microbiology. 2016;**24**(3):173-180. Available from: http://dx.doi.org/10.1016/j.tim.2015.12.001

[11] Severo MS, Stephens KD, Kotsyfakis M, Pedra JHF. *Anaplasma phagocytophilum*: Deceptively simple or simply deceptive? Future Microbiology. 2012;**7**:719-731

[12] Rikihisa Y, Lin M. *Anaplasma phagocytophilum* and *Ehrlichia chaffeensis* type IV secretion and Ank proteins. Current Opinion in Microbiology. 2010 Feb;**13**(1):59-66. Available from: http://www.pubmedcentral.nih.gov/articlerender.fcgi?artid=3251840&tool=pmcentrez&rendertype=abstract; [cited 2014 Jul 23]

[13] de la Fuente J, Ayoubi P, Blouin EF, Almazán C, Naranjo V, Kocan KM. Gene expression profiling of human promyelocytic cells in response to infection with *Anaplasma phagocytophilum*. Cellular Microbiology. 2005 Apr;**7**(4):549-559. Available from http://www.ncbi.nlm.nih.gov/pubmed/15760455; [cited 2014 Jul 23]

[14] Lee HC, Kioi M, Han J, Puri RK, Goodman JL. *Anaplasma phagocytophilum*-induced gene expression in both human neutrophils and HL-60 cells. Genomics. 2008 Sep;**92**(3):144-151. Available from http://www.ncbi.nlm.nih.gov/pubmed/18603403; [cited 2014 Jul 23]

[15] Pruneau L, Moumène A, Meyer DF, Marcelino I, Lefrançois T, VachiÃcry N. Understanding Anaplasmataceae pathogenesis using "Omics"; approaches. Frontiers in Cellular and Infection Microbiology. 2014;**4**(July):1-7. Available from: http://journal.frontiersin.org/article/10.3389/fcimb.2014.00086/abstract

[16] IJdo JW, Carlson AC, Kennedy EL. *Anaplasma phagocytophilum* AnkA is tyrosine-phosphorylated at EPIYA motifs and recruits SHP-1 during early infection. Cellular Microbiology. 2007 May;**9**(5):1284-1296. Available from: http://www.ncbi.nlm.nih.gov/pubmed/17250594; [cited 2014 Jul 23]

[17] Yoshiie K, Kim HY, Mott J, Rikihisa Y. Intracellular infection by the human granulocytic Ehrlichiosis agent inhibits human neutrophil apoptosis. Infection and Immunity. 2000;**68**(3):1125-1133. Available from: http://www.pubmedcentral.nih.gov/articlerender.fcgi?artid=97257&tool=pmcentrez&rendertype=abstract

[18] Gulia-Nuss M, Nuss AB, Meyer JM, Sonenshine DE, Roe RM, Waterhouse RM, et al. Genomic insights into the *Ixodes scapularis* tick vector of Lyme disease. Nature Communications. 2016;**7**(May 2015):10507. Available from: http://www.nature.com/doifinder/10.1038/ncomms10507

[19] Park J, Choi KS, Dumler JS. Major surface protein 2 of *Anaplasma phagocytophilum* facilitates adherence to granulocytes. Infection and Immunity. 2003;**71**(7):4018-4025

[20] Nelson CM, Herron MJ, Felsheim RF, Schloeder BR, Grindle SM, Chavez AO, et al. Whole genome transcription profiling of *Anaplasma phagocytophilum* in human and tick host cells by tiling array analysis. BMC Genomics. 2008;**16**:1-16

[21] Granquist EG, Stuen S, Crosby L, Lundgren AM, Alleman AR, Barbet AF. Variant-specific and diminishing immune responses towards the highly variable MSP2(P44) outer membrane protein of *Anaplasma phagocytophilum* during persistent infection in lambs. Veterinary Immunology and Immunopathology. 2010;**133**(15):2-4

[22] Choi K, Scorpio DG, Dumler JS. Stat1 negatively regulates immune-mediated injury with *Anaplasma phagocytophilum* infection. Journal of Immunology. 2014;**15**(10):5088-5098

[23] Rauch I, Müller M, Decker T. The regulation of inflammation by interferons and their STATs. JAK-STAT. 2013;**2**(1):e23820. Available from: http://www.ncbi.nlm.nih.gov/pubmed/24058799%5Cnhttp://www.pubmedcentral.nih.gov/articlerender.fcgi?artid=PMC3670275

[24] Choi K, Dumler JS. *Anaplasma phagocytophilum*, interferon gamma production and Stat1 signaling. Microbiology and Immunology. 2013;**57**(3):207-212

[25] Qu HQ, Fisher-Hoch SP, McCormick JB. Molecular immunity to mycobacteria: Knowledge from the mutation and phenotype spectrum analysis of Mendelian susceptibility to mycobacterial diseases. International Journal of Infectious Diseases. 2011;**15**(5):1-19

[26] Bussmeyer U, Sarkar A, Broszat K, Lüdemann T, Möller S, van Zandbergen G, et al. Impairment of gamma interferon signaling in human neutrophils infected with *Anaplasma phagocytophilum*. Infection and Immunity. 2010 Jan;**78**(1):358-363. Available from: http://www.pubmedcentral.nih.gov/articlerender.fcgi?artid=2798180&tool=pmcentrez&rendertype=abstract; [cited 2014 Jul 23]

[27] de la Fuente J, Gortazar C. Wild boars as hosts of human-pathogenic *Anaplasma phagocytophilum* variants [letter]. Emerging Infectious Diseases 2012;**18**(12):2094-2095

[28] Galindo RC, Ayllón N, Smrdel KS, Boadella M, Beltrán-Beck B, Mazariegos M, et al. Gene expression profile suggests that pigs (Sus Scrofa) are susceptible to *Anaplasma phagocytophilum* but control infection. Parasites & Vectors. 2012 Jan;**5**:181. Available from: http://www.pubmedcentral.nih.gov/articlerender.fcgi?artid=3453518&tool=pmcentrez&rendertype=abstract; [cited 2014 Jul 23]

[29] Wang X, Shaw DK, Hammond HL, Sutterwala FS, Rayamajhi M, Shirey KA, et al. The prostaglandin E2-EP3 receptor axis regulates *Anaplasma phagocytophilum*-mediated NLRC4 inflammasome activation. PLoS Pathogens. 2016;**12**(8):1-23

[30] Pedra JH, Sutterwala FS, Sukumaran B, Ogura Y, Qian F, Montgomery RR, et al. ASC/PYCARD and caspase-1 regulate the IL-18/IFN-gamma axis during *Anaplasma phagocytophilum* infection. Journal of Immunology. 2007;**179**(7):4783-4791. Available from: http://www.ncbi.nlm.nih.gov/entrez/query.fcgi?cmd=Retrieve&db=PubMed&dopt=Citation&list_uids=17878377%5Cnhttp://www.jimmunol.org/cgi/reprint/179/7/4783.pdf

[31] Chen G, Wang X, Severo MS, Sakhon OS, Sohail M, Brown LJ, et al. The tick salivary protein sialostatin L2 inhibits caspase-1-mediated inflammation during *Anaplasma phagocytophilum* infection. Infection and Immunity. 2014;**82**(6):2553-2564

[32] Dumler JS, Barat NC, Barat CE, Bakken JS. Human granulocytic anaplasmosis and macrophage activation. Clinical Infectious Diseases. 2007 Jul 15;**45**(2):199-204. Available from http://www.ncbi.nlm.nih.gov/pubmed/17578779; [cited 2014 Jul 23]

[33] Villar M, Ayllón N, Kocan KM, Bonzón-Kulichenko E, Alberdi P, Blouin EF, et al. Identification and characterization of *Anaplasma phagocytophilum* proteins involved in infection of the tick vector, *Ixodes scapularis*. PLoS One. 2015;**10**(9):1-26

[34] Contreras M, Alberdi P, Mateos-Hernández L, Fernández de Mera IG, García-Pérez AL, Vancová M, et al. *Anaplasma phagocytophilum* MSP4 and HSP70 proteins are involved in interactions with host cells during pathogen infection. Frontiers in Cellular and Infection Microbiology. 2017;**7**(July):307. Available from: http://www.ncbi.nlm.nih.gov/pubmed/28725639%0Ahttp://www.pubmedcentral.nih.gov/articlerender.fcgi?artid=PMC5496961

[35] Schlesinger MJ. Heat shock proteins: Minireview. The Journal of Biological Chemistry. 1990;**265**(21 (July 25)):12111-12114

[36] Whitley D, Goldberg SP, Jordan WD. Heat shock proteins: A review of the molecular chaperones. Journal of Vascular Surgery. 1999;**29**(4):748-751. Available from: http://www.sciencedirect.com/science/article/pii/S0741521499703290

[37] Yu A, Li P, Tang T, Wang J, Chen Y, Liu L. Roles of Hsp70s in stress responses of microorganisms, plants, and animals. BioMed Research International. 2015;**2015**:510319. DOI: 10.1155/2015/510319

[38] Vabulas RM, Wagner H, Schild H. Heat shock proteins as ligands of toll-like receptors. In: Beutler B, Wagner H, editors. Toll-like Receptor Family Members and their Ligands. Berlin, Heidelberg: Springer Berlin Heidelberg; 2002. pp. 169-184. Available from: https://doi.org/10.1007/978-3-642-59430-4_11

[39] Stewart GR, Snewin VA, Walzl G, Hussell T, Tormay P, O'Gaora P, et al. Overexpression of heat-shock proteins reduces survival of *Mycobacterium tuberculosis* in the chronic phase of infection. Nature. 2001;**7**:732-737

[40] Telford SR 3rd, Dawson JE, Katavolos P, Warner CK, Kolbert CP, Persing DH. Perpetuation of the agent of human granulocytic ehrlichiosis in a deer tick-rodent cycle. Proceedings of the National Academy of Sciences of the United States of America. 1996;**93**(12):6209-6214

[41] von Loewenich FD, Scorpio DG, Reischl U, Dumler JS, Bogdan C. Frontline: Control of *Anaplasma phagocytophilum*, an obligate intracellular pathogen, in the absence of inducible nitric oxide synthase, phagocyte NADPH oxidase, tumor necrosis factor, toll-like receptor (TLR)2 and TLR4, or the TLR adaptor molecule MyD88. European Journal of Immunology. 2004 Jul;**34**(7):1789-1797. Available from http://www.ncbi.nlm.nih.gov/pubmed/15214027; [cited 2014 Jul 23]

[42] Birkner K, Steiner B, Rinkler C, Kern Y, Aichele P, Bogdan C, et al. The elimination of *Anaplasma phagocytophilum* requires CD4+ T cells, but is independent of Th1 cytokines and a wide spectrum of effector mechanisms. European Journal of Immunology. 2008;**38**(12):3395-3410

[43] Akkoyunlu M, Fikrig E. Gamma interferon dominates the murine cytokine response to the agent of human granulocytic ehrlichiosis and helps to control the degree of early rickettsemia. Infection and Immunity. 2000;**68**(4):1827-1833

[44] Sukumaran B, Ogura Y, Pedra JHF, Kobayashi K, Flavell RA, Fikrig E. Rip2 contributes to host defense against *Anaplasma phagocytophilum* infection. FEMS Immunology and Medical Microbiology. 2012;**66**(22):211-219

[45] Sukumaran B, Carlyon JA, Cai J, Berliner N, Fikrig E. Early transcriptional response of human neutrophils to *Anaplasma phagocytophilum* infection. Infection and Immunity. 2005;**73**(12):8089-8099

[46] Kobayashi K, Inohara N, Hernandez LD, Galán JE, Núñez G, Janeway CA, et al. RICK/Rip2/CARDIAK mediates signalling for receptors of the innate and adaptive immune systems. Nature. 2002;**416**(6877):194-199. Available from: http://www.nature.com/doifinder/10.1038/416194a

[47] Akkoyunlu M, Malawista SE, Anguita J, Fikrig E. Exploitation of interleukin-8-induced neutrophil chemotaxis by the agent of human granulocytic ehrlichiosis. Infection and Immunity. 2001;**69**(9):5577-5588

[48] Magalhaes JG, Lee J, Geddes K, Rubino S, Philpott DJ, Girardin SE. Essential role of Rip2 in the modulation of innate and adaptive immunity triggered by Nod1 and Nod2 ligands. European Journal of Immunology. 2011;**41**(5):1445-1455

[49] Choi K, Webb T, Oelke M, Scorpio DG, Dumler JS. Differential innate immune cell activation and Proinflammatory response in *Anaplasma phagocytophilum* infection. Infection and Immunity. 2007;**75**(6):3124-3130

[50] Lee HC, Kioi M, Han J, Puri RK, Goodman JL. *Anaplasma phagocytophilum*-induced gene expression in both human neutrophils and HL-60 cells. Genomics. 2008;**92**(3):144-151

[51] Manzano-Roman R, Almazán C, Naranjo V, Blouin EF, Kocan KM, de la Fuente J. Expression of perilipin in human promyelocytic cells in response to *Anaplasma phagocytophilum* infection results in modified lipid metabolism. Journal of Medical Microbiology. 2008 Feb;**57**(Pt 2):159-163. Available from: http://www.ncbi.nlm.nih.gov/pubmed/18201980; [cited 2014 Jul 23]

[52] Garcia-Garcia JC, Barat NC, Trembley SJ, Dumler JS. Epigenetic silencing of host cell defense genes enhances intracellular survival of the rickettsial pathogen *Anaplasma phagocytophilum*. PLoS Pathogens. 2009 Jun;**5**(6):e1000488. Available from: http://www.pubmedcentral.nih.gov/articlerender.fcgi?artid=2694362&tool=pmcentrez&rendertype=abstract; [cited 2014 Jul 23]

[53] Wang X, Zhang J, Liang J, Zhang Y, Teng X, Yuan X, et al. Protection against *Mycobacterium tuberculosis* infection offered by a new multistage subunit vaccine correlates with increased number of IFN-γ+IL-2+ CD4+and IFN-γ+ CD8+ T cells. PLoS One. 2015;**10**(3):1-18

[54] Ojogun N, Kahlon A, Ragland SA, Troese MJ, Mastronunzio JE, Walker NJ, et al. *Anaplasma phagocytophilum* outer membrane protein A interacts with sialylated glycoproteins to promote infection of mammalian host cells. Infection and Immunity. 2012;**80**(11):3748-3760

[55] Kahlon A, Ojogun N, Ragland SA, Seidman D, Troese MJ, Ottens AK, et al. *Anaplasma phagocytophilum* Asp14 is an invasin that interacts with mammalian host cells via its C terminus to facilitate infection. Infection and Immunity. 2013;**81**(1):65-79

[56] Seidman D, Hebert KS, Truchan HK, Miller DP, Tegels BK, Marconi RT, et al. Essential domains of *Anaplasma phagocytophilum* invasins utilized to infect mammalian host cells. PLoS Pathogens. 2015;**11**(2):1-29. Available from: http://dx.doi.org/10.1371/journal.ppat.1004669

[57] Seidman D, Ojogun N, Walker NJ, Mastronunzio J, Kahlon A, Hebert KS, et al. *Anaplasma phagocytophilum* surface protein AipA mediates invasion of mammalian host cells. Cellular Microbiology. 2014;**16**(8):1133-1145

[58] Govender VS, Ramsugit S, Pillay M. *Mycobacterium tuberculosis* adhesins: Potential biomarkers as anti-tuberculosis therapeutic and diagnostic targets. Microbiology (United Kingdom). 2014;**160**(Part 9):1821-1831

[59] de La Fuente J, Garcia-Garcia JC, Blouin EF, Rodríguez SD, García MA, Kocan KM. Evolution and function of tandem repeats in the major surface protein 1a of the ehrlichial pathogen *Anaplasma marginale*. Animal Health Research Reviews. 2001;**2**(2):163-173

[60] Michelon A, Conceição FR, Binsfeld PC, da Cunha CW, Moreira ÂN, Argondizzo AP, et al. Immunogenicity of *Mycobacterium bovis* BCG expressing *Anaplasma marginale* MSP1a antigen. Vaccine. 2006;**24**(37-39):6332-6339

[61] Lin M, den Dulk-Ras A, Hooykaas PJJ, Rikihisa Y. *Anaplasma phagocytophilum* AnkA secreted by type IV secretion system is tyrosine phosphorylated by Abl-1 to facilitate infection. Cellular Microbiology. 2007 Nov;**9**(11):2644-2657. Available from http://www.ncbi.nlm.nih.gov/pubmed/17587335

[62] Niu H, Kozjak-Pavlovic V, Rudel T, Rikihisa Y. *Anaplasma phagocytophilum* Ats-1 is imported into host cell mitochondria and interferes with apoptosis induction. PLoS Pathogens. 2010 Feb;**6**(2):e1000774. Available from: http://www.pubmedcentral.nih.gov/articlerender.fcgi?artid=2824752&tool=pmcentrez&rendertype=abstract; [cited 2014 Jul 23]

[63] Xiong Q, Lin M, Rikihisa Y. Cholesterol-dependent *Anaplasma phagocytophilum* exploits the low-density lipoprotein uptake pathway. PLoS Pathogens. 2009;**5**(3):1-13

[64] Sukumaran B, Mastronunzio JE, Narasimhan S, Fankhauser S, Uchil PD, Levy R, et al. *Anaplasma phagocytophilum* AptA modulates Erk1/2 signalling. Cellular Microbiology. 2011;**13**(1):47-61

[65] Niu H, Yamaguchi M, Rikihisa Y. Subversion of cellular autophagy by *Anaplasma phagocytophilum*. Cellular Microbiology. 2008 Mar;**10**(3):593-605. Available from: http://www.ncbi.nlm.nih.gov/pubmed/17979984; [cited 2014 Jul 23]

[66] Niu H, Xiong Q, Yamamoto A, Hayashi-Nishino M, Rikihisa Y. Autophagosomes induced by a bacterial Beclin 1 binding protein facilitate obligatory intracellular infection. Proceedings of the National Academy of Sciences of the United States of America. 2012;**109**(51):20800-20807. Available from: http://www.pubmedcentral.nih.gov/articlerender.fcgi?artid=3529060&tool=pmcentrez&rendertype=abstract

[67] Goldberg MF, Saini NK, Porcelli SA. Evasion of innate and adaptive immunity by *Mycobacterium tuberculosis*. Microbiology Spectrum. May 2017;**2014**:1-24

[68] Wiker HG, Mustafa T, Bjune Ga, Harboe M. Evidence for waning of latency in a cohort study of tuberculosis. BMC Infectious Diseases. 2010;**10**:37

[69] Chan J, Mehta S, Bharrhan S, Chen Y, Achkar JM, Casadevall A, et al. The role of B cells and humoral immunity in *Mycobacterium tuberculosis* infection. Seminars in Immunology. 2014;**26**(6):588-600. Available from: http://dx.doi.org/10.1016/j.smim.2014.10.005

[70] Rao M, Valentini D, Poiret T, Dodoo E, Parida S, Zumla A, et al. B in tb: B cells as mediators of clinically relevant immune responses in tuberculosis. Clinical Infectious Diseases. 2015;**61**(Suppl 3):S225-S234

[71] Hoff ST, Salman AM, Ruhwald M, Ravn P, Brock I, Elsheikh N, et al. Human B cells produce chemokine CXCL10 in the presence of *Mycobacterium tuberculosis* specific T cells. Tuberculosis. 2015;**95**(1):40-47. Available from: http://dx.doi.org/10.1016/j.tube.2014.10.005

[72] Lindestam Arlehamn CS, Gerasimova A, Mele F, Henderson R, Swann J, Greenbaum JA, et al. Memory T cells in latent *Mycobacterium tuberculosis* infection are directed against three antigenic islands and largely contained in a CXCR3+CCR6+ Th1 subset. PLoS Pathogens. 2013;**9**(1):e1003130. DOI: 10.1371/journal.ppat.1003130

[73] Stanley SA, Raghavan S, Hwang WW, Cox JS. Acute infection and macrophage subversion by *Mycobacterium tuberculosis* require a specialized secretion system. Proceedings of the National Academy of Sciences of the United States of America. 2003;**100**(22):13001-13006. Available from: http://www.pnas.org/cgi/doi/10.1073/pnas.2235593100

[74] Sreejit G, Ahmed A, Parveen N, Jha V, Valluri VL, Ghosh S, et al. The ESAT-6 protein of *Mycobacterium tuberculosis* interacts with beta-2-microglobulin (β2M) affecting antigen presentation function of macrophage. PLoS Pathogens. 2014;**10**(10):e1004446. DOI: 10.1371/journal.ppat.1004446

[75] Larsen CG, Thomsen MK, Gesser B, Thomsen PD, Deleuran BW, Nowak J, et al. The delayed-type hypersensitivity reaction is dependent on IL-8. Inhibition of a tuberculin skin reaction by an anti-IL-8 monoclonal antibody. Journal of Immunology. 1995;**155**(4):2151-2157. Available from: http://www.jimmunol.org/content/155/4/2151.abstract

[76] Mukaida N, Harada A, Matsushima K. Interleukin-8 (IL-8) and monocyte chemotactic and activating factor (MCAF/MCP-1), chemokines essentially involved in inflammatory and immune reactions. Cytokine & Growth Factor Reviews. 1998;**9**(1):9-23

[77] Yang X, Corvalan JRF, Wang P, Roy CM, Davis CG. Fully human anti-interleukin-8 monoclonal antibodies: potential therapeutics for the treatment of inflammatory disease states. Journal of Leukocyte Biology. 1999;**66**(September):401-410

[78] Roach SK, Schorey JS. Differential regulation of the mitogen-activated protein kinases by pathogenic and nonpathogenic mycobacteria. Infection and Immunity. 2002;**70**(6):3040-3052

[79] Liébana E, Girvin RM, Welsh M, Neill D, Pollock JM, Neill SD. Generation of CD8 + T-cell responses to *Mycobacterium bovis* and mycobacterial antigen in experimental bovine tuberculosis. Infection and Immunity. 1999;**67**(3):1034-1044

[80] Shaw TC, Thomas LH, Friedland JS. Regulation of Il-10 secretion after phagocytosis of *Mycobacterium tuberculosis* by human monocytic cells. Cytokine. 2000;**12**(5):483-486. Available from: http://linkinghub.elsevier.com/retrieve/pii/S1043466699905860

[81] Gong J, Zhang M, Modlin RL, Linsley PS, Iyer D, Lin Y, et al. Interleukin-10 downregulates *Mycobacterium tuberculosis* induced Th1 responses and CTLA-4 expression. Infection and Immunity. 1996;**64**(3):913-918

[82] Fulton Sa, Cross JV, Toossi ZT, Boom WH. Regulation of interleukin-12 by interleukin-10, transforming growth factor-beta, tumor necrosis factor-alpha, and interferon-gamma in human monocytes infected with *Mycobacterium tuberculosis* H37Ra. The Journal of Infectious Diseases. 1998;**178**(4):1105-1114

[83] Widdison S, Schreuder LJ, Villarreal-Ramos B, Howard CJ, Watson M, Coffey TJ. Cytokine expression profiles of bovine lymph nodes: Effects of *Mycobacterium bovis* infection and bacille Calmette-Guérin vaccination. Clinical and Experimental Immunology. 2007;**75**(11):5127-5134

[84] Chin AI, Dempsey PW, Bruhn K, Miller JF, Xu Y, Cheng G. Involvement of receptor-interacting protein 2 in innate and adaptive immune responses. Nature. 2002;**416**(6877):190-194. Available from: http://www.nature.com/doifinder/10.1038/416190a

[85] Gandotra S, Jang S, Murray PJ, Salgame P, Ehrt S. Nucleotide-binding oligomerization domain protein 2-deficient mice control infection with *Mycobacterium tuberculosis*. Infection and Immunity. 2007;**75**(11):5127-5134

[86] Scanga CA, Bafica A, Feng CG, Allen W, Hieny S, Sher A, et al. MyD88-deficient mice display a profound loss in resistance to *Mycobacterium tuberculosis* associated with partially impaired Th1 cytokine and nitric oxide synthase 2 expression. Infection and Immunity. 2004;**72**(4):2400-2404

[87] Källenius G, Correia-Neves M, Buteme H, Hamasur B, Svenson SB. Lipoarabinomannan, and its related glycolipids, induce divergent and opposing immune responses to *Mycobacterium tuberculosis* depending on structural diversity and experimental variations. Tuberculosis. 2016;**96**:120-130

[88] Drage MG, Tsai H-C, Pecora ND, Cheng T-Y, Arida AR, Shukla S, et al. *Mycobacterium tuberculosis* lipoprotein LprG (Rv1411c) binds triacylated glycolipid agonists of toll-like receptor 2. Nature Structural & Molecular Biology. 2010;**17**(99):1088-1095. Available from: http://www.nature.com/doifinder/10.1038/nsmb.1869

[89] Gaur RL, Ren K, Blumenthal A, Bhamidi S, Gibbs S, Jackson M, et al. LPRG-mediated surface expression of lipoarabinomannan is essential for virulence of *Mycobacterium tuberculosis*. PLoS Pathogens. 2014;**10**(9):e1004376. DOI: 10.1371/journal.ppat.1004376

[90] Sethi D, Mahajan S, Singh C, Lama A, Hade MD, Gupta P, et al. Lipoprotein LprI of *Mycobacterium tuberculosis* acts as a lysozyme inhibitor. The Journal of Biological Chemistry. 2016;**291**(6):2938-2953

[91] Slama N, Jamet S, Frigui W, Pawlik A, Bottai D, Laval F, et al. The changes in mycolic acid structures caused by hadC mutation have a dramatic effect on the virulence of *Mycobacterium tuberculosis*. Molecular Microbiology. 2016;**99**(4):794-807

[92] Naffin-Olivos JL, Georgieva M, Goldfarb N, Madan-Lala R, Dong L, Bizzell E, et al. *Mycobacterium tuberculosis* Hip1 modulates macrophage responses through proteolysis of GroEL2. PLoS Pathogens. 2014;**10**(5):e1004132. DOI: 10.1371/journal.ppat.1004132

[93] Rengarajan J, Murphy E, Park A, Krone CL, Hett EC, Bloom BR, et al. *Mycobacterium tuberculosis* Rv2224c modulates innate immune responses. Proceedings of the National Academy of Sciences of the United States of America. 2008;**105**(1):264-269

[94] Madan-Lala R, Sia JK, King R, Adekambi T, Monin L, Khader SA, et al. *Mycobacterium tuberculosis* impairs dendritic cell functions through the serine hydrolase Hip1. Journal of Immunology. 2014;**192**(9):4263-4272. Available from: http://www.jimmunol.org/cgi/doi/10.4049/jimmunol.1303185

[95] Elena G, Elena RME, Scandurra M, Gafa V, Pardini M, et al. Expression of proinflammatory and regulatory cytokines via NF-κB and MAPK-dependent and IFN regulatory factor-3-independent mechanisms in human primary monocytes infected by *Mycobacterium tuberculosis*. Clinical & Developmental Immunology. 2011;**2011**:841346. DOI: 10.1155/2011/841346

[96] Remoli ME, Giacomini E, Petruccioli E, Gafa V, Severa M, Gagliardi MC, et al. Bystander inhibition of dendritic cell differentiation by *Mycobacterium tuberculosis* -induced IL-10. Immunology and Cell Biology. 2011;**89**(3):437-446 Available from: http://www.ncbi.nlm.nih.gov/pubmed/20805841

[97] Ghorpade DS, Holla S, Sinha AY, Alagesan SK, Balaji KN. Nitric oxide and KLF4 protein epigenetically modify class II transactivator to repress major histocompatibility complex II expression during *Mycobacterium bovis* Bacillus Calmette-Guerin infection. The Journal of Biological Chemistry. 2013;**288**(28):20592-20606

[98] Chandran A, Antony C, Jose L, Mundayoor S, Natarajan K, Kumar RA. *Mycobacterium tuberculosis* infection induces HDAC1-mediated suppression of IL-12B gene expression in macrophages. Frontiers in Cellular and Infection Microbiology. 2015;**5**(December):1-14. Available from: http://journal.frontiersin.org/Article/10.3389/fcimb.2015.00090/abstract

[99] Colangeli R, Haq A, Arcus VL, Summers E, Magliozzo RS, McBride A, et al. The multifunctional histone-like protein Lsr2 protects mycobacteria against reactive oxygen intermediates. Proceedings of the National Academy of Sciences of the United States of America. 2009;**106**(11):4414-4418

11

Interaction between *Mycobacterium tuberculosis* and Human Host: Role of Cytokines in Pathogenesis and Treatment Monitoring

Mikhael M. Averbakh and Atadzhan Ergeshow

Abstract

Tuberculosis is one of the most prevalent infections of human beings. According to WHO Global tuberculosis report 2016, there were 10.4 million new incidents of TB cases worldwide, and 580,000 new cases of multidrug resistant (MDR) tuberculosis. Monitoring the effectiveness of tuberculosis treatment and timely diagnosis of latent tuberculosis is an important problem for immunological research. Interaction of M. tuberculosis and the human immune system begins with phagocytosis of mycobacteria by macrophages and activate the immune response through the cytokines and chemokines release. The balance of proinflammatory and immunoregulatory cytokines and chemokines production may reflect the level of host-parasite interaction (e.g., elimination or persistence of the microbe). The review presents current clinical trends in studies on proinflammatory (IL-12, IL-1, INF-II, TNF-α) and immunoregulatory (IL-10 and TGF-β) cytokines, as well as matrix metalloproteases and hemoxygenase 1 to characterize the success of antituberculous chemotherapy. Monitoring the effectiveness of tuberculosis treatment will require the use new combinations of cytokines, chemokines, and nonspecific inflammatory factors which combinations have not yet been determined. The most promising area is studying of immunoregulatory cytokines, (e.g., IL-10, TGF-β), cell migration factors (e.g., IP-10/CXCL-10, MIG/CXCL/9), and markers of nonspecific inflammation (e.g., HO-1, SAA and MMP-1,3,9).

Keywords: *Mycobacterium tuberculosis*, immunopathology, cytokines, chemokines

1. How the TB pathogen infects the host

According to the existing scientific data based on numerous experimental studies, the macrophages and myeloid subpopulation of the dendritic cells from the upper and lower respiratory tract are first contacted with inhaled foreign antigens (including mycobacteria), phagocytize them through several receptors (mannose receptor, surfactant D, DC-SIGN-specific for dendritic cells, integrated molecule, C-lectin receptor, Nod-like molecules, and Toll-like molecules). Subsequently, some of the phagocytosed mycobacteria are transferred by dendritic cells to regional lymph nodes where they are localized through the interaction of the CCR7 receptor with the ligand CCL19/21 expressed on the endothelial cells of the lymph nodes. This was shown in an experiment using mycobacteria labeled with fluorescent protein GFP [1]. These dendritic cells have on the surface of CCR7, which binds to ligands CCL19/21, expressed on endothelial cells of lymph nodes. Here, the dendritic cells produce a sufficient amount of IL-12p40, IL-12Rβ1, and CD11c and provide the initialization of the immune response through the priming of T helper 1 in the subsequent production of effector and memory cells and their migration to the sites of invasion, where the inflammatory response provides the development the specific granuloma formation. Also, mycobacteria can be lysed in phagolysosomes or die in apoptotic macrophages, or killed with cytolytic molecules of NK- or CD8+ cells.

Mycobacterium tuberculosis, found in macrophages, has genetic deterministic mechanisms of avoiding digestion inside phagocytes and persistent persistence in the host tissues [2]. In the initial stages, mycobacterial expression of the phthiocerol dimycoceroserate molecule (PDIM) limits the recognition of Mtb through Toll receptors (TLRs) and the phenolic glycolipids (PGLs). The mycobacterial cell wall lipids prevent the fusion of MTB containing phagosomes with lysosomes through a decrease recruitment of vacuolar H+/ATPase. The mycobacterial lipids lipoarabinomannan, trehalose dimycolate, and the sulfolipids also block the phagosome/lysosome fusion. In addition, bacterial phosphatase SapM and serine/threonine kinase PknG disrupt the dephosphorylation of phosphatidylinositol 3-phosphate (PI3P) and protein kinase G (PknG) and disturb the phagosome maturation [3].

MTB has genes that prevent their death in macrophages through an aphototic mechanism. Superoxide dismutase A (SodA) interferes with the caspase-dependent mechanism of macrophage apoptosis. The nuG gene, which is part of the fourteenth operon gene and codes type I NADH dehydrogenase (NDH-1), is important for neutralizing reactive oxygen species (ROS) created by macrophage phagocyte oxidase (NOX2). The importance of the operon of the 7-gene (Rv3654c-Rv3660c) for the inhibition of apoptosis of mycobacteria is also described. This mechanism is associated with inhibition of caspase-8 pre-mRNA splicing and a decrease in this protein in macrophages [4]. Virulent mycobacteria can suppress the early stages of apoptosis by cleaves the amino terminus of annexin 1 and subsequent inhibition of annexin 1 deposition on the apoptotic membrane.

The predominance of necrotic death of macrophages results in reduced mycobacterial antigen presentation by macrophages and dendritic cells [5]. On one hand, this stimulates the further accumulation of neutrophils, monocytes, macrophages, lymphocytes, and dendritic cells in the granulomas; and on the other hand, the spread of the pathological process to the surrounding tissues. Adequate TNF-α production promotes the formation of granulomas, while excessive production of TNF-α due to stimulation with MTB tricalcium dimycolate leads to a progression of the process. Mycobacteria use their adenylate cyclase to deliver excess cAMP to the macrophage cytoplasm. This leads to suppression macrophage functions and provides a pro-granulomatous response.

Inhibition of the apoptosis process is facilitated by the region of difference 1 (RD1), and type VII secretion system (ESX) of the mycobacterium genome. This leads to activation of Calpain, and Ca^{2+}-activated protease and calcification of necrosis. The resulting tissue hypoxia contributes to the activation of the restorative regulator (DosR) of the mycobacterial genome and their transition to the dermatological state with low metabolic activity [6]. The survival of such mycobacteria occurs within the microlipid droplets that are formed when the cell membranes of the host cells are destroyed [7].

Reactivation of mycobacteria and subsequent exacerbation of the tuberculosis process usually occurs when the host's immune system is weakened or suppressed due to physiological or pathological factors. This process is provided by the Rpf system of mycobacterial genes. The production of Rpf proteins, which are structurally close to the lytic transglycosylases, leads to the hydrolysis of peptidoglycans of cell membranes and intercellular fibers, increases the permeability of tissue for blood and lymph and the inflow of nutrients. The result of these processes is activation of the mycobacteria vital activity [8].

2. Cytokines and chemokines dynamics in TB diagnosis and treatment

The pathogen and innate immunity system interaction begins with the recognition of the conservative mycobacteria antigenic structures (so-called pathogen-associated molecular patterns—PAMR). This process depends on the interaction with PPR (pathogen recognition receptors), TOL-like receptors (TOLRs), NOD-like nucleotide oligomerization domain (NOD)-like receptors, C-lectin, and mannose-binding lectin-MBL receptors. These interactions stimulate the production of pro-inflammatory cytokines and chemokines that facilitate the migration activation of cells to the sites of inflammation [9]. Microbial invasion is accompanied by host cells and tissues damage and release the parts of collagen fibers, RNA, DNA fragments, and membrane phospholipids degradation product. Such damage-associated molecular patterns (DAMP) are an additional inflammatory stimulus. Almost every cell and even platelets contains a PRR repertoire and can react to such damage factors. Interaction of microbial PAMP and endogenous DAMP causes the systemic inflammatory response (or SIRS—systemic inflammatory response syndrome) [10]. All these stimuli activate the cytokines and chemokines production and the host acquired immunity reactions. The secretion of interferons (and primarily the INF-γ) by T-helper 1 (Th1) is a key point in the control of mycobacterial infections. The strength of Th1 response does not always correlate with bacterial clearance and increased host resistance. T-helper 17 (Th17) and regulatory T cells (Tregs) subpopulations are also important. Numerous cytokines, chemokines, and other humoral factors provide the macrophages and lymphocytes interaction. This section presents the main results of experimental and clinical studies on several major cytokine families.

3. Interleukin IL-12 family

IL-12 interleukin family is represented by four heterodimeric members: IL-12p70, IL-23, IL-27 and the newest member IL-35 consisting of each of the specific subunits. These cytokines have sufficient homology in the structure of subunits and interaction with receptors, but play a different role in the generation and maintenance of reactions of acquired immunity. Heterodimeric IL-12p70 consists of two homodimeric subunits IL-12p40 and IL-12p35, which are predominantly produced and function in various immunological compartments (IL-12p40 and IL-12p35 in inflammation foci).

Heterodimeric IL-12p70 consists of two homodimeric subunits IL-12p40 and IL-12p35, which are predominantly produced and function in various immunological compartments (IL-12p40 and IL-12p35 in inflammation foci, and IL-12p70 in lymph nodes) by binding to appropriate receptors (IL-12Rβ1 and/or IL-12Rβ2 or the IL-23R). Mutations in the subunits of IL-12 or their receptors and, accordingly, inadequate character of the produced signal causes an increased sensitivity to mycobacterial infection. The presence of adequate amounts of IL-12p70 in the lymph nodes ensures a sufficient production of Th1 and production of INF-γ [11]. IL-23 and IL-27 are released in the early stages of mycobacterial infection in the lungs and in the lymph nodes. IL-23 potentiates the production of IL-17, and IL-27 promotes the production of INF-γ. Possibilities of clinical use of IL-12, as in other and other key cytokines (INF-γ, TNF-α, IL-1β, and IL-6) for diagnosis and monitoring of tuberculosis are largely limited by the presence of allelic variants of these proteins. For example, the presence of polymorphism in the IL-12B gene influences the spontaneous and antigen-stimulated production of the IL-12p40 subunit, where the patient with the AA genotype are weak, and the SS is a strong producer of IL-12p40 [12].

4. Interleukin IL-1 family

The IL-1 cytokine family is represented by 11 members, of which IL-1α, IL-1β, IL-18, and IL-33 were studied in an experiment model and patients with pulmonary and extrapulmonary tuberculosis. The available now data point to the important role of IL-1α and IL-1β. The significance of IL-18 and IL-33 for the course of the tuberculosis process has not yet been adequately studied. Unlike IL-1α, IL-1β is produced in an inactive form. Its change into the active form occurs in the inflamasomes after the cell activation (predominantly in lung macrophages and dendritic cells, and in other organs epithelial, endothelial cells, and fibroblasts) with the corresponding signal through the NLRP3 receptor on the proforma of the caspase-1 enzyme. There is another variant of the formation of the active form of IL-1β, which proceeds outside inflamasomas, after the action of other proteolytic enzymes (chymase, cathepsin, elastase). The main function of IL-1 consist of the control pro-inflammatory reactions in case of damage due to PAMP activation with viruses and bacteria, or and DAMP activation in host tissues by acting with the crystals of uric acid and adenosine-5, triphosphate [13].

IL-1α and IL-1β independently exert their action primarily through type I IL-1 receptor (IL-1R1). IL-1β causes differentiation of monocytes into macrophages and increases their phagocytic and antigen-presenting capacity [14]. The clinical IL-1α and IL-1β level significance for course of the tuberculosis process and the effectiveness of chemotherapy has not yet revealed a significant difference between the groups of patients with active and latent tuberculosis, unlike cytokines such as IL-2 and IFN-γ [15].

The significance of IL-18 for antituberculosis immunity, which, like IL-1β, is a pro-inflammatory factor, is currently at the stage of experimental studies. IL-18 plays the role of Th1 lymphocyte differentiating factor. IL-18 knockout mice are more susceptible to aerosol challenge with mycobacteria and produce less IFN-γ compared to wild-type mice [14].

5. Tumor necrosis factor family

To date, the family of tumor necrosis factors is represented by the main member TNF-α and its functional analogues LTα and LTβ lymphotoxins, among which the first factor is most significant for intracellular infections. The pro-inflammatory cytokine tumor necrosis factor (TNF-α) is produced predominantly by macrophages in response to stimuli activating through Toll-like receptors and also can be expressed by activated T, B and NK cells. TNF exists as a trimer in the form of transmembrane protein and in a secreted form in serum. Both forms act by binding to TNFRp55 and TNFRp75 receptors, the soluble form interacting predominantly with TNFRp55, and the membrane form interacting with TNFRp75.

TNF is a multipotent cytokine playing roles in the processes of apoptosis, activation, differentiation, and recruitment of cells into inflammatory foci. With regard to tuberculosis, TNF-α is involved in the differentiation of T cells secreting Th1 cytokines, the formation of tuberculous granulomas with activation of phagocytic macrophages and epithelioid cells, killing mycobacteria in cooperation with INF-γ, stimulation of macrophage apoptosis containing mycobacteria, stimulation production of chemokines (s CCL-2, -3, -4, -5, -8) and endothelial cell expression of adhesion molecules (CD54), which leads to accumulation of cells in inflammatory foci [16]. Variants of allelic polymorphism of the TNF-α molecule at positions -238, -308, -857, -863, related to sensitivity to tuberculosis are described. Based on the meta-analysis of published clinical and genetic studies on the polymorphism variants of the TNF-α molecule Yu et al. [17] suggested that substitutions in the positions of TNF-α-308G > A and -238G > A are significantly associated with susceptibility to pulmonary tuberculosis regardless of ethnic status and the presence of HIV infection. Substitutions in the TNF-α molecule at positions -308G > A, -863C > A, and -238G > A are associated with susceptibility to pulmonary tuberculosis in uninfected HIV. The Asian population of tuberculosis patients is characterized by the replacement of -238G > A, whereas for the African population -308G > A.

To date, several studies have been conducted on sufficiently large contingents of tuberculosis patients to determine the TNF-α content in serum and cell cultures supernatant stimulated by various mycobacterial antigens. Its high production in supernatants of blood cultures was revealed by stimulation of 10 μg/ml of *M. tuberculosis* H37Rv sonicate in untreated patients, preserved in the effective course of chemotherapy and decreased, while the treatment course was ineffective. However, there were no significant differences between groups of patients, depending on the extent of the tuberculous process in the lungs. The authors concluded that the level of TNF-α production correlates more with the activity of the process than with its severity [18]. When comparing the production of TNF-α in a group of patients enrolled in a repeat chemotherapy course with its level determined during the initial course, its lower culture supernatants content was revealed along with other factors (IFN-γ, IP-10, MIG, and IL-2). The of blood culture of patients with active tuberculosis stimulated by monoantigens and their combination (ESAT-6, CFP-10, ESAT-6 + CFP-10, and ESAT-6 + CFP-10 + TB7.7) was shown that these combinations of antigens cause high production of TNF-α, whereas one antigen TB7.7 is not effective [19]. However, in these studies, the authors conclude that the study of TNF-α production level is not very informative for evaluating the effectiveness of treatment of patients with tuberculosis.

6. Interferon type II

Cytokines of the interferons family and especially interferon type II (IFN-γ) are the most studied factors of antituberculosis immunity due to great importance for phagocytosis and subsequent killing of mycobacterium tuberculosis. IFN-γ is produced primarily by activated CD4+ and CD8+T cells and to a lesser extent by $\gamma\delta$ T cells, NK T cells and NK cells belonging to the innate immunity system [15]. To date, two polymorphisms of IFN-γ gene in +874 (A/T) and + 5644 (A/G) are particularly important for the output level in patients with tuberculosis, in which the former is more often associated with susceptibility to tuberculosis infection, but this fact is not absolute and varies in different geographical regions [12]. The highest level of IFN-γ gene expression is detected in Th1-activated lymphocytes which stimulate the macrophages for killing of mycobacteria, enhance the cytotoxic activity of other cells, induce apoptosis in skin and mucosal epithelial cells, regulate the expression of MHC class I and II proteins, and antigen presentation. Take into account the key role of IFN-γ in antituberculosis immunity, a large number of experimental studies have been devoted to this problem which are summarized in a number of reviews [20]. The initial clinical studies on serum IFN-γ in patients with pulmonary and extrapulmonary forms of tuberculosis was shown that the concentration of this factor was significantly higher in comparison with the same group after treatment, the group of contacts and healthy volunteers. There is also a significant individual variability in the IFN-γ concentration in all studied groups [21]. The study of the IFN-γ synthesis in lymphocyte culture stimulated with PWM (5 μg/ml), PHA (10 μg/m), and tuberculin RT (12.5 and 25 μg/ml) in patients with different clinical forms of tuberculosis and a group of contacts revealed no differences in IFN-γ production in response to mitogens and a reliable increase in production in response to stimulation with tuberculin [1]. In a similar study of patients with different clinical forms of pulmonary tuberculosis (120 patients and 144 healthy volunteers of the same place of residence), the production of IFN-γ in lymphocyte culture was determined by stimulation with *M. tuberculosis* H37Rv sonicate at a dose of 10 μg/ml before chemotherapy and up to 6 months its conduct. It was shown that the IFN-γ production in the whole patient group before the start of treatment was low, increased during chemotherapy, and was compared to the volunteer level by 6 months. However, after subdividing the patient group according to the severity of the tuberculosis process, it was shown that in patients with small and medium severity of the process IFN-γ production before treatment was significantly higher than in severe lungs changes. During the course of chemotherapy, the IFN-γ production increased in most patients, but there was a significant variability and even a drop in the concentration of IFN-γ in some patients with small and medium process severity to the initial level [18].

Since the beginning of the 2000s, several laboratory tests (interferon gamma release assays (IGRAs)) were developed for the IFN-γ revealing in the culture medium and intracellularly. The first of these was a QFT test (QuantiFERON-TB test, Cellestis Limited, Carnegie, Victoria, Australia), which used the ELISA method to determine the amount of IFN-γ secreted by cultured blood cells in response to PPD in comparison to the control antigenic stimulus of *M. avium* and saline as a negative control. However, the specificity of QFT was less than that of the Mantou skin test. The next-generation test (QuantiFERON-TB Gold—QFT-G) appeared in 2005. It used the proteins encoded by the RD1-locus of *M. tuberculosis* (ESAT-6 and CFP-10) as an antigenic stimulus. The test effectiveness t was determined as differences in the IFN-γ concentration in response to ESAT-6 or CFP-10 stimulation minus the values of spontaneous production of the factor. The ESAT-6/CFP-10 proteins are absent in vaccine strains of mycobacteria, but are present in *M. kansasii, M. szulgai,* and *M. marinum,* and sensitization with these mycobacteria can cause false-positive results of IGRA.

The next modification of the IGRAs-test (QuantiFERON-TB Gold In-Tube-QFT-GIT) was developed to more accurately determine antigen-stimulated synthesis IFN-γ which largely depended on preserving the activity of patient's blood cells samples. The blood was immediately placed in test tubes with lower antigenic stimuli in order to avoid loss of viability during transport of the samples to the laboratory. A mixture of 14 peptides copying the entire amino acid sequence of ESAT-6 and CFP-10 proteins and part of the TB7.7 sequence was used as antigenic stimuli. As a negative and positive control, test tubes with heparin and PHA were used. After a 16- to 24-h-incubation, the concentration of IFN-γ c was determined by the ELISA used in the QFT-G test. Exceeding response of the tested patient by 25–50% compared to the zero control was considered a positive indicator, less than 25% was interpreted as a negative result, while at QFT-G it was estimated as an intermediate.

The fourth T-Spot test began to use in 2008. The IFN-γ-secreting cells were determined in the 96-plate test well using the ELISpot method. The proteins ESAT-6 and CFP-10 were used separately as an antigenic stimulus. The result was determined by the difference in the number of cells (spots) compared to the control (spontaneous production by IFN-γ cells without antigenic stimulus). Because QFT-G, QFT-GIT, T-Spot, and skin tests (TST) examine various aspects of the immune response, use different antigens and have different criteria for interpreting the results, the tests are not interchangeable [22].

The development in the early 2000s of a new multiplex method of simultaneous multiple studies of genes and protein factors opened new possibilities for studying cytokines, chemokines, and the inflammation acute phase proteins in various tuberculosis clinical forms [2]. The results obtained revealed many humoral immunological criteria for active and latent tuberculosis in different age and geographical contingents of patients. Various immunodominant proteins were used as an antigenic stimulus, but mainly it was the combination of the RD1 peptides ESAT-6 and CFP-10 genomic locus of the mycobacteria. Despite some inconsistency of the results, the most informative is the combination of cytokines and chemokines (IFN-γ, IP-10, MIG, TNF-a, and IL-2), which showed the greatest differences between patients with active tuberculosis and a control group of healthy volunteers. The diagnostic significance of the combination of IFN-γ, IP-10, and MIG was the highest (96.3%). In cases of unsuccessful treatment or reactivation of the process, the concentration of this group of factors was less significant and the diagnostic sensitivity decreased by 20–25% [23]. Kellar et al. [24] identified differences in the production of IFN-γ and other cytokines and chemokines in response to stimulation of blood culture in patients with active tuberculosis with monoantigens and their combination (ESAT-6, CFP-10, ESAT-6 + CFP-10, and ESAT-6 + CFP-10 + TB7.7). The IFN-γ production was determined by ELISA, multiplex analysis, and quantitative immunomicroarray methods. The two latest methods was used to examine the production of cytokines IL-1α, IL-1β, IL-2, IL-4, IL-5, IL-6, IL-8, IL-10, IL-12, IL-13, GM-CSF, GRO, MCP-1, MIP-1α, MIP-1β, MMP-9, RANTES, TNF-α, and VEGF. The ELISA method identified significant differences in the IFN-γ production in response to ESAT-6, CFP-10, TB7.7 and a combination of ESAT-6+CFP-10, and ESAT-6+CFP-10+TB7.7 compared to the control group. The differences in the production of IFN-γ in response to ESAT-6+CFP-10 versus ESAT-6+CFP-10+TB7.7 are not reliable. The response to a mixture of antigens is always greater than for individual antigens. Multiplex analysis showed that the antigens ESAT-6, CFP-10, ESAT-6+CFP-10, and ESAT-6+CFP-10+TB7.7 stimulated production of not only IFN-γ, but also IL-2, IL-8, MCP-1, and MIP-1β in patients compared with control group. The immunomicroarray method revealed that when stimulating ESAT-6+CFP-10+TB7.7, a greater number of IFN-γ, IL-2, IL-6, IL-8, IP-10, MCP-1, MIP-1β, and TNF-α, than in the control group. The authors conclude that the determination of many cytokines improves the diagnosis of tuberculosis in comparison with the IFN-γ determination only. Four cytokines are the best diagnostic markers for mycobacterial infection (sensitivity and specificity were 100% for IL-2, IL-6, IP-10, and MIP-1β.) The sensitivity of the commercial multiplex analysis test system for IFN-γ was 91.6% and specificity of 100%.

There are studies characterizing the cytokine spectrum of the antigen-stimulated blood cells in children and adolescents patients with active and latent tuberculosis in comparison with those who do not contact the tuberculosis patients. Kellar et al. [24], using multiplex analysis, studied a spectrum of 29 cytokines and blood chemokines in a group of children and adolescents (135 people, including 46 with latent tuberculosis, 11 patients with active tuberculosis and 35 uninfected persons, age 2–15 years) after stimulation with peptides QFT-G, PPD, and recombinant ESAT-6 protein. In general, the level of cytokines after stimulation with peptides QFT-G (IFN-γ, IL-2, IP-10, and IL-13) was significantly lower in children without infection than in patients with tuberculosis, the most significant in children older than 5 years of age. Children with latent TB have a high IFN-γ, IL-2, IP-10, IL-13, and IL-5 level in comparison with uninfected children. The spontaneous and antigen-stimulated (QFT-G) TGF-β1 production was significantly higher in children with tuberculosis over 5 years of age than in the similar group with latent tuberculosis. In the age group under the age of 5 years, there was no significant difference in the cytokine production in children with latent tuberculosis compared to uninfected controls. Other relationships were obtained with PPD stimulating blood cultures. Higher IL-2, IL-13, and IL-4 production were detected in comparison with recombinant ESAT-6 stimulation [24, 25]. Armand et al.

[27] stimulated blood cultures with QFT-G test system peptides from children and adolescents aged 4–15 years with latent and various forms of tuberculosis and patients without signs of disease. The multiplex analysis of the of 14 cytokines and chemokines production revealed significant differences in IL-2, INF-γ, IL-5, IP-10 level between the control group and tuberculosis patients. There were no differences in the production of TNF-α. For patients with more severe forms of tuberculosis found no differences in the production of these factors except for a significant decrease in production of IL-5 and IL-13. The increase TNF-α production, as well as the high IL-2, INF-γ level were observed in children with lymph node form tuberculosis of the 4–15 years age group with positive skin tests Mantoux and DST [26].

7. Immunoregulatory cytokines IL-10 and TGF-β

Interleukin-10 (IL-10) is a multifunctional regulatory cytokine of inflammatory responses. Numerous studies have shown that IL-10 acts as a general inhibitor of proliferative responses of both T helper (Th) 1 and Th2 cells *in vitro* and *in vivo*. IL-10 regulates inflammation through the suppression of the production of cytokines such as IL-1α, IL-1β, IL-6, IL-8, IL-12, and tumor necrosis factor-alpha in activated macrophage and interferon gamma in T cells [27].

TGF-β is the main representative of the family, which nowadays consists of 35 factors, including 5 isoforms of TGF-β, bone morphogenic protein (BMP), growth differentiation factors (GDFs), activin, and inhibin factors. TGF-β is secreted in an inactive form (L-TGF-β) and the molecule is activated after the action of plasmin, thrombospodin-1, reactive oxygen radicals, and $\alpha V\beta 6$ integrin [28].

In the case of tuberculosis, the main producers of IL-10 and TGF-β are the regulatory antigen-specific Th1 and Th3 cells, respectively, which are activated after cooperation with dendritic cells and stipulate an optimal balance of interaction with specific effector T cells and control of tuberculosis infection for the purpose of excessive immunopathological response [29]. Nowadays, there are several studies in which the levels of IL-10 and TGF-β were determined in patients with various forms of tuberculosis and during specific chemotherapy. Jang et al. [30] found a significantly higher serum TGF-β content in patients with active pulmonary tuberculosis compare to the control group and no difference were found for serum level of IL-10. Chowdhurya et al. [31] showed a significantly higher serum production of not only TGF-β, but also IL-10 in patients with newly diagnosed tuberculosis before treatment compared to the control group of healthy volunteers. At the same time, serum TGF-β (as well as IFN-γ, TNF-α, and IL-6) level correlated with the severity of bacteremia and the radiological spread of the process. The study of TGF-β and IL-10 levels at 2, 4, and 6 months of treatment showed that within 2 months the level remained high and then gradually decreased to the fourth and sixth months, approaching the control group. Interesting results are also found for IL-6 dynamics. This factor decreased from second to fourth treatment and then did not change. The authors suggested that IL-6 can serve as a marker of the effectiveness of chemotherapy and tested the dynamics of cytokine in patients with different levels of initial bacterial release. The obtained individual curves of this cytokine content accurately reflected the effectiveness of the course of chemotherapy. Decrease in TGF-β serum production and insignificant IL-10 level at the end of the 6-month course of chemotherapy was revealed in the study by Ameglio et al. [32]. Also, there was a difference in the production of these cytokines was observed depending on the severity of fibrotic changes in the lung tissue.

8. Chemokines. CXCL-10 (IP-10)

Chemokines play a central role in the recruitment of cells into the mycobacteria infected lung, which contributes to the delimitation of the focus of inflammation from the surrounding healthy tissues. However, under specific conditions, chemokines can also cause the disproportionate inflammation and subsequent progression of the process with formation of foci of destruction of lung tissue. In humans, the balance between protective and damaging inflammation, as well as the levels of inflammation can depend on many factors, including host genotype, bacterial strain, co-morbidities, and nutritional status. Understanding the nature and the effect of these interactions between the host, mycobacteria and the environment can serve as a basis for effective therapeutic and vaccination strategies. With tuberculosis as well as other infections, the inflammatory process is regulated by a cascade of reactions, including action adhesion molecules and chemoattractant. Chemokines are a family of small proteins, which, upon binding to membrane G protein-coupled receptors, guide the gradient-driven migration of leukocytes. Chemokines are classified into the CXC-, CC-, C-, and CX3C-subfamilies according to the arrangement of four conserved cysteine residues, which are important for maintenance of their tridimensional structure. Monin [33], summarizing the available literature data, identify the positive, negative, and terrible role of chemokines in tuberculosis, which probably exists with all heavy infections. To date, the dynamics of change and the diagnostic significance of only one chemokine IP-10 have been studied most fully in tuberculosis.

Interferon gamma inducible protein 10 (IP-10), or CXCL10, is a member of the CXC family of α-chemokines that stimulate the migration and adhesion of activated Th 1 cells through binding to the CXCR3 receptor [30]. IP-10 is secreted directly by macrophage cells infected with viruses and bacteria, and even more so after T cells recognize specific peptides on the surface of antigen-presenting cells. The secretion of IP-10 is enhanced by T cell secreted INF-γ and the numerous pro-inflammatory cytokines IL-2, IFN-α, IFN-β, IL-27, IL-17, IL-23, TNF-α, and IL -1β which are secreted by antigen-presenting cells [34]. Ruhwald et al. [35] determined various sets of cytokines and chemokines in blood supernatants of patients with tuberculosis obtained by QFT-IT test using the multiplex method and revealed a high concentration of IP-10 compared to the control group. In subsequent studies in the adult contingent of tuberculosis patients, groups contacting with patients and age-matched control, it was confirmed that IP-10 is statistically higher produced in patients with tuberculosis and gives comparable results with the QFT-IT test [34].

Several studies have examined the diagnostic value of IP-10 in children aged 1–17 years in countries with high and low incidence of tuberculosis. To determine the antigen of stimulated chemokine production, the multiplex analysis method was used in comparison with the determination of the INF-γ in the QFT-IT test. It was shown that in children and adolescents, as well as in adults, spontaneous production of IP-10 was higher in children with latent and active tuberculosis, compared to the group of healthy and antigen-stimulated synthesis, gave more stable results compared with the production of INF-γ. Also, there are no age differences in the production of IP-10 [24, 36]. In the study, Ruhwald et al. [37], a cut-off point 673 pg/ml was determined for the antigen-stimulated IP-10 synthesis for the adult contingent, above which the reaction was considered diagnostically positive. Lighter et al. [19] identified a similar indicator for children and adolescents, which was 732 pg/ml. The authors showed that the IP-10 level in plasma was higher in patients with active tuberculosis than in the group of latent tuberculosis. Antigen-stimulated synthesis, on the contrary, was higher in the group of latent tuberculosis.

Studies on the dynamics changes of IP-10 in the serum and supernatant of blood cultures are single. Hong et al. [35] studied the chemokine values in 32 adult patients with pulmonary tuberculosis before and after 2 months of specific treatment. The authors showed that the initial serum level of IP-10 correlated with the degree of detection of MBT in the smear. At 0–1°, the average score was 132.5 pg/ml, and at grade 2–299.2 pg/ml. The patients studied on the basis of the severity of clinical signs were divided into groups of low and medium/severe risk of the course of the disease. The initial serum level of IP-10 groups did not differ, but in the low-risk group it significantly decreased during treatment, and remained unchanged in the middle/severe risk group. Similar trends in the change in the chemokine content during treatment are shown in the study of the antigen of stimulated synthesis in a 24-h blood culture, where the QFT-IT system was used as antigens [38].

In our studies, statistically significant increases in spontaneous and antigen-stimulated (20 μg/ml PPD and 1 μg/ml ESAT 6/CFP 10) production of IP-10 in children and adolescents with different forms of pulmonary tuberculosis were found compared with the group of latent tuberculosis. Decreased production of IP-10 revealed patients with lymph nodes form and focal tuberculosis by the third and especially by the sixth month of follow-up. In the group of patients with destructive tuberculosis, IP-10 production decreased after 3 months of treatment in patients with positive dynamics of the disease (disappearance of signs of tuberculous intoxication and cessation of bacterial release). The torpid and progressive nature of the tuberculosis process (the preservation of bacterial release for more than 6 months and the spread of the pulmonary tissue lesion) was not accompanied by a decrease in the production of chemokine IP-10 [39].

9. Matrix metalloproteases

Matrix metalloproteinases (MMPs) are a multigenic family of structurally and functionally similar Zn- and Ca-dependent endopeptidases that are able to modify all known components of the extracellular matrix, as well as many non-matrix molecules. The MMPs family consists of more than 60 enzymes, of which 20 are found in human tissues. A common feature of MMPs is the ability to hydrolyze the main components of the extracellular matrix containing Zn^{2+} ions in the active site of molecules using Ca^{2+} ions for molecular stabilization. They are secreted from the cells in an inactive form and their catalytic activity is suppressed by specific tissue inhibitors of metalloproteinases (TIMPs). Based on the MMP's primary structure, substrate specificity and cellular localization and they are classified into three groups, including six subfamilies.

10. Family I

MMPs secretory type (classical, free, soluble):

- collagenase (MMP-1, MMP-8, MMP-13, MMP-18);
- gelatinases (MMP-2, MMP-9);
- stromelysins (MMP-3, MMP-10, MMP-15);
- matrilizines (MMP-7, MMP-26).

11. Family II

MMPs associated with cell membranes (membrane type MT-MMP-14, -15, -16, -17, -24, -25).

12. Family III

Unclassified MMPs, with no relation to known subfamilies (MMP-11, -12, -19, -20).

Synthesis and secretion of metalloproteinases is realized by various blood and tissue cells (neutrophils, monocytes, macrophages, fibroblasts, osteoclasts, chondrocytes, keratinocytes, endothelial, and epithelial cells) but also by oncogene-transformed cells. MMPs induced by tissue growth factors such as epidermal growth factor, fibroblast growth factor, cytokine-TNFα, TNFβ, IL-1, IL-6, melatonin, hormones and neuropeptides, and oxidative stress. The importance of MMR for the pathogenesis and nature course of the disease is shown to arthritis, psoriasis, atopic dermatitis, atherosclerosis, neurodegenerative diseases, strokes, ischemic myocardial damage, periodontitis, primary open-angle glaucoma, thyroid gland diseases, chronic infections, and much more [40, 41]. Chang et al. [28] using the myeloid line THP-1 showed that *M. tuberculosis* and the main cell wall component LAM stimulate gene expression of MMP-1 and MMP-9 and the MMP-9 release in culture media suggesting their involvement in the digestion of collagen I to IV types, and indirect stimulation of IL-1, TNF-α. Subsequent studies showed that stimulation with virulent *M. tuberculosis* strain causes gene expression of MMP-1, -3, -7, and -10, and the expression of MMP-1 is stimulated more than with vaccine strain *M. bovis* (BCG) [7]. Similar results were obtained on the culture of blood mononuclear cells. MMP-1, -7, and -9 were found immunohistochemically in tuberculosis granuloma epithelioid and Pirogov-Langhans cells [42].

There are single clinical studies to identify MMP-1, -2, -8, and -9 in pleural fluid in tuberculous pleurisy and cerebrospinal fluid in patients with tuberculous meningitis. Parks et al. [7] conducted a comparative study of MMP-1, -2, -3, -7, -8, -9, and TIMP-1 and TIMP-2 in sputum by multiplex analysis in patients with tuberculosis during 24 weeks of antituberculous chemotherapy. The authors showed that the concentration of these factors was significantly higher in patients than in the control group of healthy volunteers except MMP-7, while the level of MMP-3 and -9 increased 15.2-fold and 14.4 times. The MMP concentration decreased during the treatment and for MMP-1. MMP-3 and MMP-8 concentration significantly different at the second, eighth and twenty-fourth weeks, while the TIMP-1 and-2 concentration increased at 2 and 8 weeks and TIMP-2 significantly by the twenty-fourth week of follow-up. Comparison of this data with microbiological indicators revealed that the concentration of MMP-2, MMP-8, MMP-9, and TIMP-2 was significantly higher in MTB positive patients before treatment. MMP-3, MMP-8, and TIMP-1 were increased significantly at 2 weeks of treatment in MBT positive patients in comparison with MBT negative. Unfortunately, the authors do not give data on the correlation of MMP and TIMP concentrations with the presence of cavernous lung lesions. The availability of such information can be useful for predicting the growth of destructive processes in lung tissue.

13. Markers of oxidative stress. Hemoxygenase 1

Hemoxygenase is a microsomal enzyme, which consists of inducible and constitutive isozymes (HO-1, HO-2) and catalyzes the decomposition of heme to CO, Fe+2, and biliverdin with conversion to bilirubin by biliverdin reductase. HO-1 is a major intracellular source of iron and carbon monoxide (CO). The investigated isoforms of HO are the products of various hmox-1 and hmox-2 genes. Hemoxygenase-1 is an inducible isoform of the enzyme, the synthesis of which is enhanced by the influence of temperature, heme components, heavy metal ions, cytokines, and reactive oxygen radicals.

HO-1 is an important part of the biological mechanism for protecting against oxidative stress and tissue damage and from excessive inflammation. The end-products of heme breakdown are potently antioxidant and anti-inflammatory, and in addition, modulation, cell proliferation and cell death, either positively or negatively, but in a manner that seems to relate to the re-establishment of a homeostasis in many diseases pathogenic mechanisms. The protective value of hemoxygenase-1 is inhibition of the synthesis of inflammatory factors (IL-1, IL-6, IL-8, TNF-α), anti-inflammatory cytokines (IL-10), and heme degradation products and their metabolic derivatives. Carbon monoxide CO reduces the production of inducible NO-synthase (iNOS), cyclooxygenase-2, the corresponding inflammatory mediators—NO and prostaglandins. More detailed information on the structure and function of HO-1 can be found in the reviews of Ryter et al. [43] and Soares and Bach [12].

Diagnosis of tuberculosis is not particularly difficult in the presence of clinical, radiological, and especially microbiological data. The presence of negative microbiological results and latent forms of infection, even with positive results of tuberculin skin (TST) or IFN-γ tests, stimulates the search for additional laboratory markers. Studies in patients with active tuberculosis demonstrated a decrease in systemic concentrations of antioxidants and increased spontaneous generation of free radicals compared to those without tuberculosis, reflecting the excessive oxidative stress associated with this disease. Increased expression of HO-1 was observed in the plasma of people with various pulmonary pathologies, including acute respiratory distress syndrome, chronic obstructive pulmonary disease, and asthma. Elevations of HO-1 levels are identified in malaria, leishmaniasis and sepsis, and plasma levels of HO-1 are often associated with the severity of many other diseases [44]. However, clinical studies of the significance of NO-1 to confirm the diagnosis of tuberculosis and evaluate the effectiveness of treatment are few.

To date, there is a single clinical study conducted on a cohort of infected *M. tuberculosis* and infected individuals from South India with a high incidence of tuberculosis. Plasma samples were collected in 97 patients with active pulmonary tuberculosis (PTB), 35 patients with extra-pulmonary tuberculosis, (EPTB), 39 people with LTBI and 40 healthy donors under the cohort study program on tuberculosis [44]. Levels of HO-1, IL-10, TNF-α, IFN-γ, and IL-17 in plasma were measured by ELISA. Levels of C-reactive protein (CRP) and Serum Amyloid Protein-A (SAA) were determined using the Bioplex multiplex ELISA system.

The authors found significantly higher systemic levels of HO-1 in patients with active pulmonary or extrapulmonary tuberculosis (medians [IQR]: 5.8 [3.2–11.6] and 3.45 [2.0–4, 5] ng/ml, respectively, $P \leq 0.01$) than persons with latent tuberculosis or healthy donors (1.3 [0.78–1.5] and 1.4 [1.0–1.9] ng/ml, respectively, $P = 0.49$). Among patients with active pulmonary tuberculosis, those with bilateral lung lesions had higher systemic NO-1 levels compared to patients with unilateral lesions detected by the chest x-ray, indicating a possible association between HO-1 and the anatomical prevalence of the disease. The systemic levels of HO-1 were higher in those with positive AFB staining in sputum than in patients with negative smears. With an effective course of chemotherapy, the elevated NO-1 concentration in the plasma returned to background levels. This was not observed in patients with a negative result of treatment, as determined by positive sputum cultures at the end of the course of drug therapy.

The authors evaluated the ability of HO-1 to distinguish between active tuberculosis and latent TB infection in combination with two other markers of inflammation, CRP and SAA, whose significance is increased with active TB [45]. Elevated levels of HO-1, CRP, and SAA have been detected in plasma in patients with active tuberculosis (PTB and/or EPTB) compared to individuals with LTBI. In addition, the authors compared the significance of HO-1, CRP, and SAA for establishing the diagnosis of PTB or EPTB. Systemic levels of HO-1 and CRP were significantly higher in PTB cases, while SAA concentrations were slightly reduced. Further analysis showed that HO-1 was the most informative parameter for recognizing pulmonary from extrapulmonary tuberculosis. It was also found that in individuals with active pulmonary tuberculosis, the levels of HO-1 positively correlated with IL-10 levels ($r = 0.59$, $P = 0.001$) and negatively correlated with TNF-a levels ($r = -0.31$, $P = 0.002$). There were no significant correlations between the levels of HO-1 and IFN-γ or HO-1 and IL-17. The correlation coefficient of HO-1 and IL-10 was higher in patients with a higher bacillary index.

14. Concluding remarks

Diagnosis of tuberculosis is not particularly difficult in the presence of clinical, radiological, and especially microbiological data. The difficulty arises from negative results of microbiological examination and minor clinical manifestations of tuberculosis. In addition, a significant problem is infected persons without clinical manifestations with a negative result of tuberculin skin (TST) or IFN-γ test results. They make up a huge reservoir of latent tuberculosis infection (LTBI). In some of these latently infected individuals, the infection becomes active and seriously affects the epidemiological situation. These two problems will stimulate the search for additional and new markers of the disease.

The scientific studies carried out to date show a significant increase in the effectiveness of IGRAs-test in combination with the determination of chemokine CXCL/IP-10 for the diagnosis of latent forms of tuberculosis. Monitoring the effectiveness of treatment of tuberculosis will require the use of other combinations of cytokines, chemokines, and nonspecific inflammatory factors. This will depend on the sensitivity and resistance (MDR-TB) of mycobacteria to antituberculosis drugs and the nature of the course of tuberculous inflammation (positive, torpid or progressive dynamics of the disease) associated with genetically determined parasite-host interactions. The optimal combination of such factors has not yet been determined, but probable search vectors indicate on the definition of dynamics immunoregulatory cytokines (e.g., IL-10, TGF-β), chemokines characterizing cell migration (e.g., IP-10/CXCL-10, MIG/CXCL/9) and factors nonspecific inflammation (e.g., HO-1, SAA and MMP-1,3,9). Comparability of the results of these studies will depend on the proximity of the methodological platforms.

Author details

Mikhael M. Averbakh* and Atadzhan Ergeshow

*Address all correspondence to: amm50@mail.ru

FSBSI "Central TB Research Institute", Moscow, Russia

References

[1] Wolf AJ, Linas BL, Trevejo-Nunez GJ, Kincaid E, Tamura T, Takatsu K, Ernst GD. Mycobacterium tuberculosis infects dendritic cells with high frequency and impairs their function in vivo. Journal of Immunology. 2007;**179**:2509-2519

[2] Orme IM, Robinson RT, Cooper AM. The balance between protective and pathogenic immune responses in the TB-infected lung. Nature Immunology. 2015;**16**(1):57-63

[3] Ruhwald M, Bjerregaard-Andersen M, Rabna P, Kofoed K, Eugen-Olsen J, Ravn P. IP-10/CXCL10 release is induced by incubation of whole blood from tuberculosis patients with ESAT-6, CFP10 and TB7.7. Microbes and Infection. 2007;**9**:806-812

[4] Butz H, Rácz K, Hunyady L, Pato A. Crosstalk between TGF-b signaling and the microRNA machinery. Trends in Pharmacological Sciences. 2012;**33**:382-392

[5] Divangahi M. The new paradigm of immunity to tuberculosis. Advances in Experimental Medicine and Biology. 2013;**783**:1-289

[6] Rohde K, Yates RM, Purdy GE, Russell DG. Mycobacterium tuberculosis and the environment within the phagosome. Immunological Reviews. 2007;**219**:37-54

[7] Parks WC, Wilson CL, López-Boado YS. Matrix metalloproteinases as modulators of inflammation and innate immunity. Nature reviews.Immunology. 2004;**4**:617-629

[8] Ke Z, Yuan L, Ma J, Zhang X, Guo Y, Xiong H. IL-10 polymorphisms and tuberculosis susceptibility: An updated meta-analysis. Yonsei Medical Journal. 2015;**56**:1274-1287

[9] Ugarte-Gil1 CA, Elkington P, Gilman RH, Coronel J, Tezera LB, Bernabe-Ortiz A, Gotuzzo E, Friedland JS, Moore DAJ. Induced sputum MMP-1, -3 & -8 concentrations during treatment of tuberculosis. PLoS One. 2013;**8**(4):e61333

[10] Akdis M, Alar A, Altunbulakli C, Azkur K, Costa RA, Crameri R, Duan Sea. Interleukins (from IL-1 to IL-38), interferons, transforming growth factor b, and TNF-a: Receptors, functions, and roles in diseases. The Journal of Allergy and Clinical Immunology. 2016;**138**(4):984-1010

[11] Coussens A, Timms PM, Boucher BJ, et al. 1a, 25-dihydroxyvitamin D3 inhibits matrix metalloproteinases induced by Mycobacterium tuberculosis infection. Immunology. 2009;**127**:539-548

[12] Soares MP, Bach FH. Heme oxygenase-1: From biology to therapeutic potential. Trends in Molecular Medicine. 2008;**15**:50-58

[13] Di Pietrantonio T, Schurr E. Host-pathogen specificity in tuberculosis. In: Divangahi M, editor. The New Paradigm of Immunity to Tuberculosis; 2013. pp. 33-44

[14] Selvaraj P, Alagarasu K, Harishankar M, Vidyarani M, Rajeswari DN, Narayanan PR. Cytokine gene polymorphisms and cytokine levels in pulmonary tuberculosis. Cytokine. 2008;**43**:26-33

[15] Sahiratmadja E, Alisjahbana B, de Boer T, Adnan I, Maya A, Danusantoso H, Nelwan RH, Marzuki S, van der Meer JWM, van Crevel R, van de Vosse E, Ottenhoff THM. Dynamic changes in pro- and anti-inflammatory cytokine profiles and gamma interferon receptor signaling integrity correlate with tuberculosis disease activity and response to curative treatment. Infection and Immunity. 2007;**75**:820-829

[16] Elkington PT, Nuttall RK, Boyle JJ, et al. Mycobacterium tuberculosis, but not vaccine BCG, specifically upregulates matrix metalloproteinase-1. American Journal of Respiratory and Critical Care Medicine. 2005;**172**:1596-1604

[17] Yu Y, Zhang Y, Hu S, Dongdong J, Chen X, Liu H. Different patterns of cytokines and chemokines combined with IFN-c production reflect mycobacterium tuberculosis infection and disease. PLoS One. 2012;**7**(9):e44944

[18] Schenk M, Fabri M, Krutzik SR, Lee DJ, Vu DM, Sieling PA, Montoya D, Liu PT, Modlin RL. Interleukin-1b triggers the differentiation of macrophages with enhanced capacity to present mycobacterial antigen to T cells. Immunology. 2013;**141**:174-180

[19] Lighter J, Rigaud M, Huie M, Peng CH, Pollack H. Chemokine IP-10: An adjunct marker for latent tuberculosis infection in children. The International Journal of Tuberculosis and Lung Disease. 2009;**13**:731-736

[20] Ehlers S. Role of tumour necrosis factor (TNF) in host defence against tuberculosis: Implications for immunotherapies targeting TNF. Annals of the Rheumatic Diseases. 2003;**62**(Suppl II):ii37-ii42

[21] Wang X, Jiang J, Cao Z, Yang B, Zhang J, Cheng X. Diagnostic performance of multiplex cytokine and chemokine assay for tuberculosis. Tuberculosis. 2012;**92**:513-520

[22] Mills KH, McGuirk P. Antigen-specific regulatory T cells-Their induction and role in infection. Seminars in Immunology. 2004;**16**:107-117

[23] Winek J, Rowinska-Zakrzewska E, Demkow U, Szopinski J, Szolkowska M, Filewska M, Jagodzinski J, Roszkowski-Sliz K. Interferon gamma production in the course of mycobacterium tuberculosis infection. Journal of Physiology and Pharmacology. 2008; **59**(Suppl. 6):751-759

[24] Kellar KL, Gehrke J, Weis SE, Mahmutovic-Mayhew A, Davila B, Zajdowicz MJ, Scarborough R, LoBue PA, Lardizabal AA, Daley CL, Reves RR, Bernardo J, Campbel BH, Whitworth WC, Mazurek GH. Multiple cytokines are released when blood from Patients with tuberculosis is stimulated with Mycobacterium tuberculosis antigens. PLoS One. 2011;**6**(11):e26545

[25] Briken V. Mycobacterium tuberculosis genes involved in regulation of host cell death. In: Advances in Experimental Medicine and Biology. Vol. 783. Springer. Divangahi M, editor. The New Paradigm of Immunity to Tuberculosis; 2013. pp. 93-102

[26] Armand M, Chhor V, de Lauzanne A, El Khourouj VG, Pédron B, Jeljeli M, Gressens P, Faye A, Sterkers G. Cytokine responses to quantiferon peptides in pediatric tuberculosis: A pilot study. The Journal of Infection. 2014;**68**:62-70

[27] Markelova EV, Zdor VV, Romanchuk AL, Birko ON. Matrix metalloproteinases:Relationship with cytokines system, diagnostic and prognostic potential. Immunopathology, Allergology, Infectology (Russia). 2016;(2):11-22

[28] Chang JC, Wysocki A, Tchou-Wong KM, Moskowitz N, Zhang Y, Rom WN. Effect of Mycobacterium tuberculosis and its components on macrophages and the release of matrix metalloproteinases. Thorax. 1996;**51**:306-311

[29] Cooper AM, Khader SA. The role of cytokines in the initiation, expansion, and control of cellular immunity to tuberculosis. Immunological Reviews. 2008;**226**:191-204

[30] Jang AS, Park SW, Ahn MH, Park JS, Kim DJ, Lee JH, Park CS. Impact of circulating TGFand IL-10 on T cell cytokines in patients with asthma and tuberculosis. Journal of Korean Medical Science. 2006;**21**:30-34

[31] Chowdhurya IH, Ahmedb AM, Choudhuria S, Sena A, Hazrac A, Pald NK, Bhattacharyaa B, Baharb B. Alteration of serum inflammatory cytokines in active pulmonary tuberculosis following anti-tuberculosis drug therapy. Molecular Immunology. 2014;**62**:159-168

[32] Ameglio F, Casarini M, Capoluongo E, Mattia P, Puglisi G, Giosuè S. Post-treatment changes of six cytokines in active pulmonary tuberculosis: Differences between patients with stable or increased fibrosis. The International Journal of Tuberculosis and Lung Disease. 2005;**9**:98-104

[33] Monin L, Khader SA. Chemokines in tuberculosis: The good, the bad and the ugly. Seminars in Immunology. 2014. DOI: 10.1016/j.smim.2014.09.004

[34] Hong JY, Lee HJ, Kim SY, Chung KS, Kim EY, Jung JY, Park MS, Kim YS, Kim SK, Chang J, Cho SN, Kang YA. Efficacy of IP-10 as a biomarker for monitoring tuberculosis treatment. Journal of Infection. 2014;**68**:252-258

[35] Ruhwald M, Bodmer T, Maier C, Jepsen M, Haaland MB, Eugen-Olsen J, Ravn P. Evaluating the potential of IP-10 and MCP-2 as biomarkers for the diagnosis of tuberculosis. The European Respiratory Journal. 2008;**32**:1607-1615

[36] Ye RD, Sun L. Emerging functions of serum amyloid a in inflammation. Journal of Leukocyte Biology. 2015;**98**:923-929

[37] Ruhwald M, Aabye MG, Ravn P. IP-10 release assays in the diagnosis of tuberculosis infection: Current status and future directions. Expert Review of Molecular Diagnostics. 2012;**12**:175-187

[38] Lighter-Fisher J, Peng CH, Tse BD. Cytokine responses to QuantiFERON® peptides, purified protein derivative and recombinant ESAT-6 in children with tuberculosis. The International Journal of Tuberculosis and Lung Disease. 2010;**14**:1548-1555

[39] Averbakh MM Jr, Panova LV, Gubkina MF. Dynamic changes of chemokine CXCL-10 (IP-10) in children and adolescents with different forms of pulmonary tuberculosis. Medical Immunology (Russia)/Meditsinskaya Immunologiya. 2016;**18**(3):279-286

[40] Chereshnev VA, Gusev EY. Immunological and pathophysiological mechanisms of systemic inflammation. Medical Immunology (Russia). 2012;**14**(1-2):9-20

[41] Peddireddy V, Sankara Narayana Doddam SN, Ahmed N. Mycobacterial dormancy systems and host responses in tuberculosis. Frontiers in Immunology. 2017;**8**:84. DOI:10.3389/fimmu.2017.00084

[42] Deshane J, Wright M, Agarwal A. Heme oxygenase-1 expression in disease states. Acta Biochimca Polonica. 2005;**52**:273-284

[43] Ryter SW, Alam J, Choi AMK. Heme oxygenase-1/carbon monoxide: From basic science to therapeutic applications. Physiological Reviews. 2006;**86**:583-650

[44] Torrado T, Cooper AM. Cytokines in the balance of protection and pathology during mycobacterial infections. In: The new paradigm of immunity to tuberculosis. Advances in Experimental Medicine. Divangahi M editor. Advances in Experimental Medicine and Biology. 2013;**783**:121-140

[45] Morse D, Choi AM. Heme oxygenase-1: From bench to bedside. American Journal of Respiratory and Critical Care Medicine. 2005;**172**:660-670

Permissions

All chapters in this book were first published in TUBERCULOSIS, by InTech Open; hereby published with permission under the Creative Commons Attribution License or equivalent. Every chapter published in this book has been scrutinized by our experts. Their significance has been extensively debated. The topics covered herein carry significant findings which will fuel the growth of the discipline. They may even be implemented as practical applications or may be referred to as a beginning point for another development.

The contributors of this book come from diverse backgrounds, making this book a truly international effort. This book will bring forth new frontiers with its revolutionizing research information and detailed analysis of the nascent developments around the world.

We would like to thank all the contributing authors for lending their expertise to make the book truly unique. They have played a crucial role in the development of this book. Without their invaluable contributions this book wouldn't have been possible. They have made vital efforts to compile up to date information on the varied aspects of this subject to make this book a valuable addition to the collection of many professionals and students.

This book was conceptualized with the vision of imparting up-to-date information and advanced data in this field. To ensure the same, a matchless editorial board was set up. Every individual on the board went through rigorous rounds of assessment to prove their worth. After which they invested a large part of their time researching and compiling the most relevant data for our readers.

The editorial board has been involved in producing this book since its inception. They have spent rigorous hours researching and exploring the diverse topics which have resulted in the successful publishing of this book. They have passed on their knowledge of decades through this book. To expedite this challenging task, the publisher supported the team at every step. A small team of assistant editors was also appointed to further simplify the editing procedure and attain best results for the readers.

Apart from the editorial board, the designing team has also invested a significant amount of their time in understanding the subject and creating the most relevant covers. They scrutinized every image to scout for the most suitable representation of the subject and create an appropriate cover for the book.

The publishing team has been an ardent support to the editorial, designing and production team. Their endless efforts to recruit the best for this project, has resulted in the accomplishment of this book. They are a veteran in the field of academics and their pool of knowledge is as vast as their experience in printing. Their expertise and guidance has proved useful at every step. Their uncompromising quality standards have made this book an exceptional effort. Their encouragement from time to time has been an inspiration for everyone.

The publisher and the editorial board hope that this book will prove to be a valuable piece of knowledge for researchers, students, practitioners and scholars across the globe.

List of Contributors

Carlo Contini, Martina Maritati, Marachiara di Nuzzo, Lorenzo Massoli, Sara Lomenzo and Anastasio Grilli
Department of Medical Sciences, Section of Infectious Diseases and Dermatology, University of Ferrara, Ferrara, Italy

Lynn S. Zijenah
Department of Immunology, University of Zimbabwe College of Health Sciences, Harare, Zimbabwe

Andra-Iulia Suceveanu, Despina Todescu, Laura Mazilu, Filippos Goniotakis Manousos, Roxana Hulea, Felix Voinea, Eugen Dumitru and Adrian Paul Suceveanu
Faculty of Medicine, Ovidius University, Constanta, Romania

Manuela Cristina Russu
"Dr. I. Cantacuzino" Clinical Hospital, "Carol Davila" University of Medicine and Pharmacy, Bucharest, Romania

Şerban Nastasia
"Dr. I. Cantacuzino" Clinic of Obstetrics and Gynaecology, "Carol Davila" University of Medicine and Pharmacy, Bucharest, Romania

Daniela Degeratu
"Dr. I. Cantacuzino" Laboratory of Pathology, Bucharest, Romania

Ruxandra Viorica Stănculescu
Department of Pathological Obstetrics, Emergency "St Pantelimon" Clinical Hospital, "Carol Davila" University of Medicine and Pharmacy, Bucharest, Romania

Kogieleum Naidoo
Centre for the AIDS Programme of Research in South Africa (CAPRISA), University of KwaZulu-Natal, Durban, South Africa
South African Medical Research Council (SAMRC) - CAPRISA HIV-TB Pathogenesis and Treatment Research Unit, Durban, South Africa

Navisha Dookie
Centre for the AIDS Programme of Research in South Africa (CAPRISA), University of KwaZulu-Natal, Durban, South Africa

Abiola Olaleye and Andy Beke
School of Health Systems and Public Health, University of Pretoria, Pretoria, South Africa

Gerardo Amaya-Tapia
Centro Universitario Ciencias de la Salud at Universidad de Guadalajara, Guadalajara, Jalisco, Mexico
Infectious Diseases Department at Hospital General de Occidente, Guadalajara, Jalisco, Mexico

Guadalupe Aguirre-Avalos
Centro Universitario Ciencias de la Salud at Universidad de Guadalajara, Guadalajara, Jalisco, Mexico
Intensive Care Unit at Hospital Civil de Guadalajara "Fray Antonio Alcalde", Guadalajara, Jalisco, Mexico

Khalid Hussain Bhat
Department of Microbiology and Immunology, University of Illinois College of Medicine, Chicago, USA

Imtiyaz Yaseen
Welcome Trust Center for Cell Biology, Scotland, UK

Vladimir López and Pilar Alberdi
SaBio, Instituto de Investigación en Recursos Cinegéticos IREC (CSIC-UCLM-JCCM), Ciudad Real, Spain

Leonardo F. Jurado
Pathology and Laboratories Department, Fundación Santa Fe de Bogotá University Hospital, Bogotá D.C., Colombia
Pathology Department, School of Medicine, National University of Colombia, Bogotá D.C., Colombia

Diana M. Palacios
Pathology and Laboratories Department, Fundación Santa Fe de Bogotá University Hospital, Bogotá D.C., Colombia
School of Medicine, Los Andes University, Bogotá D.C., Colombia
Pathology Department, School of Medicine, National University of Colombia, Bogotá D.C., Colombia

José de la Fuente
SaBio, Instituto de Investigación en Recursos Cinegéticos IREC (CSIC-UCLM-JCCM), Ciudad Real, Spain
Department of Veterinary Pathobiology, Center for Veterinary Health Sciences, Oklahoma State University, Stillwater, OK, USA

Mikhael M. Averbakh and Atadzhan Ergeshow
FSBSI "Central TB Research Institute", Moscow, Russia

Index

www.ingramcontent.com/pod-product-compliance
Lightning Source LLC
LaVergne TN
LVHW080641210926
848485LV00003B/302
* 9 7 8 1 6 3 9 8 7 5 4 2 9 *